Natural Medicine

Natural Medicine

A Practical Guide to Family Health

Beth MacEoin

BLOOMSBURY

FOREWORD

Natural medicines have come a long way since the early eighties when they came close to disappearing from the UK. Homeopathy is now regularised by an EU parliamentary directive. There is now a move afoot to integrate such disciplines as herbal medicine, osteopathy, chiropractic, ayurvedic and traditional Chinese medicine into the National Health Service. And an ever growing section of the public is vocally demanding the right to choose between symptomatic drug-based treatments offered by conventional allopathic medicine and traditional natural alternatives – what has come to be called *complementary* medicine – when seeking treatment for illness.

In no small part the progress towards making free choice available to those seeking medical treatment is due to the efforts of the Natural Medicine Society, who have lobbied long and hard for such freedom. As the only consumer body representing ordinary people who use natural approaches to health and healing – from acupuncture and anthroposophical medicine to homeopathy and herbalism – NMS only exists to protect our rights to access first-rate treatments from well-trained practitioners and to make them all more widely available. NMS continues to help guard our right to access natural health care and to improve its standing and practice through educational research.

With the publication of the Natural Medicines Society Family Health Guide another giant step has been taken to safeguard freedom of choice. Beth MacEoin, with the help of NMS consultants and NMS advisor Sato Liu, has produced a clear, well researched and practical guide to the use of natural medicine. It can not only help the reader with the ins and outs of various therapies, it even offers self-help for common problems whether they be as simple as an insect bite or a cold, or as complex as endometriosis or irritable bowel syndrome.

Beautifully organised, well informed and fascinating to read, this book is a welcome introduction to natural medicines and treatments as well as a wonderful friend to whom you can turn for help in times of trouble.

Leslie Kenton
Founding Chairperson of NMS

First published in Great Britain 1999
Copyright ©1999 by Beth MacEoin
The moral right of the author has been asserted
Bloomsbury Publishing Plc, 38 Soho Square, London, W1V 5DF
A CIP catalogue record for this book is available from the British Library
ISBN 0 7475 3023 8
10 9 8 7 6 5 4 3 2 1

Typeset by Selwood Systems, Frome, Great Britain
Printed in Singapore by Tien Wah Press

CONTENTS

Part Five: Treatment Guide to the alternative treatment of common ailments

Part Six: Chronic conditions

ACKNOWLEDGEMENTS

A book of this size, scope and vision could never have been accomplished without the advice, encouragement, and support of the following people. Sato Liu, the Natural Medicines Society's executive director and editor of this book, must be the first to be thanked for the intelligent, good-humoured and focused attention she has bought to the project as a whole. Without Sato's original concept of the potential for this book, and continued enthusiasm and input throughout the lengthy process of its being written, the whole project could have been a much more arduous and isolated undertaking.

The consultants have also done a marvellous job in being supportive, helpful and extremely co-operative and understanding when offering advice and additions to the text within a challenging time scale. Any errors that appear in the text are my own, and are not associated with the information provided by them.

I would also like to thank Alan Wherry and Kate Morris at Bloomsbury for demonstrating such commitment to an extremely challenging and demanding project, and also for being a pleasure to work with. Kate Quarry must also be thanked for her sharp and consistent editing when working with a manuscript of an unwieldy size and complicated nature.

Teresa Chris and Jeffrey Simmons also played important roles in maintaining a broad overview of this project over an extended period of time. In addition, my warmest thanks go to John Boothe who provided invaluable advice, and a calm and thoughtful perspective at a particularly stage in the writing process.

Finally, I must extend my gratitude to those who have supported me through the often turbulent time when this book was being written. Without their patience, caring and understanding I am sure I would have given up many times. My warmest love and thanks go to my husband Denis, my mother Nancy, Clare, Glynis, Paul, Lala and Samantha.

Beth MacEoin

To Beth's acknowledgements I would also like to add Rowena Gaunt who took the concept and facilitated it into becoming a reality. The following consultants who, although extremely busy, undertook to give freely of their advice and suggestions; Dr Geoffrey Douch, Teddy Fearnhamm, Sylvia Baker, Dr Harish Verma, Gopi Warrier, Suham Sidani, Christopher Turner, Julian Barnard, Judith Cresswell, Sean Doherty, Ron Bishop, Penny Woolley, Roger Groos, Dr Colin Clayton, Elizabeth Fraser, Kim Lovelace, Richard Blackwell, Andrew Chevallier, Lawrence Reemer, Simon Fielding, Ian Wiggle, Manya McMahon, Brian Daniels and Timothy Whittaker. Without their support the completion of this book would not have been possible.

My appreciation and thanks must also go to Yvonne, simon and Linda for the help and support they gave to me at the NMS office.

Finally, to Beth for agreeing to take on the authorship of this book from the original concept, I owe a great debt of gratitude especially since there were some difficult times for her through this period. I have always admired her ability to give clear and concise information in a warm, friendly manner. These are qualities she embodies and I have sincerely enjoyed working with her throughout this project...and look forward to another such opportunity.

Sato Liu

INTRODUCTION

When the history of medicine in the late twentieth century comes to be written, at least one chapter will be needed to recount the role that is increasingly being played by alternative and complementary therapies. The rise of these systems of medical diagnosis and treatment from 'fringe medicine' to tolerated adjuncts of medical orthodoxy has been rapid and relatively smooth. They deserve a place in such a history, not only because they are in themselves examples of the way in which rejected ideas can eventually earn a place in the mainstream, but because they are gradually coming to exercise a real influence on the ways we think about illness, health, and medicine.

Modern medicine has achieved a great deal, and I for one would not wish to be without it. Its great strength lies in its understanding of scientific method, its rigour, its freedom from sloppy thinking and its mastery of chemistry and technology. Its great weakness is its reductionist approach, which identifies and treats only body parts and symptoms. Alternative and complementary medicine is something of a mirror image of its established rival: it generally lacks scientific rigour and frequently bases its theories on mystical conjectures or the brain-waves of a single healer, but it can bring an individual and his or her ailments into a meaningful whole; it can think laterally, it can act on insights without the drag of an establishment, and it can effect long-lasting cures where orthodox medicine offers only palliation.

Over the past ten years or so a growing dialogue between orthodox and alternative medicine has shown that a universal system of medicine may emerge that will incorporate the strengths of both systems and, as far as possible, eradicate their weaknesses. This book provides an important contribution to this debate. In presenting alternative therapies within the structure of a regular family health guide, it can be used much as any other medical guide, for looking up symptoms or disease names and assessing what sort of treatment might be suitable. Doctors, too, can use it as a basis for comparison.

But first it may be useful to decipher some of the terms used. For example, are alternative, complementary, natural and holistic medicine all the same thing? The simple answer seems to be that these different names arose at different times to express varying aspects of the medical systems they seek to cover. It's not a bad starting point for a book like this to take a quick look at each of these expressions and how they may be used.

Alternative medicine

This is still a very popular term, although some people object to it because it suggests that non-conventional therapies want to replace orthodox medicine – something that is either thought impossible or undesirable. But as a matter of fact, a lot of practitioners will say that they can replace orthodox medicine where it's appropriate to do so. In the last century, homoeopathic doctors and homoeopathic hospitals provided comprehensive treatment for all conditions that didn't require surgery. Nowadays, they don't get much chance to do that, but they have the same powerful medicines in their cabinets.

In the case of chronic illnesses, orthodox Western medicine has very little to offer sufferers. A homoeopath, a herbalist or an acupuncturist is more likely to achieve lasting success with a condition like asthma or eczema than a conventional doctor using antibiotics or steroids. In this respect, holistic medicine provides a genuine alternative to what's on offer from your family doctor's surgery or from the hospital.

Complementary medicine

Holistic practitioners see great benefits for both patients and themselves in working alongside conventional doctors, and willingly do so where co-operation is offered (which, sadly, is still too seldom the case). Orthodox emergency treatment is unrivalled, and it is recognized that this should always be the patient's first port of call. Nevertheless, even in an emergency there can be an important role for non-conventional medications or techniques. The benefits of homoeopathy in treating burns, for example, are considerable.

Sometimes a practitioner of a major system like homoeopathy or traditional Chinese medicine may use his or her treatments alongside conventional drugs or surgery. In cases where a patient cannot safely be weaned off a certain drug or taken off essential equipment, remedies may still be used to improve symptoms.

Of course, in a properly balanced health system, the term 'complementary' has to work both ways. Holistic medicine is often the ideal primary resort, especially in chronic cases, and orthodox medicine may be most appropriate as a supplement to it. Similarly, one natural system of medicine may be used to complement another.

It should be pointed out that not all systems of natural healing are as highly developed as others. Some are, by their very nature, quite restricted and, by definition, complementary. Therapies like meta-morphic technique, chelation therapy or hopi ear candles have a limited range within which they are effective, and it would be unusual for their practi-tioners to claim to be genuinely alternative or comprehensive.

Holistic medicine

In many ways, this is the most useful term we have for describing these medical systems, though it too has its drawbacks. Many practitioners of conventional medicine argue that they too employ a holistic approach in treating their patients, for example, by helping a patient stop smoking, instead of merely continuing to treat a lung disease. Unfortunately, however well motivated, most doctors do find that, in the end, they are forced back to the prescription pad. Even non-conventional practitioners will be powerless to find jobs or willpower or love of their patients.

Nevertheless, many non-conventional practitioners do try to set every patient and every illness in a wider context. They speak of 'treating the whole person' and of harmonizing the patient with nature. A homoeopath, for example, does not treat specific conditions or symptom patterns. Every patient pres-ents a different picture. Of twenty 'arthritis' patients,

no two will be identical, and only a handful will be similar enough to require the same remedy.

Authentic holism takes the total situation into account and treats appropriately. A good holistic doctor or alternative practitioner is aware of the need to treat underlying causes, but he also recog-nizes and treats emergencies before they become life-threatening. He also appreciates that, if someone is suffering severely from even superficial symp-toms, they require rapid relief. There is much that can be done right away to alleviate symptoms, before proceeding to deeper work.

The deeper work is important, because alleviation of symptoms carries long-term risks. Asthma inhalers, antibiotics, steroids and so on never actually cure chronic conditions, and patients will often spend a lifetime dependent on one or more drugs for partial relief. The holistic approach alleviates symptoms while working towards a real cure that removes the need for treatment of any kind.

Natural medicine

This is, of course, the term on which the Natural Medicines Society based its name. On the whole, outside the USA, it's used much less widely than the others we've looked at, and probably rightly so. Of all the terms we've considered, this one is, oddly enough, the least accurate – although it's very likely that most people think it's what alternative medicine is all about.

What's wrong with it? Well, for one thing, it seems to imply that there's something inherently good about being natural, but it's obvious that not all natural things are beneficial. Cholera is natural, malarial swamps are natural, most genetic disorders are natural – if everything had been left in its natural state, there would be no civilization, no science, no art and certainly no very high levels of health. But the biggest problem in calling natural medicines natural lies in the simple fact that they aren't. Homoeopathy, for example, is entirely man-made, and acupuncture is visibly unnatural.

So why is there such an emphasis within alterna-tive medical circles on 'nature's method of cure'? In many cases, this is simple ignorance, an inability to see things as they are. More widely, however, there is a profound truth in what is said about harmonizing man with nature. Most therapies involve a concept of natural, vital energy which provides the driving force for life itself. Throughout our lives, our vital energy may get distorted – by infections, traumas, environmental pollution, synthetic drugs, too much alcohol, too many cigarettes, unhealthy food, and many other factors that challenge the vital force, much as bacteria challenge the immune systems (to which this vital force seems to be intimately related).

Alternative remedies or techniques are regarded as natural because they work in harmony with the body's rhythms and energies, bringing it back as far as possible to its original state. Orthodox drugs may be very effective in calming down symptoms, but alternative practitioners maintain that, apart from causing side effects, they tend to destabilize the system, often causing a minor condition to re-express itself in a more serious form. For example, it is thought that suppressing eczema with steroid creams may drive the original condition deeper into the body, resulting, typically, in asthma. And suppression of the asthma may result in something more serious again.

So, even though sticking needles in someone's ear is very unnatural on one level, on another it is not, in that the restoration of balance works in harmony with nature. 'Nature' here seems to mean something like 'the body's innate desire to get well'.

How does alternative medicine differ from orthodox medicine?

Orthodox medicine (or, as it's often somewhat inaccurately called, allopathic medicine) has probably done more to alleviate human suffering than any other system of health care in history. But it has its dark side, particularly major problems in three main areas. Firstly, the amount of illness directly caused by orthodox drugs, tests and surgical procedures is now reaching proportions where harm may soon outweigh benefit. Secondly, costs have rocketed to a point where even affluent societies cannot afford to provide a decent health-care service for their citizens. And, thirdly, orthodox treatments are virtually useless against chronic diseases.

Not only that, but many past 'successes' are now coming back to haunt conventional medicine as disease agents develop immunity to sulphonamides, vaccinations and antibiotics: two well-publicized examples are malaria and tuberculosis. In addition, patients are growing more and more dissatisfied with their experience of conventional medicine. Many find doctors, especially hospital consultants, impersonal, and sense that they are seen as just a bowel or a leg or an eye, and that their wider concerns and medical problems are dismissed as of no relevance.

In contrast, alternative practitioners tend to be interested in the patient as a whole person and will seek to treat not just one or two symptoms, but every aspect of the patient's ill health and perhaps their life in general; the personal takes precedence over the impersonal in almost all cases. Sessions with an alternative practitioner will tend to be time consuming, and it is not uncommon for a close bond to develop between patient and healer. Good alternative practitioners are also committed to a belief in the body's power to heal itself with as little help as possible. Using manipulation, needles, medicines or remedies is only a small part of a wider process in which the patients are empowered and encouraged to understand themselves, their bodies and their treatment.

Orthodox medicine is, of course, notorious for the side effects of its drugs, which, in extreme (but by no means rare) cases, result in conditions more serious than those they are meant to treat. By contrast, side effects with alternative medicine are rare and, in some cases, non-existent. Many herbs, given in high doses over a long period, can produce toxic effects, but if you have chosen a highly trained and experienced practitioner, this should not present a risk.

Alternative treatments have a far greater chance of effecting wholesale cure or a long-term disappearance of symptoms in chronic illnesses, and where orthodox medicine is increasingly invasive, alternatives tend to hold back as far as possible, relying on the restorative powers of the body to take the patient further on the road to recovery. This has a secondary effect in that costs can be kept low – something that is more and more difficult to do within conventional health-care systems.

Why is alternative medicine so popular?

It is almost certainly the case that the rise in interest in and use of alternative medicine is closely linked to a perception of crisis in orthodox therapy, as this introduction has already explained. And as people become increasingly dissatisfied with conventional medicine, the spreading knowledge of alternative health care – often through books, magazines, television and radio – means that they are more and more aware that alternative medicine may be able to achieve the improvement they seek so eagerly.

Of course, there are other factors influencing this growth in popularity. The orthodox medical system is overstressed, and doctors have limited time to devote to patients: the average family doctor's consultation in the UK lasts around six minutes. On the other hand, generally speaking, non-conventional practitioners practise outside the public health service and can devote more time to their patients than their orthodox counterparts. They come to their patients without a mechanistic image of the person or the illness, and are therefore more likely to be perceived as caring, understanding and empathetic.

They are trained in how to listen and observe not so much symptoms or disease indicators, but the whole person: what may seem trivial or irrelevant to a family doctor or consultant is, as often as not, the very thing that holds the key to the case for a homoeopath or a herbalist. Many have counselling skills and others work as part of a network of practitioners, ensuring that patients' concerns receive the hearing and attention they deserve.

As survey after survey has shown, patients of alternative practitioners show a very high satisfaction rate. Whatever else they do, alternative therapists seem to provide what the public want. And, in the main, what they want is to get better. When someone who has suffered for ten or twenty years from a chronic condition, like asthma or back pain, is made symptom-free, they are bound to treat it as a major event, to tell their friends and relatives, and to encourage other sufferers to try something different.

For better or worse, we live in a health-conscious age and diets, exercise programmes, health farms, personal fitness training, yoga, Pilates, saunas, massage, spas and all the rest have become part of everyday life for many. What these activities have in common is a sense of personal responsibility for the fitness of one's body and mind. For many people, this is accompanied or triggered by a feeling of insecurity: the food industry, pollution, prescription drugs, work-related stress and much else make us feel vulnerable. The only way we have of regaining control over our own bodies is to make conscious choices over what we eat and drink, how we spend our spare time, and how we treat ourselves when ill.

This attitude has played an enormous role in making alternative medicine so popular. Women in particular are increasingly opting for forms of medicine that give them freedom from a male-dominated medical system. It cannot be a coincidence that so many practitioners of alternative medicine are themselves women, or that their patients are predominantly female. However, large numbers of men, schoolchildren, truck drivers, firemen, dockers and even members of the medical profession attend alternative practices, proving their broad appeal.

Why does there seem to be such a gap between alternative medicine and medical science?

This is a difficult area, made more difficult by attitudes on either side. It has become commonplace to hear doctors and scientists make the remark that 'there is no scientific evidence for alternative medicine', as though this were a fact. Twenty years or so ago, this would have been largely (though not wholly) correct. Practitioners tended to adopt an attitude of indifference towards scientific research, pointing out that everyday experience showed that the therapies worked, and that was all that mattered. Scientists (rightly) disagreed.

In several therapies, however, there were individuals and bodies who saw the need to use scientific method as the best means of winning the approval of the medical establishment. They carried out tests, conducted trials, and investigated new research methodologies better suited to the systems of medicine involved. In particular, homoeopathy, acupuncture, osteopathy, chiropractic, herbal medicine and traditional Chinese medicine were all the subjects of an impressive range of published research, much of which has appeared in orthodox journals like the *British Medical Journal* and *The Lancet*.

Not only has the volume of research literature undergone this tremendous expansion, but the quality of the work now being carried out is higher than ever. Even in severely rigorous trials, the findings have been largely positive.

But as evidence of just how unscientific the scientific community can be, it is worth noting that the words 'no published evidence' seems increasingly to mean 'no published evidence in English'. This is particularly well demonstrated by the persistent ignorance shown by American and most European medical scientists with regard to the extensive scientific work done on herbal medicines in Germany (and reported in German journals). In Germany today, it is common for medical practitioners to prescribe herbs, because they are familiar with the published literature and comfortable with the scientific underpinning for such prescriptions. Meanwhile, their colleagues elsewhere go on pretending herbal medicine is unscientific.

While it is extremely difficult to obtain research funding for work of this kind, many practitioners of alternative medicine are their own worst enemies with respect to research. Many still hold the view that modern science is seriously flawed, and argue that intuition or other 'higher faculties' can guide us to knowledge more effectively than disciplined, controlled research, or maintain that they 'know' their therapies work, and that should be enough.

Unfortunately, it isn't. Every therapy, however weird and wonderful, has supporters claiming they 'know' it works. Science is the art of sifting claims like that and providing the public with a reasonable guide to what is and what is not verifiable. Scientific research is the key to gaining both public and government recognition.

A re-examination of easily available existing evidence for the efficacy of alternative treatments is also needed. It is usually swept aside as 'anecdotal', but the truth is that anecdotal proof is far from being a seamless fabric. There is an enormous spectrum, ranging from very, very good to wholly unreliable. Valuable evidence can be gathered from case reports in which diagnosis, prescription, previous treatment, follow-on treatment and so forth are carefully monitored and recorded, or files of patients treated on the wards of homoeopathic hospitals.

Beyond this, there is an important body of evidence that is still not taken seriously by orthodox doctors: the regular treatment of animals by vets using, in the main, homoeopathy and acupuncture. There is no obvious 'mind over matter' link that allows a herd of dairy cows to recover from mastitis just because their drinking water has been dosed with a few drops of homoeopathic medicine. And yet they do recover, as do racing horses, cats, budgerigars and hamsters.

The answer is not for supporters of alternative medicine to turn their backs on science, but instead to insist that scientists behave rationally, examine the evidence on its own merits, and set up fair and objective studies that will take us nearer to a proper understanding of this important phenomenon.

How safe is alternative medicine?

Assessing risk in any area of life is far from easy. Not many of us think twice about travelling by car, yet we often break into a cold sweat on boarding a plane, in spite of the fact that flying is statistically a great deal safer than driving. Our perception of what is safe and what is not is seldom rational. For the most part, we let ourselves be guided by rumours passed on by friends, by our feelings, and by scare stories in the media. Newspapers print scare stories because they sell copies, not because they are accurate. In the old days, alternative medicine was mercifully guarded against this sort of thing, but in recent years, scare stories of one kind or another have become commonplace in the reporting of alternative medicine. In no instance known to me has the scare element matched the real facts of the case. Many of these reports have emanated from the National Poisons Unit, and involve cases of actual or presumed poisoning from herbs, herbal teas and related substances.

In many cases, the only tenuous connection between a given poisoning case and alternative medicine was that the patient had been taking herbal remedies during the period they had been poisoned (by something else), or happened to have had a herbal tea the day before. These are tenuous grounds on which to base a presumption of serious risk.

Where problems have arisen, they have normally been the result of excess zeal or carelessness. There are patients who prefer to diagnose and treat their own illnesses. Sometimes they misunderstand the dosage or act on the assumption that natural is safe. The simple way to avoid this problem is to attend a qualified herbalist and follow their instructions to the letter.

In other cases, there have been problems with adulterated products. Most or all of these have involved herbs and other substances imported from India, China, and other 'Third World' countries. In some instances, herbs have been put together into compounds and adulterated with metals or conventional drugs. Most of the adulterated medicines tend to be used within the UK's ethnic communities, and members of those communities or anyone else visiting practitioners who may not have obtained their herbs from a reputable source should take care to check on the provenance of the remedies they are given. If in doubt, obtain a prescription to be filled at a reputable pharmacy.

Many orthodox doctors argue that, when patients attend alternative practitioners, they are denying themselves important diagnoses and possibly life-saving treatment. But the fact is, a good alternative practitioner may often be a better diagnostician than a harried family doctor or a rushed locum who has never seen the patient before.

What about conditions like cancer or AIDS? Isn't there a chance that turning to strange nostrums may delay proper treatment or even turn a patient against it? This is a difficult question to answer: if it were a black-and-white case of totally effective orthodox treatments versus wholly inadequate alternatives – as some conventional doctors would like us to believe – we would all know exactly where we stand.

But life is not that simple. In reality, the success rate of orthodox treatments for cancer has never been good and does not seem to be getting better. In 1994 one professor in this field was reported in *The Times* as saying, 'More people are getting cancer than ever before and we are losing the battle against it.' Faced with such dismal prospects of a positive outcome, it seems only reasonable for a patient with cancer to want to explore what else is available.

In practice, not very many patients abandon their orthodox treatment entirely. Many use alternative regimens to supplement conventional resources, and a much smaller group opts for a specific alternative cancer treatment – the Hoxey treatment, say, or Gerson therapy – with which it will go the whole way. We do not have good enough statistics to establish just how successful these treatments are. In many cases – perhaps a majority – the disease will already have become untreatable, and the patient turns to an alternative for help too late for any real benefit. In other cases, however, substantial results are achieved, and tumours go into remission, sometimes briefly, sometimes for long periods.

What we cannot argue with is the patient's right to make a choice. No doubt some kind of risk is involved in opting for an alternative treatment, but there are high risks in undergoing surgery, chemotherapy or radiotherapy, and every individual will want to make his or her own decision in such a crucial matter, without being railroaded in one direction or another.

In spite of all these seeming hazards, alternative medicine, when practised by qualified and experienced therapists, remains the safest body of treatments known to man.

Denis MacEoin
Chairman, Natural Medicines Society

THE THERAPIES

MAJOR SYSTEMS

Anthroposophical medicine

Anthroposophical medicine is a holistic form of medicine that aims to treat the whole person and not just the symptoms of illness. It acknowledges the importance of conventional medicine, but takes into account the fact that living beings may have a non-physical, or spiritual aspect to their existence – and, therefore, to their illnesses. Anthroposophical doctors must first train in conventional medicine before completing additional training in anthroposophical medicine.

An anthroposophical doctor believes that each person is composed of four parts: the physical body, the astral body, the etheric body and the ego, and that illness is caused by an imbalance between the etheric and astral bodies and the ego. Conventional medication may be prescribed where appropriate, but patients are often referred to other treatments including anthroposophical or homoeopathic medicines, counselling, and artistic therapies, such as music, speech, movement (eurythmy) and painting.

Historical perspectives

The word anthroposophy comes from the Greek *anthropos*, meaning man, and *sophia*, meaning wisdom. The Anthroposophical Society was founded in 1913

by Dr Rudolf Steiner (1861–1925), an Austrian scientist and philosopher. The anthroposophical movement has now developed well beyond the boundaries of Europe, and societies can be found in Australia, South America, the USA, Egypt, Japan, Israel and South Africa.

Although not a medical doctor, Steiner incorporated medical science in his ideas. He believed that the experience, structure and functioning of a living organism could not be interpreted in terms of purely physical or chemical processes, and that all living things possessed non-material elements that could not be explained by conventional medical science.

Steiner was asked by Dr Ita Wegman, a Dutch physician, to give lectures to other doctors, and they jointly wrote a book entitled *Fundamentals of Therapy*. In the early 1920s they opened the first anthroposophical clinic in Switzerland. There are now several anthroposophical hospitals in Europe and hundreds of doctors dedicated to anthroposophical medicine.

Basic background

The conventional standpoint perceives illness as having a material cause and effect, with great emphasis on finding the virus or bacteria that may be acting on the body at a molecular or cellular level. There is a general misconception in orthodox medicine that once we understand why we become ill and fight disease using the appropriate 'magic bullet', good health will ensue. This approach leads to a high degree of specialization in medicine, the ultimate goal being the search for the drug that will destroy specific diseases.

Anthroposophical medicine acknowledges the human form as fourfold, comprising:
- the physical body
- the astral body
- the etheric body
- the ego organization.

The term 'body', with reference to the etheric and astral elements is used for comparative understanding only, for they are not of a physical nature but are beyond that which is applicable to the senses. Anthroposophical medicine holds that when there is disruption or disorder between any of the four members, illness occurs.

From the anthroposophical viewpoint, orthodox medical science only gives the basic principles of anatomy, biochemistry and physiology. They have been developed in the main from studies and experiments on dissected animals, and when these principles are applied to living organisms, mistaken assumptions are usually made. Anthroposophical medicine is a medical science that recognizes living beings as having non-physical and spiritual aspects to their existence.

Anthroposophical medicine endeavours to address the non-physical aspects of illness in the patient as well as the physical.

The physical body

The anthroposophical doctor regards the physical body as belonging to the mineral kingdom only, and thereby views it as a corpse with no life of its own. It is interpenetrated by its other three counterparts from whence it sustains life, sentience and individuality. This is a radical departure from modern-day knowledge in so much as we come to know where our various seats of capability and capacity are housed.

The etheric body

The anthroposophical doctor acknowledges the human being as possessing a 'life body' or 'formative body' that architecturally and curatively maintains the physical body against decay. The supposition is that without an etheric body, the physical body returns to a corpse state, as it does in death, when the etheric has vacated the physical form. The etheric body interpenetrates the physical body from within and without. In anthroposophical medicine, the etheric body corresponds to the plant kingdom. Ultimately, the etheric body has an extremely constructive role in maintaining a state of harmony and order in the organism as a whole.

The astral body

Similarly to the etheric body, the astral body interpenetrates both the physical and the etheric bodies, with certain other capacities. The astral body corresponds to the animal kingdom in that it is sentient. It acts as a seat for everything we come to know as feelings, passions or desires, and so forth. (Thoughts arise when the ego organization 'lights up' in the astral body.)

The limitations of a purely material interpretation of existence are revealed when we consider that our feelings and subjective perception of the world around us may not be adequately explained by conventional medical techniques that attempt to examine the biochemistry and physiology of the nervous system alone, such as psychiatry, psychoanalysis and behavioural therapy.

The astral body is also regarded as having a breaking-down (or catabolic) effect. For good health and a basic sense of equilibrium to be maintained, the breaking-down potential of the astral body needs to be kept in balance with the regenerative potential of the etheric body. From an anthroposophical perspective, this essential balance must be maintained by a harmonious alternation between conscious and unconscious activity (such as the rhythm between sleep and wakefulness).

The ego

The ego is the 'I' or 'self' and should not be confused with selfishness. This part of us is the most advanced and developed part of our being. The anthroposophical doctor views the ego organization as the part that enables us to attain 'individuality', or, put another way, the ability to say 'I' to ourselves. The ego is our indestructible self, and encompasses the qualities of self-consciousness, memory and the capacity to think, all of which mean that human beings are not completely subject to the demands of instinctive behaviour. The ego does not have a predefined form as do the physical, etheric and astral bodies, but rather is present everywhere else but in us – it is everywhere outside of us, enabling us to engage with (and thereby make sense of) our inner life and the world around us.

The concept of treating the whole person

Anthroposophical doctors aim to provide a truly holistic form of treatment by considering information that relates to all four basic aspects of the human being, i.e. the physical, etheric and astral bodies, as well as the ego. From the anthroposophical perspective, illness arises as a result of imbalance or disharmony between the etheric and astral bodies and the ego. By not automatically opting for conventional medication in every case of illness, and choosing a more appropriate form of treatment, anthroposophical doctors provide a system of healing that addresses itself to the needs of the human organism on all levels, including the non-material.

Systems of the body

In anthroposophy the human organism possesses the following three main systems:

The nerve–sense system

This includes the activity of the brain, spinal cord, nerves and sense organs, and is linked to the catabolic or breaking-down processes. It is dominated by the ego and astral body, allowing consciousness, self-awareness and conscious perception to arise. It is the 'dampening' down of etheric/physical forces through catabolic activity in the nerve–sense system that allows consciousness to develop. The nerve–sense system activates the body during the day and the metabolic–limb system becomes more active during sleep. As a result, the physical and etheric bodies are restored and renewed each night, and are given the chance to repair the damage that may have occurred during the day as a consequence of the activity of the ego and astral body.

The metabolic–limb system

This encompasses the assimilation of nourishment, metabolic activity, movement of the limbs and the whole of the digestive system and metabolism. These are characteristically unconscious processes and are governed primarily by the physical and etheric bodies. The metabolic–limb system is involved in the restoring and rebuilding processes that take place in our bodies without our conscious awareness.

The rhythmic system

Although rhythm is expressed all over the body, it has a special affinity with the rhythm of breathing and the pulse, centred on the activity of the heart and lungs. The rhythmic system is especially involved in maintaining a state of harmony between the metabolic–limb and nerve–sense systems, and is regarded as playing a special role in the healing process. It is also a system that has a special affinity with feelings and emotions, which can be experienced in the response of heart and lungs to exercise or emotions.

The medicines

Anthroposophical doctors attempt to look beneath superficial symptoms of illness in order to treat the underlying cause of disease and to re-establish basic balance and harmony in the human organism. Medicines may be used from the plant, mineral or animal kingdoms in order to stimulate the organism as a whole towards cure. Medicines that are derived from plant sources are regarded as being especially related to the restorative, healing processes of the body, because, in anthroposophical medicine plants themselves have physical and etheric bodies (which have the potential for building and repair), but are considered to be without an astral body.

Anthroposophical doctors may use specially prepared anthroposophical medicines (often in a combination formula or special compounds), homoeopathic medicines, essential oils or herbal tinctures. Depending on the individual circumstances, an anthroposophical doctor may also prescribe conventional drugs chosen on a homoeopathic basis (i.e. if the patient's symptoms are similar to those known to be produced by the drug – see the homoeopathy section on pages 26–30 for a fuller explanation of this theory). However, it is noticeable that since anthroposophical doctors are generally uneasy about opting for conventional medicines as the obvious choice at the outset of illness, there tends to be less of a routine reliance on drugs that can have unpleasant or toxic side effects.

Artistic therapies

Because anthroposophical medicine works from the premise that illness arises as a result of a lack of harmony between the ego, astral, etheric and physical bodies, the aim of treatment is to regain a state of optimum balance between these elements. To support this process, artistic therapy may be prescribed, including eurythmy, a system of movement therapy developed by Steiner. Eurythmy uses specific movements in a rhythmical manner, performed in harmony with speech or music. Painting, music or other artistic activities may be used to develop an enhanced state of balance or harmony.

Art therapists work in close association with anthroposophical doctors, and treatment may be given on a group or individual basis, depending on the needs of each situation. In anthroposophical clinics and practices, art therapists work side by side with nurses, therapeutic masseurs, hydrotherapists and doctors.

The consultation

Consulting an anthroposophical doctor may initially feel much like an appointment with a conventional doctor, but extra aspects of lifestyle and diet are likely to be explored in detail. The patient may be asked to answer questions about sleep pattern and sleep quality, diet, food cravings and aversions, and emotional well-being. As mentioned above, once a diagnosis has been reached, the prescribed treatment may include a variety of medicines or therapies, depending on the requirements of each individual case. If counselling is perceived to be of potential help, an anthroposophical doctor may refer a patient to a qualified counsellor.

Conditions that may respond to anthroposophical medicine

You can consult an anthroposophical doctor for any condition, but problems that may respond particularly well to anthroposophical medicine include any of the following:

- Anxiety
- Boils
- Coughs and bronchitis
- Depression
- Digestive problems
- Ear infections
- Eczema and dermatitis
- Emotional shock or trauma
- Hay fever and allergic rhinitis
- Influenza
- Insomnia
- Muscular pains and cramps
- Physical trauma, including sprains and bruises
- Pre-menstrual syndrome and additional menstrual problems, including painful or irregular periods
- Poor circulation
- Pre-cancerous and cancerous conditions
- Sciatica and lumbago
- Sinusitis
- Tonsillitis

Ayurvedic medicine

Ayurvedic medicine is a holistic system of healing that has been practised for generations in India and neighbouring countries such as Sri Lanka. Although firmly grounded in an Asian philosophical perspective, the ayurvedic medical approach is becoming increasingly popular in the West.

In ayurvedic medicine each person's constitution is seen as being influenced by three basic *doshas* (vital energies) that are known as *vata, pitta* and *kapha*. The balance of these energies determines each individual's potential for health, as well as influencing that individual's experience of the world around them. Because health problems are thought to arise owing to a disturbance of vata, pitta or kapha energies in the body, an experienced ayurvedic practitioner will be able to assess which dosha is disturbed by an analysis of visible signs and symptoms. Adjustments in lifestyle and personal habits may be suggested as a way of re-establishing equilibrium and good health.

Basic background

The balance of the three doshas can be influenced before birth, depending on the doshas that are dominant in both parents at the time of conception. Although all three energies are likely to be present in the baby's constitution, it is only when one or two doshas dominate that constitutional weaknesses are likely to occur, leading to ill health. Additional factors that can be responsible for influencing a baby's constitution may include the physical and emotional health of the mother during pregnancy, as well as the quality of the mother's diet and the nature of the baby's birth.

From the perspective of an ayurvedic practitioner the balance and relationship between the three doshas in each person is constantly changing in response to environmental factors. Therefore, although someone may be born with a dominance of kapha in their constitutional make-up, pitta and vata doshas may come more to the fore according to the quality of that person's diet, the amount of exercise they take, or the degree of physical or emotional stress they are subjected to. Provided these changes to everyday equilibrium are not overwhelming, and positive steps are taken to protect health and well-being, good health should prevail.

The ayurvedic approach is truly holistic due to its emphasis on making a wide variety of changes in lifestyle that may incorporate adopting a more suitable diet, taking more exercise, making time to relax or meditate, or making sure we have more regular, good-quality sleep. This perspective provides us with a sharp contrast to the orthodox medical approach that tends to opt for drug treatments or surgery as an initial option, regarding more general advice about lifestyle as a secondary, adjunctive option.

Understanding the three doshas

The three doshas or energies are regarded as being responsible for all the vital processes that occur on a mental, emotional and physical level. They are essential forces that are responsible for the biological processes of growth, development and decay. Not only physical attributes, but mental potential and emotional characteristics can be interpreted within the context of the features of each dosha.

Vata characteristics

Vata combines the qualities of the two elements of ether and air, the latter being the stronger feature of the two. As a result, those who have a constitution in which a dominance of vata is apparent present a personality that may be erratic, changeable and inclined to bursts of activity.

The following key words capture the essence of vata energy:

Erratic: spasmodic, fitful, irregular and fidgety
Dispersing: scattering, evaporating and dissipating
Clear: empty, obvious and transparent
Mobile: animated, changeable and fluid
Subtle: imperceptible, sensitive or hidden
Light: fragile, thin or flimsy
Rough: coarse, irregular, husky and jagged
Dry: barren, wrinkled or shrivelled
Cold: cool, bitter or icy.

The basic functions of vata

- Creation of impulses and reflexes
- Nerve stimulation and transmitting of sensory stimuli
- Maintaining consciousness
- Circulation of blood, oxygen and nutrients
- Stimulation of digestive juices and regulation of peristalsis
- Elimination and transformation of tissues
- Ejaculation
- Expression of emotion and stimulation of tears

Vata-dominant individuals

Physical appearance

- Slim and dark with cool skin and dark, thin or coarse, curly hair
- Facial features may be long and angular with a weak chin
- Thin or scrawny neck with a narrow, small nose
- Narrow, small or sunken eyes with dull, lustreless appearance
- Small, thin mouth with receding gums

Mental characteristics

- Creative and artistic, with a tendency to be easily distracted by fresh ideas
- Capacity for great enthusiasm and vitality

Common problems

- Absence of sweat
- Fitful, light sleep
- Constipation with dry, hard stools
- Being fidgety and distracted
- Rapid depletion of energy
- Quickly expended sexual energy
- Low fertility
- Poor long-term memory
- Being fearful, insecure and anxious

Pitta characteristics

Pitta energy is related to heat and fire, arising from a combination of the two elements of fire and water, with the former element dominating. As a result, the key aspects of the constitution where the pitta dosha is uppermost may be summed up as hot, penetrating and radiating.

The following key words capture the essence of pitta energy:

Hot: burning, eager, inflamed, fiery and passionate
Light: fair, bright, radiant and glowing
Sharp: penetrating, piercing, shrill and cutting
Liquid: fluid, nebulous and flowing
Oily: greasy, smooth and fat.

The basic functions of pitta

- Maintaining a stable body temperature
- Interpreting sensory stimuli
- Regulating processes that involve transformation on mental and physical levels
- Quality, texture and lustre of eyes and skin
- Vision
- Assimilation of thoughts
- Regulating intellectual capacity and powers of reasoning

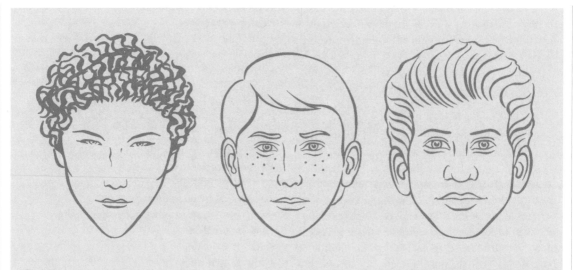

The physical characteristics of vata-,pitta- and kapha-dominant individuals can be interpreted within the context of the features of each dosha.

Pitta-dominant individuals

Physical appearance

- Fair, soft, warm skin that burns easily
- Skin that has a marked tendency to moles, freckles and inflammatory rashes
- Heart-shaped face with a well-defined, pointed chin
- The neck may be of average length and in proportion to the rest of the body
- Intense lustre to eyes

Mental characteristics

- Mental faculties tend towards being very alert and focused
- Information is readily grasped and assimilated
- Excellent memory for basic information that is connected to personal advancement, but poor for small details
- Generally ambitious and confident with a great deal of courage and enthusiasm

Common problems

- Profuse, sour-smelling sweat
- Loose stools
- Being angry, irritable and judgmental
- Ambitious with a possible tendency to over-enthusiasm and emotional, mental and physical 'burn-out'

Kapha characteristics

Kapha combines the qualities of the two elements of water and earth, with the former as the dominating element. Key characteristics of this dosha include heaviness, solidity and wetness.

The following essential features capture the essence of kapha energy:

Heavy: dense, lethargic, obese and listless
Slow: inert, lacklustre, sleepy and dull
Soft: flabby, receptive and comfortable
Static: calm, still and immovable
Slimy: mucusy, smooth, soft and slippery
Dense: heavy, firm, solid and slow
Oily: smooth, fat and greasy
Cold: cool, freezing and chilled

The basic functions of kapha

- Protection and maintenance of mucous membranes
- Lubrication of joints
- Maintenance of soft tissues of the body
- Regulation and distribution of heat in the body
- Maintenance of strength and stamina
- Regulation of cell reproduction and longevity
- Sleep pattern and quality

Kapha-dominant individuals

Physical appearance

- Pale, cold, greasy skin with thick, wavy hair
- Thick-set neck with a large, round face
- Large, round eyes and thick, full lips
- Good-quality teeth and healthy gums

Mental characteristics

- Steadiness and reliability of mind and emotions

- Slow to learn with a good memory
- Tendency to slowness and dullness of thinking with little desire for new mental challenges or stimulation
- Great capacity for caring, nurturing, fulfilment and contentedness

Common problems
- Tendency to easy sweating from little activity
- Constant chilliness
- Constipation with sluggish digestion
- Slow sexual arousal
- Inability to be rushed
- Being slow-witted with lack of mental flexibility

The balance of doshas in the individual

Although vata, pitta and kapha have specific functions in the body, it is important to bear in mind that each one does not work in isolation from the others. As a result, all three doshas are in a continual state of flux as they respond to each doshic enhancing or suppressing factor in our lifestyle or environment. From an ayurvedic perspective, we enjoy maximum health and vitality when our three doshas are balanced and in a state of optimum harmony.

Three basic constitutional types
- **Mono-types**, where one dosha is clearly dominant. In such a situation either pitta, kapha or vata is obviously visible as a constitutional trait.
- **Duo-types**, where two doshas are present in equal proportions.
- It is also possible, but quite rare, to find someone in whom all three doshas are present in equal proportion.

When the three energies are in the optimum balance for each individual, good health should follow. However, if the doshas are in a state of continual imbalance or disharmony, persistent poor health tends to be the norm, however much care is taken to try to improve matters on a superficial level. The predominant dosha in each individual is the one that is most likely to increase when the body and mind are under enough stress to precipitate a crisis. As a result, the symptoms that arise are likely to be related to that particular dosha.

The role of vata, pitta and kapha in the body

Each dosha has a special affinity with specific parts and functions of the body.

Vata is linked to functions that take place within the cavities of the body, such as the abdomen and the ear canal. The seat of vata is the colon. Subsidiary sites include the lower back, thighs, bones, ears, skin and nervous system.

Pitta is specifically related to enzyme and hormonal activity. Its seat is the stomach and the small intestine. Subsidiary sites include the liver, spleen, gall bladder, blood, perspiration, eyes and endocrine glands.

Kapha has an affinity to liquid tissues such as lymph, and maintains the balanced functioning of general secretions such as mucus and saliva. Within this framework the seat of kapha lies in the stomach and the lungs. Subsidiary sites include blood plasma, cytoplasm, the synovial membranes of the joints, subcutaneous fat, the mouth, nose and white matter of the brain.

The role of agni in digestion

For good health to be maintained chemical interactions in the body and mind must occur smoothly. These essential changes and transformations are known in ayurveda as *agni*, and it is a deficiency or weakness in agni that is regarded as being one of the chief factors in the development of disease. The primary agni is to be found in the gastric process, where food is changed by contact with secretions such as digestive juices and enzymes into substances that can be utilized by the body.

Digestive capacity and function are directly related to the vigour of agni. If agni is poor, the result is likely to be malabsorption of nutrients with digestive discomfort. Pain that occurs soon after eating while food remains in the stomach may be related to an imbalance of vata. Discomfort that sets in between two and four hours following a meal may be linked to an imbalance in pitta, while discomfort or flatulence that occur a long time after eating are likely to be an indication of a kapha imbalance.

Digestive problems may be caused by eating foods that have an adverse effect on the digestive tract when combined (such as eating fruit with cereals). Alternatively, foods that are filled with preservatives, additives or flavourings in an effort to extend their shelf-life are also considered to have a deleterious effect on the digestive process due to their lack of *prana* (life force). This can lead to fatigue and lowered vitality, as well as a general sense of sluggishness.

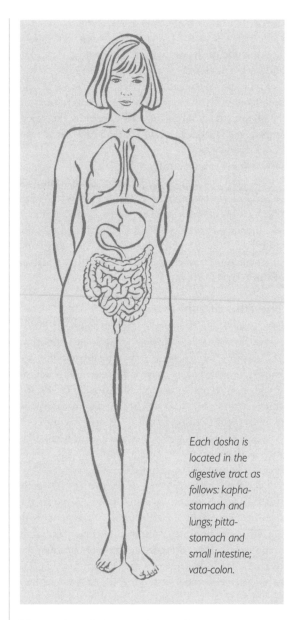

Each dosha is located in the digestive tract as follows: kapha-stomach and lungs; pitta-stomach and small intestine; vata-colon.

The role of the six 'tastes'

In ayurveda the interpretation of taste means more than the immediate perception of flavour on the tongue. There are six significant tastes, each one having an effect on the balance of doshas, the general digestive process and body tissues.

- **Sweet** reduces vata and pitta, but increases kapha.
- **Sour** reduces vata and increases kapha and pitta.
- **Salt** reduces vata and increases kapha and pitta.
- **Pungent** increases vata and pitta, while it reduces kapha.
- **Bitter** increases vata and reduces kapha and pitta.
- **Astringent** increases vata and reduces kapha and pitta.

The body is also dependent upon the healthy functioning of a network of channels that are responsible for moving a perpetual supply of nutrients and waste products around and out of the body. These channels may include the digestive tract as well as the smaller capillaries, or extremely subtle pathways of nerve stimuli. In good health, these channels should function efficiently, but in poor health may become obstructed.

Elimination of wastes

The efficient elimination of the three waste products of sweat, urine and faeces is very important in keeping the system healthy and in a state of optimum harmony. Water is kept in a state of balance in the body by the production and excretion of urine, the skin is kept moist by efficient perspiration, while the regular elimination of faeces maintains the health of the colon.

Examination of waste products can reveal a great deal about doshic imbalance. Dark stools may be indicative of a problem with vata, while yellow-tinged stools may reveal an imbalance of pitta, and mucus in the faeces may be related to problems with kapha.

Understanding disease

In ayurvedic medicine, as in traditional Chinese medicine, good health can only be achieved when all aspects of the body, mind, emotions and spirit are working in harmony. Once an imbalance occurs in one organ or system it is likely to have repercussions elsewhere, resulting in a general state of ill health. Also in common with traditional Chinese medical approaches, an ayurvedic practitioner will regard each person as operating within the context of their physical and emotional environment, which has a potentially powerful positive or negative effect on health and vitality.

Problems are likely to arise when the mind and body have been exposed to physical and emotional stress for too long, and the doshic balance has been adversely affected. Once this process is well under way, certain factors, which in a state of doshic balance are unlikely to have a profound effect on overall experience of health, may begin to contribute a negative effect. These include food, profession, nature of social interaction, seasonal changes, emotional influences, or the choice of colour of clothes.

Potential factors that can have a disturbing effect on doshic harmony may include any of the following: trauma, bereavement, surgery, accidents, accumulation of toxins, or reduced or compromised agni.

AN EXCESS OF VATA

Specific factors that may accentuate an imbalance of vata include any of the following:
- Becoming chilled
- Lack of routine
- Skipping meals
- Poorly regulated exercise
- Excess of alcohol or convenience foods
- Use of stimulants
- Reduction in good-quality sleep
- Neglecting to moisturize the skin
- Repression of fear, anxiety or worry
- Change of season to autumn or early winter

If a dominance of vata is diagnosed, the following items should be avoided:
- Raw foods
- Dry foods
- Leafy vegetables
- Cold or frozen foods

The following may help establish a favourable balance of vata:
- Warm, dense, oily, moist foods
- Spices

AN EXCESS OF PITTA

An imbalance of pitta may be accentuated by:
- Consumption of red meat, or excessively spicy or salty foods
- Eating sporadically
- Antibiotic treatment
- An excess of alcohol
- Exhaustion
- Excessive exposure to heat
- Repression of anger, irritability or hatred
- Change of season to summer

If the pitta dosha is dominant, the following items should be avoided:

- Salty, sour or spicy foods
- Alcohol
- Meat
- Fatty, fried foods

The following may help balance pitta:
- Salads
- Cooling spices and herbs

AN EXCESS OF KAPHA

An imbalance of kapha may be accentuated by:
- Becoming too cold
- Excessive amounts of meat, fats, dairy products, fried foods or sweets
- Too much salt or water
- Overeating
- Too little exercise
- Oversleeping
- Lack of stimulation
- Sedative or tranquillizing drugs
- Becoming withdrawn and inward-looking as a result of lack of confidence
- Change of season to late winter and spring

Where kapha is dominant, the following items should be avoided:
- Sweet foods
- Salty foods
- Dairy products
- Fried foods
- Frozen foods

The following may help balance kapha:
- Vegetables
- Salads
- Light, dry-textured foods
- Spices

Phases of the disease process

From an ayurvedic perspective, the process of illness tends to build up over a fairly extended period of time. Within this timescale the following stages are likely to occur:

- **Accumulation** may take the form of mild discomfort in a particular area or system of the body. Where there is a dominance of vata this may take the form of too much wind, dryness of the mouth, constipation, chilliness or mild anxiety. In a predominantly pitta constitution this stage may manifest itself in symptoms of burning in various parts of the body, acidity of the stomach, or a general state of irritability. Those who have an imbalance of kapha may experience a general state of fatigue, reduced appetite and a pervasive sense of sluggishness.

• **Provocation** sees an increase in the severity of symptoms. Where the vata dosha is dominating, this may take the form of production of excess wind and constipation, chilliness of hands and feet, and a state of dehydration. Excess pitta at this stage may lead to acid indigestion, burning pains and a general tendency to be overcritical. An imbalance of kapha may produce a general state of distension, queasiness, drowsiness and increased production of saliva.

• **Spreading** occurs when the dominant dosha makes itself felt by affecting the tissues of the body, especially in areas of weakness or vulnerability. Symptoms may change at this point, or there may still be a vague sense of unease in the body, without being able to identify a specific problem in an isolated location. Where an excess of vata dosha exists this may lead to a general state of lethargy, relief of bloating, increased mental and emotional restlessness, as well as fear and anxiety. A dominance of pitta may lead to corrosive sensations on passing stools or urine, pale or yellow-coloured bowel movements and general digestive discomfort. On the other hand, excess kapha at this stage may result in generalized water retention, excess mucus production, vomiting and an overwhelming sense of sluggishness.

• **Deposition** occurs when the dominant or imbalanced dosha settles in the vulnerable tissues, creating toxic by-products.

• **Manifestation** can be identified when the results of the previous stage become more apparent and severe. At this stage, doshic balance can still be achieved by making positive adjustments in order to improve general lifestyle, especially if the latter is combined with treatment and advice from a ayurvedic practitioner.

• **Differentiation** occurs when the imbalanced dosha has upset the checks and balances of the system as a whole. Once this process has taken hold, an identifiable disease is likely to appear, with corresponding symptoms. At this point, even if appropriate measures are taken to rectify the doshic imbalance, there is a likelihood that the body will remain vulnerable or weak in this area. On the other hand, if the dominant dosha is not treated, and the symptoms are treated on a superficial level, there is a strong risk that the imbalanced dosha will do further damage in other tissues of the body and additional complications may arise in the future.

Although the first few stages of illness described above may be improved considerably by adopting self-help measures and making appropriate positive adjustments to general lifestyle, once the later stages are well under way, it is essential to seek qualified ayurvedic help in order to promote the best chance of a favourable outcome.

Dietary guidance

The following general guidelines are considered to have a beneficial effect on health and vitality from an ayurvedic perspective:

• Eat when genuinely hungry rather than from boredom or in response to a need for comfort.

• Avoid eating until your stomach has emptied itself of the last meal.

• Eat moderately, avoiding tendencies to under- or overeat.

• Concentrate on fresh, wholefoods, avoiding those that are undercooked, overcooked, burnt, unripe or overripe.

• Convenience foods or any items that have a long shelf-life should be avoided.

• Avoid drinking iced liquids immediately before or after a meal.

• Relax when eating a meal, concentrating on chewing each mouthful thoroughly. Avoid eating when the mind is distracted by other activities, such as reading or watching television.

• Always stop eating once your stomach feels satisfied.

The consultation

When determining the state of health of a patient ayurvedic practitioners make use of their powers of observation as well as a profound knowledge of the way the body functions. Questions will be asked about one's personal and professional life and eating habits, and a full medical history will be taken. The pulse is taken and the eyes, skin, tongue and nails may be examined.

On analysis of this information, an ayurvedic practitioner will decide on a course of therapeutic action. This could consist of the prescription of medicines made from herbal, mineral or vegetable origin, advice on dietary modifications, and the use of breathing techniques, steam baths, massage, oil treatments, meditation, exercise, relaxation, fasting, or deep cleansing through the use of enemas, purgatives and emetics.

Patients do not have to wait until they experience symptoms of illness before they consult an ayurvedic practitioner, since this is a system of healing that is particularly suited to the prevention as well as the treatment of illness.

Although ayurvedic treatment is much more accessible in India, where conventional doctors and ayurvedic practitioners work side by side, this system of healing is gaining popularity in the West. In the UK and the USA treatment may be obtained from Indian-trained practitioners or orthodox doctors who have undergone additional training in ayurvedic medicine.

Biochemic tissue salts

Biochemic tissue salts (also known as mineral tissue salts) are prescribed with a view to preserving or re-balancing the natural mineral salts found in the body. From the biochemic perspective, good health is dependent on these mineral salts remaining in a balanced and harmonious relationship with the body and each other.

There are twelve tissue salts, each one being identified by its chemical name, number and potency (strength). The latter is usually the 6x homoeopathic dilution (see page 87), and the tissue salts are taken in the form of small white tablets. In addition to the twelve primary tissue salts, there are also combination formulas that are suitable for the treatment of specific conditions such as hay fever, heartburn and acidity, or coughs and colds. The combination formulas are prepared and manufactured in the same way as the single salts and are taken in exactly the same way.

Historical perspectives

The development of the theory and practice of biochemic tissue salt therapy is attributed to a German physician, Dr William Heinrich Schuessler, who was born in 1821, and practised medicine in Oldenburg, Germany. Schuessler became intrigued by the work of the homoeopathic physician, Samuel Hahnemann (see page 27) and decided to incorporate the use of homoeopathic medicines into his practice. Although he initially employed the full range of homoeopathic medicines, he slowly began to focus on the use of inorganic substances in homoeopathic dilution.

Schuessler's decision was motivated by his growing belief that the organs of the body required support from optimum amounts of inorganic substances in order to maintain their structure and function. This view was explored in 1873 when he published his *Shortened Therapeutics*, and further expanded in a later range of articles a cohesive explanation of mineral tissue salt therapy. By conducting a series of experiments in which he observed the effects of the salts in some naturally occurring minerals on the body, Schuessler's method for experimentation resembled that of Samuel Hahnemann, since he proceeded to administer doses of his mineral salts and then take note of any changes or effects in health.

The basis of Schuessler's theory rested upon the idea that ill health resulted from an imbalance of essential minerals in the cells of the body. Once this balance could be rectified by administering the appropriate mineral salt, the problem would be solved as the optimum cell balance was re-established. As Schuessler came to develop and refine his ideas, he isolated the twelve vital mineral salts that came to form the basis of current mineral tissue salt therapy. These medicines are understood to act 'biochemically' by balancing and harmonizing chemical changes at a cellular level in the body, thereby treating illness by rectifying a basic mineral deficiency.

After Schuessler's death in 1898, Dr Julius Hensel, a fellow German, continued the development begun by Schuessler by publishing a number of books on minerals which he had started in the 1880s. This included material on both the agricultural and medical potential of minerals.

In common with the spread of homoeopathic ideas, Schuessler's therapeutic concepts were readily imported to the USA, largely as a result of the work of Dr H.C.G. Luyties, an American who translated Schuessler's texts into English. Further links were also established with the homoeopathic system of medicine when the eminent American homoeopathic physician Dr Constantine Herring published a text that dealt with tissue salts as a system of healing.

Basic background

When biochemic tissue salts are prepared, the active ingredient must be diluted with lactose (milk sugar). The desired proportions are one part of active tissue salt to nine parts of lactose base. These are ground together for a considerable period of time in a process called *trituration*.

The mixture continues to be diluted by adding nine parts of lactose to the mixture until the final stage has been reached. At each stage of dilution, the potency of the product is regarded as being increased. Therefore, in the same way that homoeopathic medicines are regarded as becoming more powerful as they go through progressive stages of dilution, biochemic tissue salts may also be regarded as becoming stronger as they are triturated and diluted further.

Most tissue salts are available in the 6x potency, which means that they have gone through the process of trituration six times with a ratio of one-in-ten dilution (see page 87).

The consultation

Biochemic tissue salts may be prescribed as an adjunctive treatment by a range of therapists such as naturopaths, herbalists or homoeopaths. However, most of the mineral tissue salts that are used are likely to have been bought in a self-help capacity, since they are readily available in pharmacies and health-food shops. They are generally very user-friendly because their labelling clearly identifies the condition they are likely to help, and dosage instructions are easy to follow. Acute conditions (see page 74 for a definition of 'acute'), self-limiting conditions such as colds, cuts and minor burns are most suitable for treatment, although some long-standing conditions such as hay fever may be temporarily relieved by using the appropriate tissue salt formulation.

Biochemic tissue salts are non-habit forming and should not give rise to any side effects. However, those who suffer from an intolerance to lactose (milk sugar) should bear in mind that tissue salt tablets are lactose-based.

Conditions that may respond to biochemic tissue salts

- Anxiety
- Arthritis
- Asthma
- Boils
- Bronchitis
- Catarrh
- Chilblains
- Colds
- Coughs
- Digestive problems
- Hay fever
- Headache
- Migraine
- Muscular aches and pains
- Neuralgia
- Painful periods
- Poor circulation
- Sprains and strains
- Stings

Homoeopathy

Homoeopathic medicine is a system of healing that was established approximately 200 years ago. It is practised by both conventionally trained doctors and professional homoeopaths in a wide variety of countries. In experienced hands, homoeopathic medicine provides a way of restoring the sick patient to health in a gentle, thorough and effective way.

This approach to healing is particularly attractive to those who are interested in tackling ill health at a fundamental level. Unlike conventional medical approaches that attempt to suppress symptoms of disease, homoeopathic treatment aims to stimulate the self-healing mechanism of the body by the use of appropriately prescribed homoeopathic medicines.

Historical perspectives

The word 'homoeopathy' originates from a Greek source, and can be loosely translated to mean 'similar suffering'. In other words, a substance that causes disease symptoms in a healthy person if given in detectable, material doses can be used in a therapeutic way. The substance works therapeutically when given to a sick person in the form of a minute, energized dose, provided the symptoms experienced by the patient resemble those that are known to be produced by that substance.

This idea of using similar substances in order to stimulate cure, rather than medicines that would have the opposite effect, is an idea that dates from the time of the ancient Greeks. However, it was the eighteenth-century German physician, Samuel Hahnemann (1755–1843) who developed the basic concept into the modern medical theory of homoeopathy. By doing so, he established the theoretical and philosophical basis of a radically original medical system.

In the process, Hahnemann put forward an extremely controversial interpretation of the understanding of health and disease that ran completely at odds with the popular medical ideas of his day. Although a large gulf still exists between conventional medical approaches and the homoeopathic perspective, we are gradually seeing the emergence of explanations for the proof of the efficacy of homoeopathy from an orthodox scientific perspective. However, a large proportion of conventional physicians have great difficulty in accepting the validity of homoeopathy as a system of healing.

At the age of thirty-nine Hahnemann abandoned his career as a conventional doctor, feeling he was inflicting rather than alleviating suffering. Since he was a gifted linguist, Hahnemann chose to translate foreign medical texts, while he continued to conduct experiments into gentler ways of restoring sick patients to health. He gained a major insight while translating the work of the Scottish herbalist William Cullen, who offered an explanation for the effectiveness of cinchona bark in treating the symptoms of malaria. In Cullen's opinion, the medicinal effects of cinchona were related to the astringent or bitter qualities of the bark. Hahnemann, however, was unsatisfied with this reasoning, since he could cite examples of other astringent medicines that did not ease malaria symptoms. As a result, he decided to conduct his own experiments in order to see if he could find a more appropriate answer.

Hahnemann proceeded to take regular doses of cinchona himself, recording the effects that arose. The results of this experiment proved to be both fascinating and of crucial importance, allowing Hahnemann the insights that were needed in order to establish a fresh perspective on the healing process. What he discovered was that while he continued to take cinchona bark he experienced symptoms that resembled malaria, but once he stopped taking it, the symptoms subsided. This discovery became the cornerstone of homoeopathic theory which involves giving patients 'similar' medicines.

Although the theoretical and practical origins of homoeopathy lie in Germany, the therapy rapidly gained popularity in the UK, spread with enthusiasm to the USA by the nineteenth century, and had firmly established itself in India by the beginning of the twentieth century. Homoeopathic medicine also has a high profile in France and continues to gain ground in a number of other countries such as Mexico, Argentina, Brazil, Australia, South Africa, New Zealand, Holland and Greece. There are also hopeful signs of positive development in Eastern Europe and Russia.

Basic background

'Similar' medicines are understood to stimulate the healing process only when they are given to a patient whose disease symptoms closely resemble those that are triggered when the same substance is repeatedly given to a healthy person. As he developed these ideas further, using an increasing range of substances, Hahnemann began to consider how he might lessen any adverse effects caused by the administration of these medicines. In his quest for the gentlest and most humane form of treatment, Hahnemann used more and more dilute forms of each substance.

As he was working with increasingly dilute medicines, Hahnemann made a quantum leap in his thinking by adding the systematic repetition of vigorous shaking or 'succussion' at each stage of dilution. He discovered that dilution and succussion must be carried out in order for a medicine to fulfil its curative potential, a process that came to be known as 'potentization'.

As Hahnemann observed the effects of these potentized medicines in action (provided they were prescribed on the basis of 'similar' selection), he became increasingly aware that his observations ran

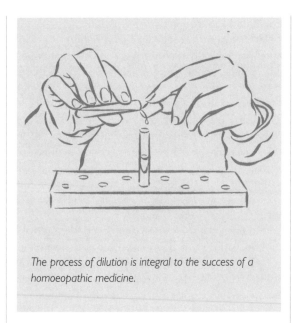

The process of dilution is integral to the success of a homoeopathic medicine.

totally at odds with anything that could be explained by the scientific theories of his day. From the reactions he witnessed in his patients, the more dilute and succussed a medicine became (even to the point where there were no molecules of the original substance remaining), the more powerful the medicinal effect appeared to be on the patient.

Homoeopathic 'provings'

In order to establish the effects of a substance on a healthy individual, Hahnemann proceeded to carry out a series of controlled experiments – like his cinchona experiment – on himself and a small circle of volunteers. These experiments were called 'provings' and involved each person taking tiny amounts of a substance repeatedly and recording its effects at emotional, mental and physical levels in minute detail.

It was very important that the people selected for the experiments should be in good health and free of obvious symptoms. They also had to be prepared to observe and record very precisely any marked variation in their physical, mental or emotional health for as long as the experiment continued.

Concepts of vital energy

As Hahnemann refined and developed his ideas, he came to the conclusion that there must be some fundamental intelligence that governs the smooth functioning of the human body in a state of good health. When this basic intelligence or 'vital force' comes into conflict with a stressful stimulus that cannot be resisted, symptoms of illness or disease appear. This lack of resistance, different in each individual, is called susceptibility and may occur for a variety of reasons, including genetic inheritance and the weakening effect of conventional drugs. Hahnemann concluded that these symptoms are a sign of the body's dynamic, but inconclusive attempt to establish self-healing, thus giving vital clues as to the nature of the imbalance, while also providing essential information that can lead towards the selection of the most appropriate homoeopathic remedy.

The single dose

Although it is common practice in some areas to give more than one homoeopathic remedy at a time in the form of a combination formula, it is also usual among classical homoeopathic practitioners to give one remedy at a time to the patient. This is important on a practical level alone, since it can be very difficult to assess how effective each remedy has been if more than one has been given at the same time.

It is also important to bear in mind that the wealth of information we possess about each homoeopathic remedy has been gathered as a result of experiments using single remedies rather than multiple formulas. Consequently, we have no reliable information on the specific action of combination remedies.

On the other hand, special circumstances do exist in which the use of combination formulas can be helpful. These include situations when an untrained person is self-prescribing, or where it may be extremely difficult to obtain sufficient individualizing or characteristic symptoms from a patient (this can happen, for example, when prescribing for babies or small children). When this problem occurs, it can be practically very difficult to differentiate between the choice of one homoeopathic remedy over another. For example, it can be helpful in this type of situation for a homoeopathic practitioner to give a homoeopathic travel-sickness formula that may contain up to half-a-dozen appropriate remedies. On the other hand, the practitioner should bear in mind that if an obviously indicated remedy emerges after considering the main features of the patient, it is always worthwhile going for the single remedy first.

Treating the whole person

Homoeopathic and conventional medical practitioners work in very different ways when gathering relevant information on which to base an appropriate prescription. An orthodox doctor is interested in symptoms classed in the relevant disease category, and as a result of this diagnosis, a specific course of action may consist of drug therapy, conducting further tests or considering surgery. A homoeopath, on the other hand, is much more likely to show interest in symptoms that communicate something of the individuality of the patient.

This may be illustrated by the following simple example. Two patients consult a homoeopath, having both been given a diagnosis of osteoarthritis. The first patient experiences severe joint pains that are most troublesome on waking, improving progressively as the limbs become more mobile through the day. The pains are much more severe at night, leading to terrific physical and mental restlessness with an accompanying sense of despondency and depression. However, a warm bath does a great deal to ease the pain. The second patient, although suffering from the identical condition, experiences joint pains that feel much easier when lying in bed or keeping as still as possible. Becoming too warm results in increased discomfort and overall distress and irritability, while cooling down brings marked relief.

From this simple comparison we can appreciate that although two patients may be given the same diagnosis, each one experiences their illness in their own individual way. Although information about general symptoms can be useful in reaching a diagnosis, it is the uncommon or peculiar symptoms that convey a sense of the patient's individuality to the homoeopath, rather than common features of the condition such as pain, swelling or inflammation.

In order to understand how an individual patient is affected by their symptoms it is essential for a homoeopath to have a detailed grasp of the problem. If the major symptom that the patient is suffering from is severe pain, the homoeopath must question the patient very closely in order to gain as much information as possible about the specific sensations experienced by the patient. Questions may include: How long has the pain been present? What makes it better or worse? Is it static in location or does it move around from place to place? What emotional response does the patient have to the pain? and What is the nature of the pain? (e.g. stinging, burning, cutting, stabbing, throbbing or aching.) The homoeopath will also explore general effects on the mind and body, and investigate the possible factors that may be linked to the onset of the problem.

By working along these lines, a homoeopath can build up a detailed picture of the patient's problem and place it within the broad context of the patient's mental, emotional and physical health. This is known as the 'symptom picture'. Once this information has been obtained and analysed, the practitioner can choose the most appropriate homoeopathic remedy for his or her patient.

The consultation

Many patients are surprised to discover that their initial consultation with a homoeopath lasts an hour to an hour and a half. This interview needs to be lengthy because of the thoroughness of the questions, which are likely to include detailed questions relating to the current problem, general quality of health, current orthodox medication and the patient's full medical history. The homoeopath gains as accurate a picture of the patient's psychological and emotional well-being as is possible within the constrictions of time available. A conventional doctor who practises homoeopathic medicine may also want to conduct appropriate tests or physical examinations.

Once a full and detailed case history has been taken, your homoeopath will want to analyse the

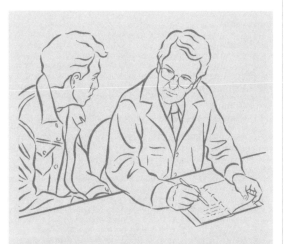

The first homeopathic consultation may last up to an hour and a half, during which a detailed history of the patient's mental, emotional and physical health is taken.

information, in order to identify the unifying or characteristic features that run through your symptoms. Once this analysis has been completed, your practitioner will select an appropriate homoeopathic medicine that matches your symptoms most closely on mental, emotional and physical levels.

The remedy may be given as a single tablet or a short course of tablets that may be taken daily. Other possible methods of administration include powders, liquids, granules or globules. Once your reaction to the treatment has been established, a decision will be made whether to watch and wait, repeat the remedy, choose a higher potency (stronger dose) or change the prescription.

You are likely to need to return for follow-up appointments at intervals of four to six weeks for the initial few months in order to give your homoeopath a chance to assess the progress you are making.

Conditions that may respond to homoeopathy

As with anthroposophical and herbal medicine, homoeopathy can be used for a wide range of health problems. However, conditions that may respond well to homoeopathic treatment can include any of the following:

- Allergies
- Anxiety
- Asthma
- Cystitis
- Depression
- Digestive problems
- Eczema
- Menopausal problems
- Menstrual problems
- Osteoarthritis
- Recurrent infections
- Rheumatoid arthritis
- Strains and sprains
- Tension headaches and migraines
- Thrush

Naturopathy

Naturopathy is a holistic system of healing that seeks to increase the body's inherent ability to maintain its equilibrium and fight off disease. Naturopaths view ill health as an indication that the body is struggling to return to a state of good health. Instead of attempting to suppress symptoms, a naturopath seeks to discover the source of the problem and offer advice that will support the body in overcoming illness. As a result, when naturopathic treatment has been effectively completed, the patient's whole system should have been strengthened. Naturopathic treatment can include dietary change, controlled fasting, as well as hydrotherapy and relaxation and stress-management techniques.

Naturopaths regard ill health as something that affects the whole person, including their physical, emotional and mental well-being. As a result, treatment is seldom targeted at a specific symptom or organ in isolation, but is much broader and far reaching in scope.

Basic background

Naturopathy is different from conventional medicine in that it does not seek to identify a specific disease agent and subdue it with an appropriate drug. The conventional approach is not generally interested in building up the body's capacity for self-healing, with the unfortunate result that problems tend to recur after drug therapy has been completed, often because the patient's underlying predisposition – due to an unhealthy diet, an excess of physical or mental stress or a drastic lack of exercise – to the condition has remained untouched.

Naturopaths believe that the symptoms of illness retreat when the body, mind and emotions are functioning in optimum balance for each individual. In order to reach this balanced state, they seek to stimulate a natural healing mechanism (very similar to the homoeopathic concept of 'vital force' or Chinese concept of qi). This mechanism may be stimulated in any of the following ways.

The nutritional perspective

Restoring optimum health through dietary and nutritional measures is a vital part of the naturopathic approach. Controlled fasting, use of fresh vegetable and fruit juices, raw foods and unprocessed foods are often recommended by naturopaths in order to cleanse or detoxify the system. Naturopaths regard many illnesses as arising from a build-up of toxic waste in the body, so encouraging efficient elimination of these toxins through dietary measures is thought to increase the body's resilience and resistance to disease. It, is interesting to note that the general consensus of opinion about what constitutes a healthy diet has moved much closer to a naturopathic perspective, since the bulk of current nutritional advice stresses the need for a high-fibre, low-salt, low-fat and low-sugar diet. Convenience or 'junk' foods are increasingly associated with a poor state of health due to their high proportion of chemical additives such as preservatives, colourings and flavourings. Since they also often include surprisingly large amounts of 'hidden' fats, sugars and salt, they can also be detrimental to those people who suffer from heart disease, high blood pressure, diabetes or arthritis. Convenience foods are also often very low in fibre due to their highly refined nature, and may be extremely low in vitamin and mineral content. When viewed in the light of this information, the naturopathic perspective makes a great deal of sense, with its emphasis on the need for food to be as fresh and wholesome as possible in order to aid the body's capacity for resilience and renewal.

The physical perspective

Some naturopaths may offer soft tissue manipulation (massage) or osteopathic techniques in order to promote optimum alignment of the spine, and suppleness and lack of rigidity of the muscles. In addition, hydrotherapy techniques such as alternating hot and cold sitz baths (see pages 314-15), compresses, packs, wraps, sprays or douches may be recommended in order to stimulate circulation and balanced nerve function. The water used may be either hot or cold, or may alternate. In health hydros the therapeutic benefits of sea water (thalassotherapy) in the form of jet sprays or massage techniques when bathing in a shallow amount of sea water may be recommended. In addition, seaweed body wraps and bathing in mineral-rich mud may also be advocated.

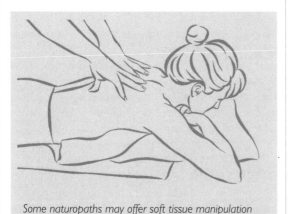

Some naturopaths may offer soft tissue manipulation (massage) in order to promote optimum alignment of the spine.

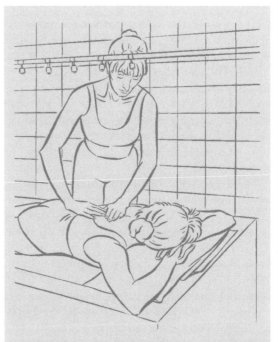

The therapeutic benefits of sea water can be used as part of hydrotherapy massage.

The psychological perspective

Naturopaths offer a system of healing that may be used as a preventative measure, in promoting the self-healing potential of the body, as well as a treatment for disease. They acknowledge the important link between the state of mind of a patient and their overall experience of health – in other words, they realize that bereavement, stress or prolonged anxiety can have a detrimental effect on the body's ability to keep illness at bay, while prolonged pain or chronic illness can also result in feelings of depression and despair. In such situations naturopaths may make use of counselling skills, relaxation techniques and stress-management skills when treating their patients.

Historical perspectives

Naturopathy can be regarded as a Western form of Far Eastern or Asian systems of holistic medicine that emphasize the positive role played by herbalism, dietary adjustments, exercise and relaxation in supporting the body in fighting illness. In many ways, there are strong parallels between the naturopathic approach and traditional Chinese and ayurvedic medicine.

Although the basic guidelines of naturopathy were laid down by the Greek physician Hippocrates approximately 2500 years ago, it only became fully developed in the nineteenth century, when it was extremely fashionable to visit the spa towns of Europe and 'take the waters'. Mineral-rich waters could be taken internally or externally, and were regarded as having beneficial therapeutic qualities because of their purity or health-enhancing properties, such as their content of zinc, calcium or sodium.

Therapists such as Vincent Priessnitz, in Germany, emphasized the healing potential of water, developing the concept of hydrotherapy. This involved hosing or sprinkling the body with water, as well as advocating the pursuit of walking barefoot in damp grass. Priessnitz set up the first hydrotherapy establishment in Bohemia (now part of the Czech Republic) in the early part of the nineteenth century and similar establishments were opened in Austria and England later in the century.

By the close of the nineteenth century, naturopathy was brought to the USA by Benedict Lust, a patient who had been treated successfully in Europe by the naturopathic approach. Although naturopathy has waxed and waned in popularity over the course of the last hundred years, it appears to be enjoying a healthy upsurge of interest as we approach the close of this century.

The consultation

The initial consultation with a naturopath is likely to take roughly an hour, during which all aspects of a patient's health will be explored. The patient will be questioned about his or her full medical history, working environment, eating patterns, sleep quality, digestive symptoms, including bowel movements, quality of relationships and energy levels. Blood pressure, lungs, heart, joints, muscles and body reflexes may be assessed in a range of routine tests, and blood and urine samples may be taken for analysis. Mineral imbalances or toxic metal accumulations may be established by examination of the iris, while samples of blood or hair may be sent off for analysis for the same reason.

If any conditions requiring surgery or further medical examination are apparent, your naturopath should refer you to your family doctor in order to arrange for a more detailed assessment. If, on the other hand, your condition is of a more straightforward nature, your naturopath will give advice about positive adjustments to your lifestyle. These may include dietary changes, fasting, hydrotherapeutic techniques or relaxation exercises. In addition, any of the following treatments may be offered in order to speed up the healing process: acupuncture, osteopathy, herbalism or homoeopathy.

The length of treatment will be related to each individual's potential for progress. As improvement occurs, experience of overall health should improve steadily, sometimes punctuated by occasional relapses or 'healing crises'. When symptoms reappear, they often occur in reverse order of their appearance, and move from more internal levels to the surface. As a result, digestive or respiratory problems will usually clear up before a skin disorder, which may be the last symptom to leave.

Conditions that may respond to naturopathic treatment

Although naturopathy may not be a cure-all, patients suffering from many common conditions may respond well to this kind of treatment. These problems may include any of the following:
• Allergies

- Asthma
- Bronchitis
- Constipation
- Cystitis
- Diverticulitis
- Eczema
- Indigestion
- Irritable bowel syndrome
- Menstrual problems
- Migraine
- Osteoarthritis
- Post-viral syndrome and ME
- Psoriasis
- Recurrent colds
- Rheumatoid arthritis
- Thrush

Naturopathy is holistic in approach and will encourage the natural healing mechanism to create balance, harmony and health in the body, mind and spirit, so all 'symptom' labels can be addressed at some level. However, a properly qualified and responsible naturopath will always be aware of 'disease crises' as well as 'healing crises', and in these cases will liaise with the medical profession.

Age should not be a barrier to treatment, since babies and the elderly may benefit from naturopathy. On the other hand, it can be helpful to adopt a naturopathic approach as early as possible in the development of illness, ideally before the situation may have become complicated through the use of suppressive drug treatment. Conventional drugs have the dual disadvantage of creating possible side effects that may become difficult to differentiate from the symptoms of the original problem, and they can also weaken or suppress the functioning of the immune system if used in large doses over an extended period of time. Since the naturopath encourages the body to strengthen its own defences, it is clear that the sooner treatment begins, the better.

It is also helpful to bear in mind that naturopathy can be extremely beneficial when used as a preventative treatment to keep the body in optimum condition. As a result, it is quite appropriate to consult a naturopath before symptoms of illness have developed.

TRADITIONAL CHINESE MEDICINE

Traditional Chinese medicine is a holistic system of healing that attempts to restore the whole being to health, rather than concentrating solely on the removal of symptoms of illness. As a result, practitioners of TCM acknowledge the importance of maintaining a harmonious interaction between mind and body if a genuine state of good health is to be experienced. Strong emphasis is also put on the interdependence of bodily systems and organs, with attention being drawn to the way that an imbalance in one organ will often result in a chain reaction in others that eventually destabilizes good health.

Although many people may be most familiar with acupuncture as a form of TCM, the latter also embraces the practice of Chinese herbal medicine, and systems of movement such as qi gong, which can be regarded as forming a bridge between meditation and exercise.

Because TCM puts strong emphasis on the need for preventing the development of disease in the first place, practitioners of this branch of medicine are also likely to give clear advice on the need for changes in diet or lifestyle that are supportive of good health. In this way, the patient is encouraged to see himself as playing a positive role in achieving and protecting a state of positive good health once the immediate problem has been taken care of. As a result, relapses should not be a frequent occurrence, nor should it be necessary to embark on a permanent course of treatment in order to keep symptoms at bay.

Historical perspectives

Chinese medicine has its roots in the distant past,

with traces of its practice dating back 4000 or 5000 years. This is not particularly remarkable: many ancient civilizations have built up impressive bodies of herbal lore, usually linked to a belief in evil spirits and malign forces as the causes of sickness. We still have sometimes detailed accounts of the medical practices of the Babylonians, Egyptians and others.

Where China stands out is in the creation of a corpus of medical texts within which a living tradition of medical theory and practice has been preserved and developed for around 2500 years. Some 8000 medical texts are recorded and accorded the status of 'national treasures'.

Chinese medicine gradually moved from an early reliance on superstition and shamanism towards a codified, naturalistic understanding of sickness and health, linking specific imbalances in the patient's physical system or environment to specific counter-balances in the form of herbs, acupuncture or exercise. The subsequent development of the system owed much to the relative stability of Chinese civilization. A steady output of more or less canonical books culminated in the sixteenth-century *Ben Cao Gang Mu*, written by Li Shizhen. This text, *The Outlines and Branches of Herbal Medicine*, came to be regarded as the most important treatise on the subject, and by the time it was written, contact between China and the West had already begun.

Europeans first came into contact with Chinese medicine in the fifteenth century as a result of Jesuit activity in the Far East. By the sixteenth century some Chinese herbs were imported to Europe, while a form of inoculation against smallpox was introduced to England in the early part of the eighteenth century. This inoculation developed by the Chinese involved inserting powdered smallpox scabs into the nostrils on wads of cotton wool. The nose was plugged and left for a number of days. Unfortunately, this method was not risk free: some children died as a result, although many more survived.

In the nineteenth century, some hospitals using Western medical approaches and drugs were set up in the cities, while the use of TCM was relied upon by the vast rural population. After the nationalist takeover in 1911, the Government attempted severely to restrict the practice of TCM as part of its drive towards modernization. However, TCM retained its popularity and, in addition, by the 1940s it had become apparent that there were far too few doctors trained in Western conventional medicine to meet the needs of the Chinese population as a whole. As a result, the Communist leader Mao Tse-tung announced in 1950 that all medical resources should be pooled together so that patients could benefit from the best of TCM and Western medical techniques. The aim was to train health workers called 'barefoot doctors' in basic medical care so that simple but effective treatment could be given in the country areas. In practice, the system did not work as well as it could have done. Learning was under attack – one of the slogans of the time was 'The more books you read, the stupider you get', and untrained and unqualified people were sent out to practise medicine. If this anti-learning bias had not existed it is conceivable that the barefoot doctor scheme could have become a model for primary health care in the Third World.

In many ways, the greatest publicity coverage given to TCM was in the early 1970s, when a US journalist covering Richard Nixon's state visit to China required emergency surgery to remove his appendix. The operation was done using acupuncture for pain relief instead of a general anaesthetic, so that the journalist remained fully conscious for the duration of the operation. When his account of his experience of acupuncture was given worldwide coverage, the attention focused on this method of anaesthesia was immense. Suddenly, questions were asked in the West about the possible explanations that could be given for the effectiveness of acupuncture as a pain-reliever, and investigations made into how widely it was used within Chinese hospitals. As a result of this media coverage, the Western world was introduced to the concept of acupuncture on a large scale.

The development of TCM in China has continued to the present day with research units conducting scientific studies into tongue examination, pulse-reading and acupuncture. Strenuous efforts have been made to amalgamate Western medicine and TCM, so that a patient admitted to a Chinese casualty department is likely to find their pulse and tongue examined in the traditional way, while a victim of a heart attack may find themselves being given an intravenous drip of red sage and black aconite as well as topical herbal treatments and acupuncture.

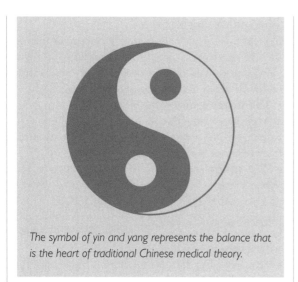

The symbol of yin and yang represents the balance that is the heart of traditional Chinese medical theory.

Basic background

The theory behind traditional Chinese medicine is one of the most profoundly holistic approaches to medical treatment in existence. Not only are individual parts of the body viewed as relating to and being dependent upon others for their balanced and healthy functioning, but the human organism is seen as part of a greater whole that is affected by the rhythms of nature and climatic changes. In this way, each human being can be viewed as operating within a broader context that includes social relationships and environmental factors such as reactions to pollutants, weather changes and so forth.

The concept of balance (Tao, as it is often called) is at the heart of traditional Chinese medical theory with two opposing but complementary aspects that make up a perfectly balanced whole. These two principles are called *yin* and *yang*. Yang is associated with qualities such as heat, fire, light, restlessness and dryness, and is outgoing and extrovert. Yin qualities are related to cold, dampness, tranquillity, earth and darkness, and are reflective and inward-looking.

In good health these two principles should be in balance, with neither dominating the other. However, once ill health manifests itself, a traditional Chinese physician is likely to discover that either yin or yang is dominant, creating an unhealthy imbalance that may be expressed in symptoms of physical and/or emotional unease. Within this context, health can be positively or adversely affected by internal and external factors that can result in body fluids or vital fluids becoming excessive, diminished, stagnant, chilled or heated.

As a result, in TCM practitioners may speak of chill affecting the circulation in the same way that extreme cold may cause the water of a river to freeze, or excessive heat of the blood resulting in inflammation, high temperature or the formation of boils or abscesses. Although this language may sound rather strange and unscientific to Westerners when we first encounter it, we may begin to grasp these concepts more readily if we regard them as expressing disorders of the body in terminology that would normally be reserved for describing seasonal influences and changes in our external surroundings.

The concept of harmony

The notion of balance and harmony is central to traditional Chinese medical perspectives, and the concept of harmony may be expressed in three ways.

Harmony with nature

This involves the necessity of being in tune with nature and its seasonal ebbing and flowing. Within this context, the diet should consist of foods that are in season, and advantage should be taken of longer summer days and good weather by taking more exercise in the fresh air. On the other hand, the shorter, colder days of winter are a good time to enjoy longer periods of rest and relaxation.

Internal harmony

This emphasizes the need for the five major organs (the heart, lungs, liver, kidneys and spleen) to work

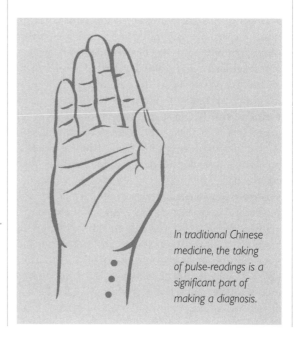

In traditional Chinese medicine, the taking of pulse-readings is a significant part of making a diagnosis.

in harmony with each other and with the stomach, gall bladder, intestines and bladder.

Physical and mental harmony

Balance and harmony must be maintained on mental and emotional levels to ensure physical health. In the same way that physical disorders can affect the mental outlook and state of mind, an overpowering emotional experience can have an adverse effect on physical health. In this way, mind and body are regarded as being inextricably interlinked.

The five substances

These are regarded in TCM as the elements that make up a human being.

• **Shen** is related to consciousness, mental faculties, spiritual experience and memory, and a disturbance on this level may result in lethargy, anxiety, difficulty in concentrating, sleep problems or hysteria, depending on the nature of the imbalance. A deficiency that affects the shen may result in depression, melancholia or lack of energy, while shen obstruction could lead to more serious mental illness such as manic depression or schizophrenia.

• **Qi** is similar to the homoeopathic concept of vital energy: the unseen force that animates the mind and body. A deficiency of this element may result in weak muscles, exhaustion, lack of appetite, recurrent infections and easy bleeding. Stagnation of qi may lead to stress-related problems, irritability and digestive disorders.

• **Jing** may be understood as our inherited constitutional experience of health and energy: in other words, our optimum level of well-being. A deficiency of this substance may result in retarded development in children, poor bone density, mental slowness, infertility and failure to thrive.

• **Body fluids**, such as perspiration, saliva or gastric juices. A deficiency of these fluids may lead to chronic dryness of the skin, hair or mucous membranes, while an excess may result in fluid retention.

• **Blood** nourishes and irrigates the various parts of the body. A deficiency of this element would lead to light-headedness, blurred vision, numbness, trembling and pallor. Stagnation would lead to signs of poor circulation such as purple tinges to the nails, lips and tongue and a tendency to dark, clotted menstrual bleeding. Heat in the blood could result in inflammation, skin rashes and heavy bleeding.

The major organs

In TCM the organs manufacture, store and distribute the five substances. As a result, the relative strength or weakness of an organ will have a profound effect on the production of an essential substance.

• **The heart** regulates the blood and blood vessels, as well as storing the shen. If the shen is out of balance we may experience problems with insomnia that are connected to palpitations and anxiety.

• **The lungs** are related to the regulation of qi. When the qi is functioning well we should experience smooth, regular, deep breathing, but, if we have problems with the regulation of qi as a result of poor lung function, we may suffer breathing disorders, asthma or recurrent coughs.

• **The liver** has the dual function of regulating the smooth flow of qi as well as storing the blood. Problems with the flow of qi might result in irregular periods, breathing problems, poor digestion and mood swings, while disturbance in the latter could lead to dizziness on standing, pins and needles, muscle cramps or heavy or light periods.

• **The spleen** is responsible for transporting and transforming food and drink into energy or qi. If these functions are poor, symptoms such as loss of appetite, heavy sensations after eating and loose bowel movements are likely to occur. Weakness in the spleen can lead to heavy and drooping sensations in the abdomen, a tendency to prolapse of the bowel or uterus, problems with hernia and seepage of blood from the blood vessels.

• **The kidneys** are particularly important, because all other organs are dependent on the kidneys for their yin or yang energy. As a result, TCM practitioners always pay a great deal of attention to whether the kidneys are functioning well by examining the pulse and tongue. Because of the strong relationship between the kidneys and the jing element, problems with the kidneys may emerge as jing-deficiency symptoms, such as retarded development, premature ageing or impotence.

External influences

These can provide the final part of the puzzle and enable a TCM practitioner to reach a diagnosis of the 'pattern of disharmony' in each patient. There are five external influences in total, all of which can be resisted when we remain in vigorous good health. However, when we are under par, we may be vulnerable to any of the following climatic influences.

• **Wind** may be combined with cold to form a chill that can penetrate the body, giving rise to ill health. Wind symptoms may arise with rapidity and often take on an intermittent nature (such as pains that move from joint to joint). Areas of the body most vulnerable to problems from wind include the lungs and the skin.

• **Cold** can penetrate the body, leading to pains in the joints, stomach, intestines or uterus that may respond well to topical applications of heat.

• **Damp** can become a problem when the body is exposed to wet domestic or working conditions for an extended period of time. It can encourage accumulation of body fluids and it can also obstruct the free movement of qi. Damp can also occur in the body if body fluids are not circulating with the necessary vigour. Symptoms that may arise as a consequence of this kind of stagnation include poor appetite and a tendency to feel full soon after eating. This situation may be aggravated further by eating foods that have a reputation for aggravating internal damp, such as dairy products or fried foods.

• **Fire and heat** are associated with inflammatory states. Heat may be associated with superficial problems such as the common cold, especially if it is associated with mild feverishness and a sore throat. Fire, however, is an internally generated problem that may occur as a result of a deficiency of body fluids. Common symptoms that arise as a result of this state include a flushed face, high temperature, boils, marked thirst, a bitter taste in the mouth, easy bleeding, disturbed sleep and irritability.

• **Dryness** has some similarities with heat, since it is manifested as a deficiency of body fluids, and may cause dryness of the lips, nostrils, tongue, stools and skin.

Methods of application

When consulting a practitioner of traditional Chinese medicine any of the following treatments may be used:

• Chinese herbal medicine
• Acupuncture
• Systems of movement such as qi gong.

Since each of these forms a discipline in its own right, it is best to examine each branch of TCM independently to get a general perspective on how each facet of this holistic medical system complements the others.

Chinese herbal medicine

A Chinese herbal medicine practitioner places great importance on the examination of the pulse and tongue, and will closely question a patient, as well as using keen powers of observation. A combination of dried herbs prescribed to help re-establish harmony in the system. Although it has been employed in China for over 2000 years, the use of Chinese herbs has only recently gained much publicity in the West, due to the effective treatment of skin conditions such as eczema.

Basic background

A Chinese herbalist gathers information about a patient through a combination of verbal communication and detailed physical observation. A diagnosis and plan of treatment will be decided upon after the herbalist has identified the patterns of the illness suffered by each individual. It is important to remember that the resulting diagnosis is unlikely to sound anything like that which a conventional Western physician would give, since a Chinese herbalist will make use of a different vocabulary. For example, one patient may be described as experiencing 'heart blood deficiency', while another may be regarded as suffering from 'liver qi stagnation'. (For a simple explanation of this terminology see page 36.)

A diagnosis can be reached only after the Chinese herbalist has put together a wealth of information from the patient that is gathered as a result of keen observation and subtle questioning. The latter may involve asking detailed questions about the nature of the main health problem, including its duration, intensity, location and persistence. Additional questions may be asked about factors that make it better or worse, and if there is a pattern to the onset of the

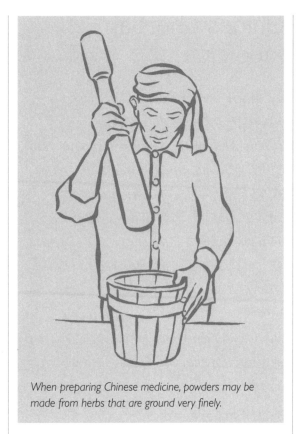

When preparing Chinese medicine, powders may be made from herbs that are ground very finely.

problem (for example, if there is any time of day when the condition seems most apparent).

Some time may also be spent investigating potential triggers of illness that may have been present immediately before the onset of the problem, such as a period of extreme physical, emotional or mental stress. Aspects of a healthy or unhealthy lifestyle are also likely to be explored, including areas such as diet, exercise and relaxation.

A system of head-to-toe questioning may be employed in order to establish the various parts of the body that are vulnerable to illness and infection, exploring each of these problems in detail. Special attention may be given to questions relating to the functioning of the digestive organs and the kidneys, focusing on patterns of thirst, food preferences and aversions, as well as the regularity of bowel movements and the amount of urine that may be passed. Sleep quality may also be explored, as well as information regarding reactivity to heat and cold, and tendencies to be vulnerable to recurrent infections.

By putting this information together, a Chinese herbalist will get a picture of his patient's full medical history, including details of inherited weaknesses and drug treatment, including current conventional medical treatment.

The significance of the pulse

A Chinese herbalist will also want to take the patient's pulse and examine his tongue. Reading the pulse in this context is different from the pulse-taking that may be part of a conventional medical examination. This is because a practitioner of traditional Chinese medicine will be able to glean far more detailed information about the general condition of his patient by a close examination of the pulse. While he will be interested in the number of beats per minute (in common with an orthodox medical practitioner), he will go beyond this to examine its regularity, strength, and whether it can be felt with a light touch or requires deeper examination.

In traditional Chinese medicine, reading the pulse has a major role to play in diagnosis, since there are twenty-eight pulse qualities, each one giving strong hints of underlying clinical conditions. A herbalist will use each wrist in turn when obtaining a pulse reading, placing his fingers in three positions on each wrist.

The significance of the tongue

Examining the tongue is also an important aid to diagnosis, since a great deal may be revealed by its colour, shape and texture. A tendency to cracking or coating of the surface of the tongue will be noted as well as its thickness and general shape. The condition of the tongue in TCM is regarded as revealing more than the health of the digestive tract, since specific areas of the tongue relate to certain parts of the body. For example, the tip of the tongue corresponds to the heart and lungs, the edges to the liver and gall bladder, while the centre reveals the condition of the stomach and spleen. Therefore, any furrowing or wrinkling of these parts of the tongue indicate a disorder in the corresponding organ or part of the body. An enlarged tongue that takes the imprint of the teeth would suggest that there might be problems with the kidneys or spleen, leading to a tendency to water retention or swelling.

The role of general observation

A TCM practitioner will also be able to glean a great deal of information from additional signs such as the sound of the voice of his patient, as well as observing the general appearance and noting any marked odour that may be present.

The tenor and inflexions of the voice can reveal whether the patient is weak, hesitant, decisive, anxious or depressed. The practitioner's sensitivity to subtle body odour, on the other hand, may give clues about specific disorders affecting individual organs or the body as a whole. For example, a fetid smell may suggest problems with the digestive tract, while vomit that gives off a fishy odour may point to the possibility of a pulmonary abscess, or the scent of rotten apples may suggest the presence of diabetes as a problem.

The colour and texture of the patient's skin and the appearance of the eyes may reveal additional information about his general state of health. The eyes may lack lustre in illness, and sparkle in good health. The skin can be moist or dry, and touching the patient's skin can also give a Chinese herbalist an impression of whether localized pain is eased or intensified by light or firm pressure.

Dispensing Chinese herbal medicines

Once a diagnosis has been reached, a Chinese herbalist will decide on a prescription of herbs that will be given in the form of pills, powders, tinctures or decoctions. A decoction is made by putting a mixture of dried herbs into a pan of water that is simmered for roughly twenty to thirty minutes. The liquid is strained off and drunk. This process can be time consuming and slightly cumbersome for the patient, with the additional major drawback that the taste of the herbal formula can also be rather unpleasant.

With the former considerations in mind, the herbalist may choose pills in preference to a decoction. Because of their slower rate of absorption, pills may be most appropriate for treating long-standing problems, as opposed to shorter-lived, acute conditions that require a fast response.

Powders may be made from herbs that are ground very finely, or from a concentrated decoction that has been dried to a fine powder. The formula may be dissolved in hot water and taken as a decoction, or some powders may be encased in a gelatinous capsule. Medicines in this form are absorbed quickly and are generally faster acting than pills. They may also be used as external applications when mixed to a paste with water, sesame oil or alcohol, placed on a clean piece of cloth, warmed and applied to areas of

pain or discomfort. Granules are much the same as powders, and can be used in a similar way. The advantages of granules include a long shelf-life, rapid absorption and strong concentration.

Chinese herbs may also be obtained in a liquid form called a tincture. This is made by dissolving the herbs in a wine or alcohol solution and may be taken daily in measured doses of a recommended number of drops. This method of administering Chinese herbs has the dual advantage of being easy to use, as well as being absorbed quickly by the body.

Substances used by a Chinese herbalist

Although we speak of Chinese herbal medicines as a group, a TCM practitioner has a wide range of medicines at his disposal, including fruits, minerals and animal parts, as well as herbal ingredients. Although only a small proportion of animal ingredients may be used in comparison with the common prescription of roots and fruits, it is important for vegetarians who seek TCM treatment to know that there are appropriate plant substitutes for these animal parts. Those who are concerned about the welfare of animals should also bear in mind that practitioners who are included on the UK Register of Chinese Herbal Medicine do not use animal ingredients from any endangered species, and restrict their prescription of animal substances to an absolute minimum, or may avoid them altogether.

Self-help treatment

Although Chinese herbs may be obtained by the self-prescriber, there are certain disadvantages when untrained people use these herbs. Misunderstanding of the nature of an illness is one hazard, since the wrong herbs may be chosen by the untrained prescriber, with a potentially problematic result. This is most likely to occur where someone may be concentrating on trying to eliminate individual symptoms without having understood the way that a Chinese herbalist would attempt to rectify subtle imbalances or 'patterns of disharmony' in the body. A trained practitioner will be familiar with the way a change in function in one organ in response to a course of herbs may have a knock-on effect on another. The herbalist may adjust the prescription accordingly as the case is proceeding, something the home prescriber is most unlikely to be able to do.

In addition, it is important to know that there have been a few rare problems with Chinese herbs. Often these have occurred due to problems linked to poor quality control or because the herbs have been prescribed by unqualified practitioners in non-traditional ways. Although these difficulties can be avoided by consulting a fully trained and qualified practitioner, perhaps one person in 10,000 can experience an adverse reaction to a herbal formula. If you feel unwell or have flu-like symptoms, nausea or diarrhoea while taking the herbs, stop immediately and contact your practitioner. A good practitioner will always be available if you need to contact them in such circumstances. Because these rare adverse reactions involve the liver, you should tell your practitioner if you consume a lot of alcohol, or if you have ever suffered from a liver disease such as jaundice or hepatitis.

The consultation

The pages above (00–00) discuss in detail how a Chinese herbalist makes a diagnosis and decides upon a prescription, but you should have certain minimum expectations of a consultation. These include the following:
• A full medical history should be taken, including a detailed description of physical, emotional and mental symptoms.
• General questions should also be asked regarding lifestyle and diet.
• The pulse should be taken.
• Examination of the tongue should take place.

Conditions that may respond to Chinese herbal medicine

Although its success in treating eczema may have attracted the main focus of attention in the UK, remember that Chinese herbal medicines are by no means restricted to treating skin conditions, but can be used as an appropriate way of rectifying a broad spectrum of physical and emotional problems. The following are suggestions of some of the wide-ranging problems that can be helped by Chinese herbal medicines:
• Acne
• Anxiety
• Asthma and bronchitis
• Coughs and colds
• Cystitis
• Digestive disorders, including irritable bowel syndrome, indigestion and diverticulitis
• High blood pressure

• Insomnia
• Irregular periods
• Menopausal symptoms
• Painful periods
• Poor circulation
• Post-viral syndrome and ME
• Pre-menstrual syndrome
• Psoriasis
• Stress-related symptoms

Acupuncture

Acupuncture is a healing system that involves the insertion of extremely fine needles into specific points on the surface of the body called acupuncture points. These are thought to be located on energy pathways or channels that run along the body called meridians.

Many of us may be aware of the existence of acupuncture as a result of its effectiveness as a pain-reliever. However, this is just one, limited aspect of this system of healing.

Historical perspectives

The origins of acupuncture go far back before the time of recorded history, with the earliest form of needles being made from stone and bone, with later refinements involving the use of bamboo, gold, silver and copper. The needles that we currently make use of are manufactured from stainless steel with copper handles.

Basic background

An acupuncturist works from the basis that ill health results from an imbalance of vital energy or qi (see page 36). When this energy flows smoothly and in a harmonious way we experience good health on mental, emotional and physical levels. However, when this smooth passage of energy is disrupted or the energy is deficient, symptoms begin to appear, drawing our attention to the imbalance that has developed.

From the perspective of an acupuncturist, apply-

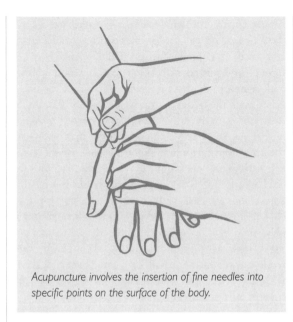
Acupuncture involves the insertion of fine needles into specific points on the surface of the body.

ing pressure or inserting needles into the surface of the body directly influences and affects internal conditions. The internal and external parts of the body are regarded as being connected by invisible tracks or pathways that are located beneath the surface of the skin. These channels, called the meridians, are arranged in a continuous loop of main and subsidiary pathways that travel over the whole body.

There are thirty-five of these channels in total, and the twelve main pathways are connected to the lungs, large intestine, stomach, spleen, heart, small intestine, bladder, kidneys, pericardium (the membrane that shrouds the heart), the 'triple burner' or 'heater' (see page 42), gall bladder and the liver. The main channels radiate along the arms, legs, torso and head and have superficial pathways that lie under the surface of the skin, as well as channels that lie on a deeper, more internal level of the body.

These are the pathways upon which the qi travels as it supports the body fluids and blood, maintaining the optimum harmony of yin and yang (see page 35), as well as protecting the body in its fight against disease. It has been estimated that there are a total of 365 traditional acupuncture points on the surface of the skin that form connections with the vital organs, and that allow for the stimulation of qi through inserting needles. Research has suggested that there are a larger number of acupuncture points (as many as 2000 in total), but a significant proportion of acupuncturists still favour the traditional points.

An acupuncturist will interpret a patient's problem within the context of an imbalance of the five substances (see page 36). Once this imbalance has been identified, the acupuncturist can diagnose the 'pattern of disharmony' affecting the patient. Within the context of Chinese medicine, the heart is related to the function of the blood and houses the spirit or shen. As a result, an acupuncturist does not see an imbalance in the heart as being restricted to a heart complaint in the same way that a conventional doctor would understand a cardiac problem. From the perspective of an acupuncturist, disharmony affecting the heart can be related to a wide variety of symptoms, including emotional imbalances, such as depression, sleep disturbance, problems with memory or disorders that relate to poor circulation, such as chilblains. As a result, these conditions need to be treated by working with acupuncture points along the heart channel, which begins at the armpit and extends to the little finger.

Problems with the lungs may result in disharmony affecting the whole respiratory system, including the sinuses, throat and the chest, as well as being related to emotional problems that may be the result of problems with the smooth flowing of qi. Poor circulation of qi may result in mental, emotional and physical apathy, as well as physical complaints such as recurrent colds, coughs, asthma, or weakness or loss of the voice. These problems may require treatment along the lung channel, which begins 5cm (2in) from the nipple, running along the length of the arm and ending in the thumb.

The liver is also closely related to governing the smooth passage of qi and has a strong affinity to the functioning of the eyes. Problems with qi may give rise to menstrual irregularities, as well as digestive problems or severe mood swings and stress-related symptoms. In TCM eye problems are thought to arise as a result of poor storage or regulation of the blood, symptoms of which can be conjunctivitis or sore, tired eyes. Eye disorders and problems with qi may require acupuncture treatment along the liver channel, which begins at the big toe and radiates up the outside of the ribcage under the nipple.

On the other hand, digestive problems that are linked to poor assimilation of nutrients from food and drink, low energy levels, or general symptoms of poor muscle tone giving rise to prolapse of the womb, bowel, or prolapse leading to hernia, may need treatment along the spleen channel, which plays a vital transforming (converting food and drink into energy) and transporting (moving food through the digestive tract) role in the body. The spleen channel begins at the big toe, runs up the centre of the leg and travels along the side of the abdomen until it reaches the ribcage.

In TCM theory the kidneys regulate not only urine, but other body fluids, including seminal fluid and hormonal secretions. As a result, problems arising from an imbalance in kidney energy may include sexual problems, infertility, premature ageing or growth deficiencies. Because of their pivotal importance, an acupuncturist will want to check whether the kidneys are functioning well through an examination of the tongue and pulse. Imbalanced functioning of the kidneys may respond to work on the acupuncture points on the kidney channel, which originates on the sole of the foot and runs to the area beneath the collarbone.

The channel that relates to the pericardium is referred to as the protector of the heart. Because of the pericardium's enveloping and embracing function, treatment of the pericardium channel is often regarded as being more appropriate and effective in the case of heart problems, chest pains and palpitations than using acupuncture points on the heart channel itself. The pericardium channel begins at the level of the nipple, running up to the shoulder and down the arm until it reaches the middle finger.

The channel of the large intestine may be used to treat digestive imbalances such as constipation and diarrhoea, as well as other conditions linked to the process of detoxification, such as skin problems or sinusitis. The channel of the large intestine starts at the tip of the index finger, runs up the arm and across the shoulder to the opposite side of the nose. The channel of the small intestine, on the other hand, is paired with the heart and has a regenerative function that affects both emotions and physical functions, and may be used to treat problems with frequency of urination, and jaw, neck and shoulder pain. This channel begins at the little finger and runs up the arm and across the shoulder to the ear.

Problems with self-confidence and self-image are related to imbalanced functioning of the gall bladder and are likely to be treated by using acupuncture points along this channel. This begins at the outer corner of the eye, running in a zigzagging movement across the trunk, down the leg and ending at the fourth toe. Other conditions that may respond to similar treatment include arthritis, menstrual disorders, headaches and eye problems. The rather exotically termed 'triple heater' or 'triple burner' may be loosely interpreted as relating to the action of the endocrine glands, with its main function being associated with the body's thermostatic system. Although it is not exactly an identifiable organ, the triple burner has its own treatment channel that begins at the ring finger, running along the back of the arm and side of the neck until it reaches the temple. In cold weather it is the job of the triple burner to adjust the internal body temperature to suit the changing external conditions. It is also brought into play when chill or fever occur, in order to regularize the system as quickly as possible. As a result, the triple burner channel will be treated when dealing with an illness that involves high temperatures or severe chills or shivering. It may also be implicated in problems such as neuralgic pain, paralysis, migraine or tinnitus.

The stomach channel will be used to treat some digestive problems, including irregularities of bowel function. In addition, psychological problems relating to food may also be helped by treating the stomach channel, such as anorexia or bulimia nervosa. This channel begins underneath the eye, travelling down the side of the body and leg until it ends in the second toe.

The bladder channel is related to the kidneys and it shares the detoxifying function of regulation and distribution of body fluids. This channel originates at the inner corner of the eye, travels over the head, running down the back and leg and ends in the little toe.

The consultation

An acupuncturist gathers information from his patient in a very similar way to a Chinese herbalist. In other words, examination of the pulse and tongue will take place and detailed information will be obtained about the current problem and interpreted within the context of the patient's general medical history.

In addition, the ears and abdomen may be examined, and the meridians may be tested by warming the tops of the fingers and toes with an item that looks rather like an incense stick. Alternatively, a custom-made electrical device may be used for this purpose.

Once an acupuncturist has reached a broad diag-

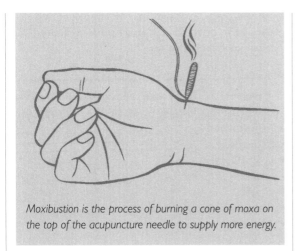

Moxibustion is the process of burning a cone of moxa on the top of the acupuncture needle to supply more energy.

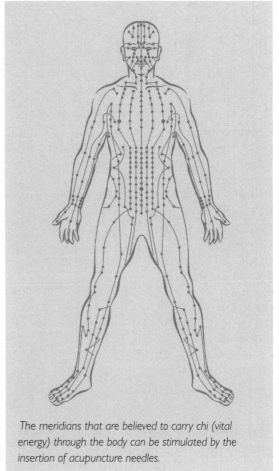

The meridians that are believed to carry chi (vital energy) through the body can be stimulated by the insertion of acupuncture needles.

nosis, he will insert the chosen number of acupuncture needles into the appropriate points on the body. In addition, extra energy may be supplied by burning a cone of moxa on the top of the acupuncture needle. Moxa (the dried leaves of the plant *Artemesia vulgaris*) is thought to act as an additional stimulant, providing further impetus to the body's self-healing mechanism. This process is called moxibustion, and may be used for a number of chronic conditions either with or without needles.

After an initial sensation on insertion of the needles there should be no further discomfort once they are in place. They may be left in position for anything between fifteen and thirty minutes, with the acupuncturist assessing which ones should be rotated or electrically stimulated in order to act as a tonic or dispersing effect on the flow of energy through the body.

When it is time for the needles to be removed there should be no pain and very little or, ideally, no bleeding. The patient will be given advice about activities that should be avoided immediately or soon after an acupuncture session, which may include eating a heavy meal, or engaging in strenuous exercise or sexual activity, for a minimum of six to eight hours after treatment. Advice on dietary adjustments, exercise and relaxation techniques that may be helpful in stimulating the mind and body towards an improved state of health may also be supplied.

For those who are wary of the idea of having needles inserted into their skin as a result of negative experiences with vaccinations or blood tests, it is important to stress that acupuncture needles are extraordinarily fine: as a result, insertion should not

feel distressing or very painful. The acupuncturist will use thoroughly sterilized needles or disposables that can be discarded after one session.

The sensations described by those who have experienced acupuncture include any of the following: slight aching or tingling on insertion of the needle, sometimes followed by a warm sensation or tingling flowing along the meridian that is being treated. Stronger sensations may be experienced on occasion, and some people do find acupuncture uncomfortable. Most people, however, are pleasantly surprised by their experience of this therapy.

Conditions that may respond to acupuncture

These include any of the following:
- Acid indigestion
- Acne
- After effects of stroke

- Allergic rhinitis
- Anxiety
- Arthritis
- Asthma
- Back pain
- Bronchitis
- Constipation
- Cystitis
- Depression
- Diarrhoea
- Eczema (only sometimes responds well to acupuncture alone)
- Facial paralysis
- Headache and migraine
- Menstrual problems
- Neuralgia
- Psoriasis
- Reduced libido
- Sciatica
- Shingles
- Sinus headaches
- Sleep disorders
- Tendinitis
- Tennis elbow
- Vertigo

ACUPUNCTURE IN RELATION TO OTHER THERAPIES

It is usually possible to receive treatment from an acupuncturist as well as enjoying the benefits of additional alternative therapies or conventional treatment. However, there are certain limited situations that might interfere with the effectiveness of acupuncture treatment. These include the following:
- Engaging in vigorous exercise, sexual activity or eating a heavy meal within six hours of treatment.
- Receiving physiotherapy, chiropractic, shiatsu or massage within six to eight hours of an acupuncture session.
- Using conventional drugs such as steroids, tranquillizers, or antidepressants may slow down or inactivate positive responses to acupuncture treatment due to interference with the secretion of endorphins. Endorphins are chemical secretions that can be stimulated during acupuncture treatment, with resulting analgesic and antidepressant effects.
- Using homoeopathic remedies immediately before or after an acupuncture session. Your

responses to the therapies may become confused, meaning that you and your practitioner will not be able to judge their efficacy.

The following are quite compatible with the use of acupuncture, but the usual period of six-to-eight-hours' grace should be given either side of treatment:
- Aromatherapy
- Reflexology
- Hydrotherapy
- Shiatsu
- Yoga*
- Therapeutic touch
- Alexander technique
- Meditation*
- Relaxation techniques*
- Herbal treatment

(Therapies marked with a * do not need the six-to-eight-hour interval.)

Qi gong

Qi gong is a form of meditation in movement that is thought to balance the flow of qi (see page 36) through the body along the meridians (see pages 41–42). Those who can stimulate the balanced flow of qi throughout the body by using the power of the mind in qi gong are believed to be able to achieve a similar balancing effect on the systems and organs to that of a proficient acupuncturist.

The words 'qi gong' can be loosely translated to mean 'the cultivation and conservation of vital energy'. Qi gong may be seen as the precursor of the traditional Chinese medical approach because its central concept is the importance of promoting the balanced flow of life energy or qi. This idea was further developed by those working within the systems of acupuncture and Chinese herbal medicines.

One important aspect of qi gong is the emphasis

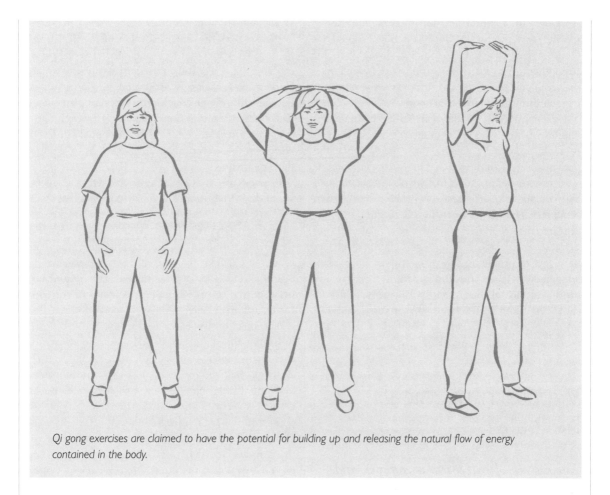

Qi gong exercises are claimed to have the potential for building up and releasing the natural flow of energy contained in the body.

placed on the need for balance and awareness of the centre of the body. Once this sense is highly developed and a fine sense of balance and solidity has been achieved, it is thought that the flow of qi is, correspondingly, perfectly harmonized. Once this state is reached, energy levels should flow at their optimum level, while mental, emotional and physical well-being should be maximized.

Basic background

Because of the strong emphasis in Chinese philosophy on the need for prevention of illness, one's personal responsibility for promotion of emotional, mental and physical well-being is seen as a central feature of life. If a person lives according to the rules of the Way of nature (the Tao), it is possible to achieve a healthy, long and serene life.

To enjoy the benefits of this positive perspective on life the three cavities of the body in which three essential qualities are stored (the three 'treasures') must be protected and nurtured. The three cavities are located in the head, the centre of the abdomen and the lower abdomen, while the three 'treasures' are regarded as shen, qi and jing (see the section entitled 'The Five Substances' on page 36 for an explanation of these terms). In order to experience a sense of optimal well-being and vitality it is essential to guard against depletion of these substances by avoiding overwork, excess of stress, poor diet and lack of exercise. On the other hand, these substances are thought to be enhanced by the practice of qi gong or the use of acupuncture.

In qi gong, certain points on the body are regarded as being of central importance and significance. These include the crown of the head, the brow, the tongue, the heart, the navel, the palms of the hands, the kidneys, the perineum and the soles of the feet. Also, controlling the inhalation and exhalation of breath is believed to enhance physical strength as well as mental and emotional stability.

Although to a Westerner this may sound rather fanciful, research carried out in a Beijing hospital has demonstrated that it is possible to slow down and strengthen the heartbeat, improve circulation, reduce blood pressure, and increase assimilation of oxygen through the use of qi gong.

Hospitals using traditional Chinese medicine employ doctors who use qi gong to transmit their qi to their patients by passing their hands above the patient's body. Conditions that may be treated in this way include any problem that involves chronic pain and discomfort, such as back problems or frozen shoulders. Those who learn to practise qi gong may also use the technique to ease stress-related disorders, tension headaches, migraines, joint disorders or digestive problems. However, the practice of qi gong is not to be recommended if there is any history of mental illness, and a full medical history should be taken before beginning qi gong classes in order to check that there is nothing to make the practice of qi gong inadvisable.

Western medical herbalism

The history of herbalism is complex and fascinating due to its multifaceted nature as a healing art. Although in the West we may be more familiar with the aspects of herbalism that have developed into Western medical herbalism, it is important to realize that Far Eastern and Asian communities have also developed their own interpretation of this therapy (see Chinese herbal medicine and Ayurvedic medicine on pages 37–40 and 18–25).

The general impact and significance of herbal medicine can be appreciated when we consider that the World Health Organization has estimated that herbalism is three or four times more likely to be practised on a global basis than orthodox medicine. It is also important to note that until the last 200 years, herbalism was the accepted form of medical treatment in Western countries. The link between herbalism and the conventional medical treatment we are familiar with today is illustrated by the way that doctors still rely on a high proportion of plant-based drugs when treating their patients. However, these drugs are manufactured in a fundamentally different way from the methods used by herbalists to produce their medicines.

In principle, it is possible to claim that all plants are herbs with potential culinary or medicinal qualities. In theory, the leaves, stems, flowers and roots of a bewilderingly wide range of plants may be used as flavouring, colouring or preservative ingredients in foods and drinks, as well as having medicinal or health-giving properties. Indeed, the boundaries between the use of plants as medicines or for food has traditionally been flexible.

The links between the need for a healthy, nutritious diet and the use of herbal medicine are strong and many medical herbal practitioners are acutely aware of the need for plants to be grown in optimal – essentially organic – conditions, and prefer not to choose overly cultivated herbs that might be compromised by artificial chemicals. Herbalists are also aware of the nutritional properties of plants and their ability to rectify imbalances of mineral and trace elements in the body. Dietary advice is often given as part of a consultation with a practitioner of ayurvedic medicine or a Chinese herbalist, due to the links that exist between food and medicine as part of a holistic approach to healing.

Historical perspectives

The history of herbalism goes back to the beginning of civilization, as we can see from surviving historical records from ancient Egypt and China, which list the use of specific plants in treating disease. The use of plants as food, cosmetics, medicines and colourings is something that has been employed on a worldwide basis, with less technologically developed societies being able to hold on to this knowledge more effectively than those of us who have moved into a more high-tech environment.

Many discoveries that were made regarding the medicinal properties of plants occurred on an instinctive or trial-and-error basis. As a body of knowledge was built up, it was recorded in books known as herbals written in Europe in classical times and later, in the sixteenth and seventeenth centuries. A great deal of inspiration was drawn from ancient Greek and medieval Islamic material. By the eighteenth century, as well as traditional herbalists, a new breed of commercial apothecaries began to emerge in urban centres who were open to criticism from an emerging profession of 'chymists'. The latter were busily developing compounds that became very attractive to those who felt organic medicines did not sit well with the development of surgical techniques and the new technological advances that were associated with the Industrial Revolution in Europe.

As scientific medical developments occurred as part of general technological progress, a campaign against the use of 'ineffective' herbal medicines gained ground, with the result that herbs fell into disrepute and lost popularity in urban centres. The most significant moment in this development was the discovery in 1785 by the English physician William Withering of the medicinal effects of the foxglove leaf on the heart. Herbalists were already aware of the positive potential of the foxglove in the treatment of dropsy (water retention) but were also aware that the use of the plant could lead to unwanted toxic effects.

Withering discovered that the principal effect of the plant was on the heart, which then stimulated the kidneys to flush out the excess fluid that led to fluid retention. Once this discovery had been made, Withering concluded that small and strictly measured doses of the foxglove leaf (*digitalis*) could be used to treat heart failure. This was the beginning of a process of standardization of drugs that eventually led to the use of active medicinal agents such as digitoxin and digoxin, now commonly used in conventional medicine to treat heart problems.

As a result of this discovery, conventional medical practitioners argued that effort must be put into isolating the active ingredients of plant medicines that should only be given in strictly measured doses. This led to the development of a range of drugs manufactured from plants that were already in common use in the hands of herbalists.

In the nineteenth and twentieth centuries, many herbal preparations were abandoned, not because they were ineffective or inappropriate, but mainly because they did not fit comfortably into the practical and theoretical framework that conventional medicine was building. As a result, plants were increasingly omitted from pharmacopoeias (books that list and describe the medicinal properties of drugs), even though they were used as the base material for developing modern drugs. It is nonetheless estimated that 25 per cent of drugs prescribed today in conventional medicine are herbal in origin.

The tradition of modern medical herbalism owes a great debt to the emigrants who moved from Europe to America in the last two centuries. These people were thrown into a situation where they were forced to cope with a minimum amount of health care. As a result, they had to depend on their memories of traditional herbal treatment, combined with those of the native North Americans. Throughout the nineteenth century the hybrid that was formed from the meeting of these two strands of herbalism was imported to the UK, where it was incorporated into the surviving herbal tradition. In the UK, the practice of medical herbalism had been established for centuries in the rural areas, while it also became established in the urban centres that developed as a result of the Industrial Revolution.

A move was made to protect and define the term 'medical herbalist' under the remit of the Medicines Act of 1968. Since then, a new generation of medical herbalists has been trained, greatly raising standards within the profession.

Basic background

The establishment of the training of medical herbalists is a development that bridges the gap between orthodox medicine and more traditional home-based approaches to herbal treatment. However, it is important to bear in mind that medical herbalists differ from conventional physicians in prescribing only whole herbs, as opposed to isolated chemical compounds (as in conventional drugs). Herbal medicines prescribed by a medical herbalist are given with the intention of stabilizing deep-seated biochemical or nutritional imbalances in the body. As a result, they may take longer than conventional drugs to achieve the required effect.

Although it can be a problem to test herbal remedies along similar lines to orthodox drugs (using the double-blind technique of the clinical trial), some efforts have been made to demonstrate the safety and efficacy of herbal preparations in order to satisfy governmental requirements in various countries. Unfortunately, testing programmes for the vast majority of herbal remedies commercially available would be prohibitively expensive for most herbal manufacturers. However, if a practical solution could be reached in order to solve this problem, the results could be beneficial to both herbal manufacturers and pharmaceutical companies alike.

The value of using the whole plant

Although there may be obvious practical advantages to using measured, concentrated doses of drugs obtained from a natural plant source, the concentration can cause unwanted complications. Consider aspirin, for example. Salicylic acid was initially obtained from the flowerbuds of the meadowsweet as well as from willow bark in 1838. By 1899 a drug company formulated a new pain-relieving drug (acetylsalicylic acid) that they called aspirin, which is known to cause stomach irritation, and even bleeding. It is interesting to note that the name is derived from the old botanical name for the plant meadowsweet, since the latter is used in herbal practice as an anti-inflammatory to ease the pains and stiffness of rheumatism.

However, unlike a conventionally produced extract of the plant, a herbal medicine is produced from the whole plant, and has a balanced effect on the body. For example, the anti-inflammatory action of the salicylates contained in the plant eases the discomfort of rheumatic pain, while the tannin and soothing mucilage content effectively act as a buffer against the effect of the salicylates that can cause stomach bleeding and irritation when given in isolation. Consequently, giving the medicine in which the whole plant is used can guard against the problems that can arise when an isolated compound is given. This is often referred to as the 'synergistic' effect of plants by medical herbalists: in other words, a whole plant is regarded as being much more than the sum of its individual parts. By using these parts in isolation we are likely to be limiting their healing potential. The multifaceted type of healing action is by no means restricted to meadowsweet, since most plants used by herbalists will have their own synergistic pattern of action.

Basic aspects of the herbal medical approach

At the centre of herbal medicine, in common with other holistic approaches such as traditional Chinese medicine, lies the concept that there is a fundamental vital force or principle that animates the human form. The human organism is regarded as a self-regulating, self-healing mechanism that functions well in good health and falls into disharmony when illness sets in. This basically adaptive quality is reflected in the way that the human body can readjust to rapid changes in temperature. Effective and appropriate treatment is seen as supporting and re-establishing the body's self-healing mechanism whenever it shows signs of vulnerability through the appearance of symptoms of illness.

Herbal treatment is very much aimed at restoring harmony and equilibrium at a fundamental level in the human body as a whole, rather than concentrating on superficially improving the situation through suppression of symptoms. As a result, a tendency to recurrent infection may be treated by administering herbs that have a cleansing action on the body, supporting the body in fighting infection. This approach may be contrasted with the use of conventional drugs such as antibiotics that may temporarily clear the problem, but often leave the body open to further infection in the near future.

When herbal medicines are appropriately prescribed they can produce a range of protective reactions from the body. They may be used to soothe irritated and inflamed skin and mucous membranes, either when taken internally or applied locally. They may also be given to set up gentle irritation in order to encourage effective elimination and detoxification of the body. Circulation may be encouraged to work more vigorously where necessary by the use of stimulants, and the functioning of the digestive system may be improved through the use of herbs that stimulate digestive reflexes.

Herbal remedies can have a powerfully detoxifying effect on the body, encouraging efficient functioning of the eliminatory organs such as the kidneys, bowels, lungs and sweat glands. The herbal approach can also support the digestive organs in neutralizing potentially toxic substances in the diet.

The consultation

A Western medical herbalist is likely to gather information regarding the general lifestyle of his patient, including quality of diet, and the level and nature of physical and emotional stress. In addition, he will ask questions to establish the health of the main systems of the body, including the functioning of the lungs, digestive organs and the nervous system. The pulse and blood pressure may be monitored, as well as urine and blood tests and a number of other physical examinations. Some herbalists may choose to use

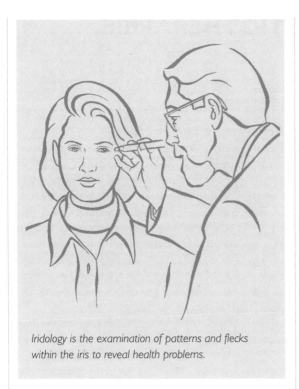

Iridology is the examination of patterns and flecks within the iris to reveal health problems.

adjunctive tools of diagnosis such as iridology (the examination of patterns and flecks within the iris to reveal health problems).

Once this material has been assimilated and analysed, herbal treatment can begin. The main emphasis is likely to be put on using herbs to encourage the body to begin self-healing. Herbs with antibacterial or anti-inflammatory properties may be used to relieve symptoms, as well as stimulants, tonics or relaxants to encourage a greater state of balance in the body as a whole.

The herbalist may also give dietary advice, recommendations for exercise, or relaxation techniques in order to support the body as it returns to health. A herbalist will probably aim to keep the course of treatment as short as possible, with the most positive result being the renewed ability of the body to take over and maintain normal body functions as soon as possible. Additional supportive measures might include breathing techniques that encourage efficient detoxification.

Dispensing Western medical herbal treatments

Herbal preparations containing a variety of different herbs are commonly prepared and dispensed by the herbal practitioner. The herbalist will tailor the prescription to the needs of the individual patient rather than being content with routine prescribing for the symptoms of the disease alone. Medicines may be prescribed in the form of **t**inctures (herbal essences prepared by steeping the required herbs in an alcohol and water base), capsules (gelatine or plant-based casings that are filled with finely ground herbs, juice extract or oils), tablets (powdered herbs or oils that are mixed with gum or sugar into lozenge or tablet form), teas, creams, oils (extracted essential plant oils that may be used as inhalants or diluted with an appropriate base oil for massage), or ointments (tinctures or herbs that are mixed with a beeswax or oil base for local application to the skin).

Conditions that may respond to Western medical herbalism

Most conditions respond favourably to Western medical herbal treatment, unless they fall into any of the following categories:

• Serious, life-threatening conditions that require emergency orthodox medical treatment.

• Conditions that need help from a 'hands on', manipulative approach such as osteopathy, chiropractic or acupressure. These may include sciatic pain or discomfort that originates from a mechanical source such as a displaced vertebra. However, the pains of sciatica and all forms of arthritis may be eased by herbal medicine in combination with a manipulative treatment.

• Some psychiatric problems, epilepsy or emotional disorders. Depression, anxiety and stress-related problems may respond well to herbal treatment.

• Conditions where conventional drugs have been used over an extended period of time (such as the need for long-term insulin in a diabetic). However, herbal medicines can sometimes be used to supplement or gradually replace orthodox drugs in a controlled programme of reduction, ideally directly involving the support and consent of the patient's family doctor.

• Any diseases that are associated with legal restrictions and restraints, such as notifiable illnesses (for example, typhoid).

POPULAR HOLISTIC THERAPIES

Acupressure

In many ways, we all enjoy a simple form of acupressure when our instincts instruct us to rub or apply pressure to a painful or injured part of our bodies. As a development of this basic awareness, the ancient Chinese discovered that there were specific points on the body that could be pressed in order to relieve pain, tension or discomfort.

From its beginnings in China over 5000 years ago, the art of acupressure has developed in a primarily instinctive and practical way, with the clinical experience of practitioners contributing to increasing knowledge about the subject over time. Acupressure exists within an extremely fluid framework that allows for additional information to be incorporated as practitioners evolve fresh techniques within traditional boundaries.

Basic background

Although acupressure and acupuncture use the same points in order to stimulate the balanced flow of vital energy (known in traditional Chinese medicine as qi, see page 36) through the body, acupuncturists apply stimulation through the use of fine needles, while those who practise acupressure make use of their hands or feet in order to apply gentle pressure. Although some of the points used in acupressure relate to the specific location where pain may be felt, they are also associated with relief of pain in other parts of the body that are physically remote from the pressure point.

In traditional Chinese medicine, acupressure was employed along with dietary prescriptions, breathing techniques and the use of herbs as a non-invasive, gentle way of improving health and well-being and encouraging the body to fight ill health. Acupressure is especially well adapted to encourage the body to relax muscular tension and relieve persistent symptoms of stress.

Acupressure and stress

When dealing with muscular tension, a practitioner using acupressure will select a single or a number of pressure points that are known to relieve muscular tension. These points are located along energy channels called meridians, the pathways along which vital energy is conducted. An acupuncturist sees tension as a condition of stagnation affecting the blood vessels, nerves, lymphatic channels and meridians. Factors that may influence this state of stagnation include anxiety, physical and emotional stress, or the repression of emotions that are struggling to be released. If these stresses and tensions go on for long enough, they can result in blockages of vital energy occurring within the body as a whole. When this happens, the body's capacity for self-regulation and self-healing can be adversely affected, leading to recurrent health problems or a compromised ability to fight off infections. Unlike conventional painkillers that suppress acute pain on a short-term basis, acupressure is believed to work directly on the tense muscles, releasing constricted areas, while also encouraging the body to correct the imbalanced response to stress.

Understanding acupressure

Acupressure and acupuncture work by stimulating chemicals called endorphins within the body. Endorphins have pain-relieving and antidepressant qualities and are believed to encourage a state of relaxation and well-being.

By stimulating specific points on the skin by applying pressure, practitioners of acupressure believe they are stimulating the flow of vital energy in the body. By encouraging this energy to move more freely, they encourage the body to function in a more balanced way on emotional, mental and physical levels. The suggestion that endorphin production may be stimulated during acupressure treatment enables Western scientists to investigate and examine an identifiable biochemical process during that treatment. This is clearly more appealing to Western medical scientists than an explanation that involves

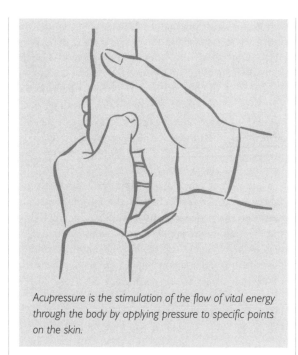

Acupressure is the stimulation of the flow of vital energy through the body by applying pressure to specific points on the skin.

the acceptance of an energy force that cannot be identified and examined through a series of tests.

However, even in Western scientific circles, links are being explored between stress and physical illness as part of the developing science of psychoneuroimmunology, which is beginning to recognize that our emotional and mental well-being can have a profound effect on our physical health. When viewed from within this context, acupressure may be understood to work by relieving pain (through the production of endorphins) and aiding the self-regulating mechanism of the body through easing the tense areas that may eventually compromise the efficient working of the immune system. Acupressure is, therefore, a holistic treatment that encourages the body to adjust more easily to environmental changes and pressures, and enhances the ability of the body to fight illness.

The physical effects of acupressure may include general relaxation, improved circulation and increased efficiency of the disposal of toxins and waste products from the tense or contracted area. By improving circulation, oxygen and other vital nutrients are conveyed more freely to previously tense areas of the body, which can then throw off illness faster and more decisively, limiting the frequency and duration of episodes of illness. Additional positive effects of improved circulation include greater vitality and well-being.

The consultation

In common with most forms of alternative medical consultation, the initial appointment is likely to begin with your case history. The practitioner will ask questions relating to your lifestyle, quality of diet and degree of stress. As part of your initial assessment, your practitioner may also want to read your pulse (in a similar way to an acupuncturist).

Once treatment begins, you may be asked to lie on a firm surface (such as a treatment table or a futon on the floor) or you may be asked to sit up. As with a shiatsu session, there is no need to undress, but it is helpful to make a point of wearing unrestrictive, loose-fitting clothes. You will quickly notice that your therapist may use a range of different techniques of applying pressure, depending on whether the objective is to energize or to subdue energy levels. While this is being done, your practitioner may use the pads of his thumbs or fingers, or his palms, elbows, knees or feet.

While the pressure is being applied you may feel a temporary sense of tenderness or coldness, but discomfort should not linger. The treatment may last anything between thirty and sixty minutes, and you are likely to be asked to return at weekly intervals at first. Once a specific problem or series of problems has improved, you may want to return for treatment on a less frequent basis as a general preventative measure.

Although self-help acupressure can be very useful for minor problems, when suffering from any chronic condition it is best to seek treatment from an experienced practitioner (this is especially important for anyone who is pregnant). If you would like to learn how to use acupressure for self-help situations at home, it is invaluable to attend a beginners' class run by a trained and experienced practitioner. In addition, you can buy acupressure devices for straightforward treatment of short-lived nausea associated with travel sickness: these are usually towelling wrist bands that are positioned at nausea-relieving points.

Conditions that may respond to acupressure

- Arthritic pain
- Constipation
- Cramp
- Emotional stress and tension
- Fibrositis

- Insomnia
- Lower back pain
- Muscle aches and tension
- Muscle strains
- Recurrent stiffness of the neck
- Sciatica
- Sinusitis
- Tendinitis
- Tension headaches

Fractured bones, severe osteoporosis or degenerated discs should not be treated with acupressure. In addition, those who suffer from severe low back pain, back pain during pregnancy, or sciatica should seek advice from an osteopath, chiropractor, medical specialist or physiotherapist before embarking on a course of acupressure.

Aromatherapy

Aromatherapy is an increasingly popular and accessible therapy that employs the use of highly concentrated essential oils obtained from plants and trees. Its application has an excitingly broad potential, and essential oils are used to improve quality and experience of health and well-being on physical, emotional and mental levels.

A trained aromatherapist can treat a range of chronic problems such as recurrent headaches, painful periods or skin disorders, while more acute or short-lived problems may be dealt with effectively at home. However, those who make use of aromatherapy oils at home should ideally have attended an introductory course on the subject.

There is evidence that aromatic oils were used in the process of embalming in ancient cultures, as well as being incorporated in incense, perfumes, medicines and cosmetic preparations. Aromatic essences that were known to be used include cinnamon, juniper, myrrh, sweet flag and cedar wood.

The ancient Greeks appear to have appreciated the importance of fragrant flowers and plants even more strongly than the ancient Egyptians, who were also known to use them. The ancient Greeks recorded specific advice on the mood-enhancing qualities of flowers such as the rose, hyacinth and narcissus, and also used perfumes, healing ointments, massage and aromatic bathing in health-promoting regimes. This emphasis on the health-giving properties of scented massage and bathing was also a strong feature of Roman life.

However, a particularly significant moment for aromatherapy was reached in the eleventh century AD when the process of distillation was perfected by the Persian physician Avicenna, who advocated a particularly holistic approach to healing. The Middle East also played a significant role by using the scent of aromatic oils to act as fumigants. Rose water, sandalwood and camphor were in common use as purifying agents for clothes and skin in order to help the body keep disease at bay. This knowledge was imported to Europe by the Crusaders on their return from the Middle East.

The body/mind link and its treatment by the use of essential oils was developed in the 1920s by two Italian physicians, Cajola and Gatti, who concluded that essential oils could have a profound effect on the nervous system. The credit for the development of modern aromatherapy is usually given to the French scientist René-Maurice Gattefossé. He conducted research into the healing properties of essential oils, becoming especially interested in their anaesthetic and antiseptic qualities, as well as their cosmetic potential. Gattefossé personally experienced the healing potential of essential oils when his hand was severely burned in a laboratory accident. After the topical application of lavender essential oil, his hand healed extremely well with no complications of infection or scarring. He was the first to use the term 'aromatherapy' in 1937.

As a result of Gattefossé's work, a great deal of interest was generated in aromatherapy in France. Ex-army surgeon DriJean Valnet treated the wounds of soldiers fighting in the First World War with essential oils, as well as exploring the use of aromatic essences in helping patients with long-term psychiatric problems. This avenue continued to be explored fifty years later in the 1970s, in Italy at the university of Milan, when professor Paolo Rovesti explored the application of essential oils in relieving emotional problems.

By the 1950s the idea of using essential oils was combined with the healing art of massage by the Austrian, Marguerite Maury. She developed the idea of diluting essential oils in a carrier oil before massaging them into the skin, and also emphasized the need to tailor the prescription of oils to the individual client and their physical and emotional requirements.

Today, interest in aromatherapy has grown to the point where it is included in the syllabus of some medical schools or is practised by trained aromatherapists who do not have a conventional medical background. Practitioners may be found in the UK, Spain, Italy, Canada, South Africa, Japan, the USA, Australia, New Zealand, Scandinavia and Iceland.

Basic background

Essential oils are volatile, highly complex and concentrated substances that contain a wide range of chemicals such as alcohols, aldehydes, esters and terpenes (for an explanation of these terms, see the box below).

It is because of their very complexity that essential oils have such a broad spectrum of action. As a result, a single essential oil can combine antibacterial, antidepressant, sedative, analgesic and antiseptic properties. Because of their minute molecular structure they can make contact with the bloodstream as a result of absorption through the skin, or through reaching the lungs by the process of inhalation.

Essential oils may be found in petals, roots, bark, seeds, resin or the leaves of plants and trees, as well as in the rind of citrus fruits or the bulbs of edible items such as garlic. They are unusually volatile, evaporating readily when left open to the air, so it is never a good idea to leave the top off a bottle of essential oil. Some oils may be very fluid with an easy-pouring consistency (for example, peppermint), others may be quite sticky and thick (for example, myrrh), while some may be semi-solid at room temperature, requiring warmth to make them liquid (for example, rose otto).

COMMON CHEMICAL COMPONENTS OF ESSENTIAL OILS

Aldehydes are chemicals that have a combined sedative and uplifting property. They are to be found in lemon-scented essential oils such as citronella or lemon grass.

Phenols have bactericidal properties and are also reputed to stimulate the central nervous system. Those essences that contain a high proportion of phenols can be irritating to the skin and mucous membranes (these include clove, thyme and oregano).

Alcohols are linked to antiseptic and antiviral properties. Good examples include lavender and geranium.

Oxides may be found in a broad range of essential oils, for example eucalyptus and tea tree, and have an expectorant effect.

Terpenes have an extremely broad-ranging action that includes antiviral, antiseptic, antibacterial and anti-inflammatory properties. Good examples include lemon and pine essence.

Ketones are mentioned with caution since some of them are known to be toxic. As a rule, essential oils that contain toxic ketones should be avoided by self-prescribers. They include sage, wormwood and mugwort, which are not available over the counter. However, non-toxic ketones are to be found in jasmine and sweet fennel. Ketones reduce congestion, encourage the easy flow of mucus and can be of particular value in treating problems of the nose and throat.

Esters have sedative and fungicidal effects and are to be found in plant essences such as lavender and Roman chamomile.

How essential oils and absolutes are produced

There are only two methods of producing pure essential oils.

Distillation

This is a very well-established method of producing essential oils which involves placing plant material in a still where it is heated up by contact with concentrated steam. This process creates an aromatic vapour that travels along a number of glass tubes cooled by cold water. The resulting essence is siphoned off through a container with a narrow neck.

Expression

This is a method that may be used to extract citrus essential oils such as lemon, lime or bergamot. Although the process can be done by hand (by squeezing the rind and collecting the oil in a sponge),

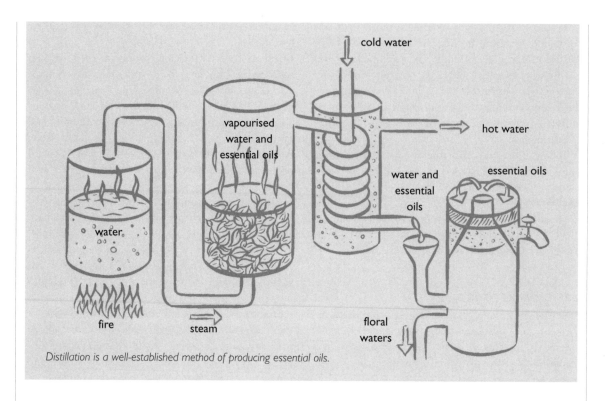

Distillation is a well-established method of producing essential oils.

cold water

hot water

vapourised water and essential oils

essential oils

water and essential oils

water

fire

steam

floral waters

custom-built machines are now available that collect the essential oil using centrifugal force.

Other methods used to extract essential oils include:

Volatile solvent extraction

This method is widely used by the perfume industry. During volatile solvent extraction, plant material is exposed to a volatile solvent such as hexane, benzene or petroleum ether. On contact with the solvent, a waxy substance is produced called a concrete, which is then treated with alcohol a number of times in order to render an aromatic liquid obtained after a process of evaporation using a gentle vacuum. The oil that is left after this process is complete is called an absolute.

Liquid carbon dioxide extraction

This method was introduced in the early 1980s when it was seen as being a milestone in the development of methods of extraction. Sadly, the cost involved in this method is high, with the result that its use is generally restricted to the production of very expensive extracted oils.

During this process carbon dioxide gas is used at extremely high pressure to dissolve essential oil from the plant material. As the pressure falls the aromatic oils can be collected as a mist.

Hydrodiffusion/percolation

This system is similar to steam distillation, with the exception that the steam is produced above the plant material and allowed to percolate through it. When plants are used this process is quicker than distillation, although barks and woods take longer to produce their oils.

The phytonic process

The development of this technique has been regarded as the most significant breakthrough since the discovery of distillation. This process makes use of a new type of solvent called phytosols that make it possible to obtain aromatic oils at room temperature. This is a tremendous advantage, since the heat-sensitive ingredients of an essential oil can be preserved during the process of extraction.

The consultation

Aromatherapists are trained to have an understanding not only of essential oils and their action, but also of the way the body functions, and part of their training is the study of anatomy and physiology. After taking a thorough case history exploring mental, emotional and physical symptoms, the aromatherapist will select one or a blend of essential oils most likely to suit the patient. The chosen oils

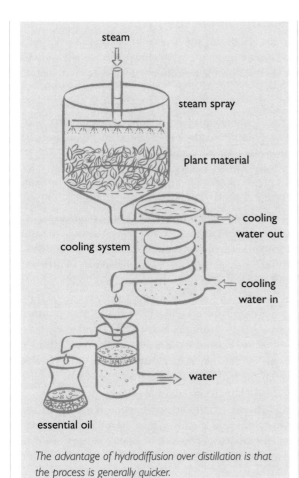

The advantage of hydrodiffusion over distillation is that the process is generally quicker.

Aromatherapists may be trained primarily in aromatherapy with adjunctive knowledge of anatomy and physiology, or they may be trained primarily in conventional medicine with additional qualifications in aromatherapy. As interest in complementary medicine grows, increasing numbers of nurses and midwives are becoming familiar with aromatherapy as an invaluable therapy to help patients reach an enhanced state of health.

Conditions that may respond to aromatherapy

Aromatherapists may be called upon to treat a variety of problems including any of the following:

- Anxiety
- Arthritis
- Asthma
- Back pain
- Constipation
- Depression
- Fluid retention
- Headaches
- High blood pressure
- Insomnia
- Irritable bowel syndrome
- Menopausal problems
- Menstrual problems
- Muscle strain
- Poor circulation
- Stress-related disorders

may be applied to the skin in aromatic massage, inhaled or given to the patient for home use.

Aromatherapy is a holistic treatment. A skilled aromatherapist will seek to improve the overall health of the patient rather than treating specific symptoms. It is for this reason that some time is likely to be spent in the initial consultation exploring issues such as general lifestyle, diet, exercise regimes and sleep pattern and quality.

For example, an aromatherapist is likely to treat muscular aches and pains that spring from muscle tension by prescribing a blend of oils that can act specifically on tense muscle tissue, but that may also be equally appropriate in easing stress. Further advice may also be given about general ways of reducing stress, such as increasing physical activity, taking up a relaxation technique, and reducing consumption of foods and drinks that make a negative contribution to an overstressed mind and body.

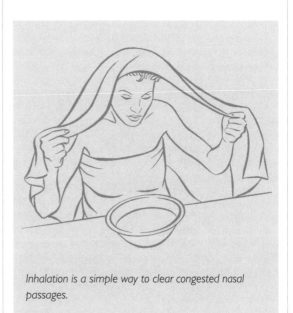

Inhalation is a simple way to clear congested nasal passages.

Chiropractic

Chiropractic is the art of manipulation of the spine and other joints. A chiropractor uses his hands to make gentle adjustments to the spine and joints to correct joint fixations (see below), gently encouraging the body to carry out its functions in a balanced way as the spine returns to normal alignment.

In true holistic fashion, a chiropractor will consider each person's unique experience of health or health problems in the context of their general lifestyle, and will probably suggest general changes and adjustments that will help the patient to support and speed up the healing process. For example, if an excessive amount of strain is being placed on the spine and the whole body by excess weight, an effective weight-loss programme will be recommended. In this case the weight loss will allow the chiropractor to make progress in returning an overworked, weak spine into a strong, resilient, healthy one.

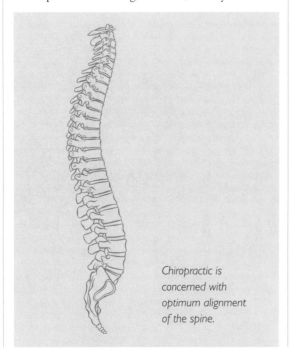

Chiropractic is concerned with optimum alignment of the spine.

Historical perspectives

In the UK during the nineteenth century practitioners who used manipulative techniques to rectify musculoskeletal problems (often referred to as bonesetters) were extremely popular. Bonesetters found themselves in brisk competition with surgeons, with many patients preferring the gentler approach of manipulation to the more radical techniques of the physicians and surgeons.

In common with osteopathy, chiropractic also emerged during the last half of the nineteenth century from the USA. Both chiropractic and bonesetting were concerned with optimum alignment of the skeletal system. It was developed as a system of manipulation of the spine by D.D. Palmer in 1895. Palmer recognized the merit of spinal adjustment and manipulation when he treated a patient who had suffered from loss of hearing for seventeen years. By manipulation of the vertebrae in the neck, Palmer was able to restore the hearing of his patient.

On the basis of experiences of this kind, Palmer came to the conclusion that the basis of ill health could be traced to abnormal movement in specific joints, which he called 'subluxation' or 'fixation'. It was Palmer's opinion that fixation interrupted the flow of nervous impulses, ultimately adversely affecting health throughout the whole system. Palmer declared that a misaligned (or subluxed) vertebra or joint was responsible for 95 per cent of all diseases. As a result, he believed that most illness could be affected by restoring the vertebrae to their optimum state of alignment.

Because of the extreme claims made by Palmer regarding the potential curative application of chiropractic, the orthodox medical establishment in the USA reacted with hostility and disbelief. However, today chiropractors have gained the right to grant licences in each state of the USA and Canada, and many of the primary medical insurance companies will cover chiropractic treatment for a wide range of medical conditions. As a result, chiropractic is now part of the mainstream health-care system in the USA.

Chiropractic, in common with osteopathy, has been steadily establishing its credentials in the UK, with increasing co-operation developing between chiropractors and conventional doctors for the treatment of back pain and joint problems. However, most doctors would have problems in referring patients with more general conditions, such as asthma, diabetes or psoriasis, for chiropractic treatment.

Basic background

Chiropractors regard most of the problems affecting the spine as related to excessive strain being exerted on intervertebral joints. The chiropractor may be alerted to the problems by examining the patient or the patient may already be experiencing physical pain, restricted or excessive movement, swelling or weakness of the affected area, perhaps occurring as a result of accident, injury, stress, trauma or strain. Poor postural habits are also thought to contribute to the problem, especially in situations where they may put too much strain on the joints of the vertebrae. This may in turn affect other joints or muscles, or even other organs and tissues. Within this context, minor fixations may not be the cause of illness, but may have the effect of exaggerating it. Therefore, migraines or dizziness may be aggravated, but not caused by a problem in the cervical vertebrae of the neck.

The notion that the condition of the spinal column is linked to diseases affecting organs in other parts of the body has generated controversy from the earliest days of the development of chiropractic. However, opinion has modified with emerging evidence, suggesting that the healthy functioning of the spine and other joints may influence processes elsewhere in the vital organs of the body.

The consultation

During the initial consultation with a chiropractor a full medical history will be taken, and he is likely to question you about any traumas, accidents or injuries that may have happened in childhood or as an adult. Aspects of general lifestyle, such as working conditions, amount of exercise taken, and degree of stress experienced may also have a bearing on the current problem. An X-ray may be necessary in order to establish any underlying conditions.

The aim of the examination is to identify whether the patient is suffering from a problem that stems from a mechanical cause or from an underlying organic condition relating to a specific organ. Once the chiropractor is satisfied with his diagnosis he will explain it, together with the proposed treatment plan. The standard treatment is manipulation, unless it is inappropriate for your condition. Your practitioner will usually ask you to remove your clothes,

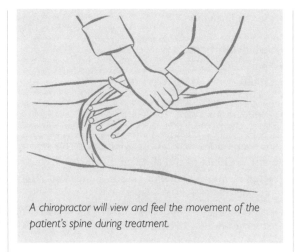

A chiropractor will view and feel the movement of the patient's spine during treatment.

excluding your underwear, and wear a gown that opens down the back to allow him to view and feel the movement of the spine during treatment. Throughout treatment you will sit or lie on a specially designed couch.

During chiropractic manipulation the practitioner applies precise, short, thrusting movements to appropriate parts of the spine and other joints. He may also need to manipulate soft tissues, applying regulated, sustained pressure to ligaments or massaging muscles with a view to easing pain or muscle spasm. Massage techniques may be especially valuable in preparing the affected area for manipulation. In addition, he may use heat treatment, and may advise on dietary changes, exercise or general postural adjustments.

Conditions that may respond to chiropractic

Patients suffering from any of the following may benefit from consultation with a chiropractor:
- Back pain
- Chest pain
- Digestive problems
- General neurological disorders
- Headaches
- Limb pain
- Localized rheumatic pain
- Lumbago
- Migraines
- Neck pain
- Neuralgia
- Numbness
- Osteoarthritis

- Pins and needles
- Sciatica
- Spondylitis
- Sports injuries
- Strains
- Tennis elbow
- Whiplash injury

Some conditions may not be appropriate for chiropractic treatment, and if examination by a chiropractor identifies underlying disease, or a condition for which chiropractic treatment is inappropriate, the patient will be immediately referred to a family doctor or specialist. However, chiropractic can be used in some cases to provide relief of symptoms, even when manipulation may be inappropriate.

Flower remedies

The thirty-eight flower remedies are gaining an increasingly popular profile in alternative self-help circles. This is partly due to their growing availability and accessibility in retail outlets such as health-food shops. This is especially true of the Rescue Remedy five-flower formula, which has become extremely popular as a non-addictive, gentle medicine for the treatment of symptoms arising from trauma, stress or accident.

Apart from self-help use, alternative therapists, such as herbalists, homoeopaths, aromatherapists or naturopaths, prescribe flower remedies as a useful supplement to their therapy.

Historical perspectives

The flower remedies were discovered and developed by Dr Edward Bach in the early years of the 1930s. Although a conventional physician by training, Edward Bach became disillusioned by the way that orthodox medicine was unable to do more than palliate or temporarily suppress the symptoms of illness. As a result, Bach came to regard conventional medicine as being singularly ill-equipped to deal with the problems of chronic disease.

Initially working as a respected immunologist and bacteriologist, Bach began working with vaccines based on various forms of intestinal bacteria in an effort to discover a treatment that would relieve the problems of chronic disease. He was pleased to find that many patients responded well to this approach, with improvements occurring in those with symptoms of headaches and arthritis in particular, who also reported more general improvements in health.

By 1919, Bach became interested in the work of the founder of homoeopathy as a medical system, Samuel Hahnemann (see page 27). In many ways, Bach's own motivation and development parallel Hahnemann's, since both began their careers as orthodox doctors but became disillusioned with the limitations of conventional approaches and began experimenting with extremely dilute forms of medication in an effort to diminish the occurrence of side effects as much as possible.

As a result of familiarizing himself with Hahnemann's theories of health and disease, Bach began to prepare his vaccines in homoeopathic dilution (see page 87) so that they could be given in oral form, called nosodes, to his patients. The vaccines were well received by both medical doctors and homoeopaths alike, but Bach remained unsatisfied, and felt that he was still limiting himself to the treatment of physical symptoms, rather than addressing the basic issues of promoting good health and curing disease. He came to the conclusion that ill health was the consequence of lack of harmony between physical, mental and emotional states, with disease emerging as a result of negative states of mind. It came to Bach's attention that symptoms of deep disharmony in the patient, such as anxiety, despair or aggression, could be draining to the body's natural ability to resist infection.

By thinking along these lines, Bach gained inspiration from the ideas of the Greek 'father of medicine', Hippocrates, the Swiss physician, Paracelsus (1493–1541) and Hahnemann. Modern researchers such as Dr Hans Seyle, who pioneered work on stress and the immune system, and Carl Simonton, who introduced the use of positive imaging into cancer care in the USA, have developed these concepts further in their work, which examines the links between physical health and emotional imbalance. The exciting emerging field of psychoneuroimmunology explores the relationship between emotional and mental states, and the reasons for the emergence of all sorts of health problems, from colds to cancer. In this context, Bach's preoccupation with finding ways of balancing emotional and mental states as a way of improving overall health and easing disease symptoms makes a great deal of sense.

Bach visited Wales in 1928 where, working along purely intuitive lines, he began to experiment with preparations of the wild flowers impatiens, mimulus and clematis. By 1930 he had abandoned his laboratory in London, spending his time in Wales and the south of England refining his system of treatment by flower essences. It has been reported that for several days before finding a remedy, Bach would experience intense physical and mental symptoms. He would then go into the fields and, it is claimed, use his extremely refined intuitive sense to lead him to the appropriate plant or flower that would provide symptom relief.

The information relating to the thirty-eight flower remedies Bach discovered was written up and published in contemporary homoeopathic journals during his lifetime, while information was also made available to the public in the form of popular pamphlets. Bach also continued to practise using his flower remedies, moving to Oxfordshire for the final years of his life, until his death in 1936. His work has continued since then through the establishment of the Bach Centre at Mount Vernon in Oxfordshire. Today the Bach flower remedies are prepared in strict accordance with Bach's own methods, with flowers being used from the original locations. A regular newsletter is published, and practical questions may be answered by the staff who work at the centre.

Basic background

Edward Bach believed implicitly in treating the sick person rather than the disease. This conviction, coupled with his intense religious belief, led Bach on a search for a system of healing that would address physical, mental, emotional and spiritual imbalances that he regarded as being at the root of the development of disease. He took an uncompromising view of illness, regarding it as arising from the patient's lack of ability to listen to their intuition and follow positive instincts. He viewed the human being as becoming vulnerable to illness if a basic resistance acted as an obstruction to the personality's true development. The resistance could take the shape of emotions such as anxiety, anger or rigidity of mind, since these might be sufficient to blight the positive potential of a balanced personality.

In common with Samuel Hahnemann, Bach viewed symptoms of illness from a positive perspective, since they can alert us to the fact that changes are needed. These might involve rectifying excesses in diet, addressing deficiencies in basic lifestyle such as lack of exercise or relaxation, or attending to negative thought patterns that might be undermining health. However, Bach went many steps further than Hahnemann in his interpretation, since he developed a highly symbolic approach to the understanding of physical symptoms. For example, he saw stiffness of the joints and muscles as being reflective of rigidity of mind, while asthmatic symptoms might be interpreted as the smothering of emotional reactions to trauma.

It is interesting to note that here we have a marked contrast between Hahnemann's and Bach's approaches to developing a coherent medical system. Although both began from similar basic principles, Hahnemann laid great emphasis on the need for observation of the clinical data that could be verified by conducting controlled experiments (this has been continued in clinical trials that explore the efficacy of homoeopathic remedies). Edward Bach, on the other hand, appears to have been much more attracted by the use of intuition and symbolic interpretation of the symptoms of disease, making the boundaries between religious experience and the healing of illness extremely fluid.

Bach regarded orthodox drug therapy as counterproductive, as physical symptoms were temporarily suppressed while the root of the problem remained untreated. If the constitutional weakness remained unchecked, Bach maintained that the inevitable result would be progression to more serious illness in the future. He saw the role of doctor as one of adviser and counsellor, assisting the patient in taking increasing responsibility for his or her own health, and the Bach flower remedies have a very similar function. As well as supporting patients in times of stress and ill health, the flower remedies can be used before the first symptoms of illness have appeared as a form of preventative therapy to be taken when feeling generally run down or unfit.

How a flower remedy is made

The mother tincture is prepared either by a method of exposing plants and water to sunlight or using a boiling technique. The former is considered suitable for flowers that bloom during the late spring and summer when the sun is at its strongest. Boiling is used for the preparation of flowers and twigs of trees, bushes and plants that bloom at other times of the year when sunshine can be in short supply.

The solar method

• Flowers should be picked when blooms are freshly opened (around 9am) when they will already have had exposure to some hours of sunlight.

• The selected flowers are floated on the surface of pure spring water in glass containers, and left exposed to sunlight for a number of hours.

• After the required time the flowers are removed from the surface of the water and the 'impregnated' liquid is decanted into bottles with brandy added in order to preserve the tincture.

The boiling method

• A pan should be three-quarters filled with flowering sprays, twigs and leaves of the selected plant or tree.

• The contents of the pan are covered with spring or mineral water and brought to the boil.

• The flowers and twigs are pressed beneath the water at periodic intervals as the liquid boils for half an hour.

• The pan is removed from the heat, and left to stand until the liquid has a chance to cool. Once this has happened, all the leaves, twigs and flowers are removed, and the liquid is left to stand for a little longer in order to allow the sediment to settle.

• The liquid is then passed through filter paper and mixed half-and-half with brandy.

• Since tree flowers and twigs produce a great deal of sediment, it is sometimes necessary to filter the liquid twice. Even if this is done, further sediment may appear at the bottom of the container. If this occurs, the liquid should be refiltered and rebottled.

Conditions that may respond to flower remedies

Flower remedies may be of help in easing a number of problems including any of the following:

• Anxiety
• Burn-out
• Depression
• Eating disorders
• Fainting
• Grief and bereavement
• Headaches and migraines
• Insomnia
• Panic attacks
• Phobias
• Shock and trauma
• Stress-related disorders
• Travel sickness

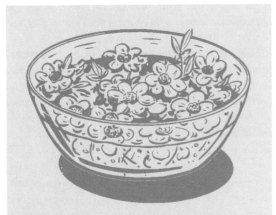

Using the solar method for preparing a flower remedy, the selected flowers are floated in spring water and left for several hours in the sun.

Massage therapy

Massage is one of the most immediate, accessible and pleasurable complementary therapies. Therapists claim that it can play an important part in easing a wide range of health problems, especially when used in combination with other appropriate systems of healing such as herbalism, homoeopathy, naturopathy and traditional Chinese medicine.

In essence, massage consists of using rhythmic, firm or light stroking, kneading or tapping movements that may cover the whole body from head to foot, or may be restricted to the head, face, back, shoulders, hands or feet. In this way it is an extremely flexible therapy that may be adjusted to the needs or mood of the person being massaged.

Historical perspectives

Massage in one form or another is one of the oldest forms of health-care disciplines. Massage therapy is referred to in a Chinese medical manual that is at least 4000 years old, and was used in Japan and India, while the ancient Greeks and Romans also regarded it as an invaluable form of therapy for health promotion.

Massage became especially popular in Europe in the nineteenth century when the system of Swedish massage was formulated by Per Henrik Ling (1776–1839). A gymnast by training, Ling combined knowledge of previously existing massage practices with exercises that he believed would have a beneficial effect on the muscles and joints.

Although this form of massage rapidly spread to the USA, where it gained significant popularity, general enthusiasm for massage therapy went into decline as conventional medicine became established in the twentieth century. During this time only a small number of massage therapists continued their work, but the tide began to turn in the early 1970s when *The Massage Book* was published by the American, George Downing. A massage therapist by training Downing stressed the need to regard massage as a whole-person therapy that could assist in easing a range of mental, emotional and physical problems. This fitted in extremely well with the general mood of the decade, with its emphasis on self-development and the need for each person to take responsibility for their own health.

This trend has continued, and now massage therapy is regarded as an especially valuable tool in helping those suffering from stress-related problems. Indeed, the benefits of massage are now widely recognized – to the extent that certain airlines provide in-flight aromatherapy massage for the head and shoulders for passengers, while more forward-looking companies also acknowledge the role massage and other stress-reduction techniques can play in protecting the health of their staff.

Basic background

Massage therapy works by stimulating the body's basic functions, and is a holistic system of healing, with similarities in approach to homoeopathy, acupuncture, ayurveda and herbal treatment. By encouraging the body's self-healing mechanisms to function efficiently, massage helps maintain a state of good health.

Massage therapy relieves symptoms of stress partly because of its effect on the autonomic nervous system, which governs the involuntary movements of the heart, glands and smooth muscles, affecting circulation and digestion. Massage helps to improve the circulation of blood and lymph, and promotes efficient drainage of waste products. When these systems are working inefficiently, feelings of stress and lethargy are intensified, and the metabolism may slow down.

Stimulation of the nerve endings promotes feelings of relaxation which in itself encourages deeper breathing, correcting the balance of oxygen and carbon dioxide in the body, while massage can also reduce muscular tension, increasing flexibility and relieving the discomfort of stiff muscles.

Massage strokes

The following are some of the most common strokes that are used during a massage:

Effleurage

These are rhythmical, slow strokes that are done with the hands close together and the thumbs about 2.5cm (1in) apart. The pressure may come from the fingertips or palms of the hands for a light massage movement, or from the knuckles or thumbs for more vigorous pressure.

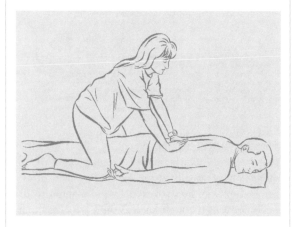

Petrissage

This movement consists of grasping and squeezing areas of muscle in a motion that rather resembles kneading dough. The hands move steadily over the area that is treated, with the flesh being rhythmically rolled and released. This has the effect of stimulating the circulation and draining the lactic acid deposits that can settle in the muscles after exercise. Kneading the skin in this way helps to relax hard, tight muscles as well as discouraging cramp.

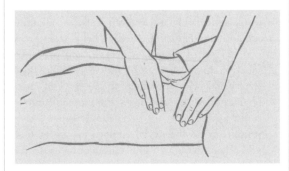

Friction

This consists of making small, circular movements with the fingers, pads of the thumbs, or heel of the hand. This may be especially helpful where strains or sprains have occurred, since the movement enables joints to move more freely and stimulates the circulation in the area being treated. However, massaging injured or bruised areas in this way should be avoided by the non-professional.

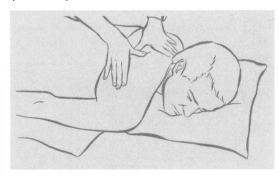

Percussion

This fast, rhythmic movement is also sometimes called *tapotement* (which can be translated as 'drumming'). It is usually done using the sides of the hands, applying the strokes in a rapid manner to the fleshy areas of the body such as the buttocks, shoulders, waist or tops of the thighs. However, although this is a movement that is briskly done, it should not result in pain or discomfort, just a pleasant sensation of stimulation.

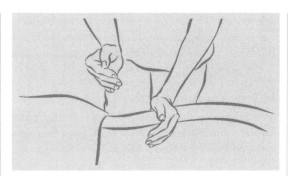

Wringing

This is particularly suitable for treating the fronts and backs of the thighs. One hand may be placed on the client's outer thigh with the other hand resting on the inner part of the muscle. The hands should slide firmly and slowly towards each other, applying steady pressure to the muscle so that it is lengthened as the hands cross each other. The stroke is then repeated in the other direction as the masseuse works her way down the thigh.

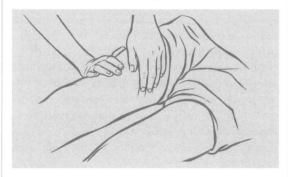

Feathering

This is an extremely light stroke that is done by softly stroking the length of the large muscles of the back. This movement is so delicate that only the tips of the fingers should make contact with the skin.

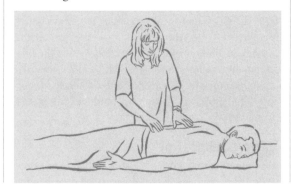

Because of its light and soothing nature, this is a movement that is often used to finish a body massage.

The consultation

Although simple massage skills can be learned by most people through introductory courses and following self-help manuals, it is best to consult a trained therapist when suffering from any of the chronic conditions listed on page 75.

A consultation is likely to last roughly sixty to ninety minutes. At the beginning your therapist will take details of your medical history to establish if you are suffering or have suffered from any medical conditions that might render massage therapy inappropriate. He or she will also want to establish if there are specific areas of discomfort or tension in your body that need to be taken into account.

Once the basic information has been gathered you are likely to be asked to remove your clothing after your therapist has temporarily left the room. Since most massage techniques require the hands of the therapist to make contact with your body, it is helpful if you remove as much clothing as you feel comfortable with. Jewellery should also be removed.

Once this has been done, your body will be covered with a towel or blanket that can be moved appropriately as your therapist works on each part of your body. In this way, contact may be achieved without the privacy or comfort of the client being compromised. The room should be comfortably quiet and warm, feeling neither stuffy nor chilly. If you begin to feel uncomfortably cold, always tell your therapist, as muscles contract and become tense when they become chilled.

The surface you are lying on should feel pleasantly firm, neither so hard that it causes discomfort, nor so soft that it sags. Practitioners may work on the floor using a futon, or a custom-made massage table that provides sufficient support for the whole body. Extra comfort may be derived from putting a pillow under the upper body in order to protect the chest and stomach from uncomfortable pressure, while a rolled-up towel placed under the ankles will take potential strain from the feet. Some massage tables have an oval space to rest the face in, which when the client is lying prone, keeps the head, neck and chest in optimum alignment.

Most practitioners use oil to lubricate the skin and enhance the flowing movements of the hands on the body. Vegetable oils such as almond or grapeseed are most likely to be used in preference to those that are of mineral origin, since the latter can clog the pores of the skin. Oil should never be poured directly onto the skin, but should be warmed in the practitioner's hands before making contact with the body. Quite often, scented oils may be used to enhance the relaxing or stimulating effect of the massage, depending on the individual needs of the client. In some situations talcum powder or lotions may be used in massage in preference to oil.

It is quite common to feel extremely relaxed or energized after a treatment, depending on the way the massage has been given. Generally speaking, it is advisable not to get up quickly after treatment, since slight dizziness may occur. Once you feel ready, it is best to roll onto one side rather than sitting straight up, which is less stressful for the spine.

After massage it can be very beneficial to relax for half an hour and to drink plenty of mineral water to support the detoxifying action of the massage. If essential oils have been used, avoid showering immediately after having a massage so that the oils have enough time to be absorbed through the skin. This process takes at least thirty minutes to get under way, but once essential oils have made contact with the bloodstream, the effects may last for anything up to eight hours.

The effects of massage vary greatly from person to person, and often from one massage to another. Possible reactions during and following massage may include euphoria, a profound sense of being at peace, tearfulness, tiredness, slight soreness or increased energy.

Conditions that may respond to massage

There appear to be very few situations for which massage is inappropriate (see below), since most people are likely to benefit from some form of massage. Age should not be a barrier, since babies, toddlers and the elderly can all respond well to some form of soothing therapeutic touch. In fact, since many elderly people find themselves living alone and suffering from a sense of loneliness, sensitively given massage can do a great deal to ease feelings of isolation. Massage therapy is being used for similar reasons in some hospital intensive-care units, where patients can benefit greatly from soothing physical contact.

Problems that may respond well to massage therapy include any of the following:

- Anxiety
- Back pain
- Circulatory problems*
- Depression*
- Digestive problems such as indigestion and constipation
- Fatigue
- General feelings of physical and emotional stress and tension
- Headaches
- High blood pressure*
- Menstrual pain
- Muscle strains
- Pain in the neck and shoulders
- Postnatal problems
- Repetitive motion disorders
- Sciatica
- Sinus congestion
- Sleep problems

Disorders marked with a * mean that you should always seek conventional medical advice before embarking on treatment. Be sure to tell your massage therapist that you suffer from any of these problems.

Massage is inappropriate for:

- Advanced osteoporosis (brittle bones)
- Feverishness
- Open wounds
- Phlebitis (inflammation of the veins)
- Thrombosis (blood clotting)
- Varicose ulcers
- Varicose veins

Nutritional therapy
by Roger Groos

An average human in the West consumes over 500kg (1100lb) of food every year, and the significance of this large consumption for health and well-being is obvious. Indeed, the saying 'you are what you eat' sums it up very aptly. From this basic perspective, we can see that nutritional therapy may be one of the most fundamental strategies we can adopt to improve our sense of health and vitality. Beyond that, we can use it as a therapy that can ease the symptoms of illness.

During approximately the first fifteen years of human life food fuels active growth and some change of form in the body; thereafter, there is no change in form, with the result that all food consumed goes towards energy production, cellular repair, regulation and reproduction.

Historical perspectives

During the million or so years of human evolution, our collective biochemistry has changed to handle the food we eat. A good example of this is our present-day inability to synthesize ascorbic acid (vitamin C). This may be due to a historically large dietary intake, which sets us apart from virtually all other mammals, who can synthesize this vitamin. Hunter-gatherers were forced by limited technology and seasonal adjustments to eat a broad, mixed, whole-food diet, as were early agriculturists and pastoralists, and much evidence points to plant foods being the main source of energy for all of them. Sometime during our evolution, the metabolic ability to produce vitamin C was lost because it became possible to have a plentiful intake of the substance.

Dietary manipulation forms an important part of several ancient medical systems: Oriental medicine classifies the energy of foods in terms of yin and yang, ayurvedic medicine by how suitable foods are for the three constitutions, kapha, pitta and vata (see pages 22–23). Both use diet to restore bodily balance. In ancient Greece, Hippocrates gave dietary prescriptions for treatment, and was credited with the saying 'let food be your medicine and medicine be your food'.

Most religions impose dietary restrictions, and some recommend or demand periods of fasting. In practice, however, not all of these regimes contribute to the healthy functioning of the body. Their true function is regarded as spiritual rather than therapeutic. In the Middle East and elsewhere, for example, the fast of Ramadan involves long periods without food or water, normally followed by enormous meals after sunset, and can cause an immense strain on

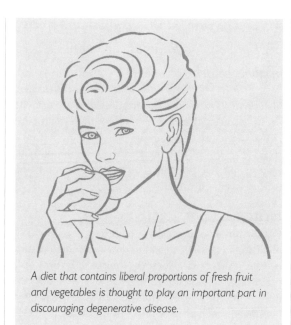

A diet that contains liberal proportions of fresh fruit and vegetables is thought to play an important part in discouraging degenerative disease.

manual workers and others.

In the West, from the Middle Ages down to the seventeenth century, physicians employed the humoral system of viewing the body, which held that the balance of four bodily fluids (blood, phlegm, yellow bile and black bile) determined emotional and physical disposition. They would then make use of dietary recommendations in order to correct the hot, cold, dry and moist imbalances in the patient.

The rise in popularity of nutritional therapy as a means of treating health problems in the West owes much to our diet and lifestyle. The scourges of modern affluent society – chronic conditions such as coronary heart disease, rheumatic disease, constipation and the like were rare before 1900. A great deal of blame for their upsurge has been logically attributed to diet, a perspective that has been partly supported by epidemiological studies.

In the 1920s some obsessive dietary therapeutics were practised in the USA in health-farm settings, using fasting, rigid diets, enemas and the like, but this approach waned in the face of a more rational, scientific approach. The latter has mainly been championed in the USA by several doctors and researchers who actively promote the use of specific nutrients in high, pharmacological doses for the active treatment of a broad range of diseases. Dr Roger J. Williams expounded 'biochemical individuality', a concept now commonly recognized by present-day nutri-

tional therapists to be a key for assessing and balancing the body through diet and supplementation.

Basic background

Modern nutritional therapy is scientifically based and draws upon extensive research into individual nutrients, as well as some of the older practices, such as fasting, the biochemistry of which is now well understood. The difference between this kind of scientifically regulated fasting and earlier religious-based regimens is quite considerable.

The scope for employing nutrition therapeutically in the treatment of many health conditions is very wide, and interventions may be made at the following levels:

• Food source: e.g. wholefood, refined, organic, gluten-free, etc.
• Food preparation: e.g. raw, cooked, minced, liquidized, boiled, etc.
• Digestion: e.g. food-combining diets, chewing thoroughly.
• Absorption: e.g. food quality, regularity of meals.
• Metabolism: e.g. vitamin and mineral therapy, diets tailored for individual types of metabolism, etc.
• Excretion: e.g. low- or high-residue foods.

In addition, consideration is given to the exposure to antinutrients (e.g. environmental pollutants, heavy metals, antibiotics, hormones, alcohol, etc.), the level of fluids in the body, the status of the gut flora and food sensitivities. If negative factors are present, nutritional measures should be taken to improve the situation.

While we may talk in general terms about dietary recommendations, the personal constitution or specific make-up of the individual is paramount in assessing the action to be taken. As a result, an individually based set of recommendations is usually made for each person. This is often of crucial importance, because involving an individual in their own healing through dietary measures can give a sense of empowerment, which in itself is beneficial.

A wide range of conditions may be treated alone or in part with diet, or through specific nutrients. Although classic nutritional deficiencies like beriberi (a deficiency of vitamin B1, common in many 'third world' countries) are obvious but uncommon in the West, subclinical deficiencies are much more likely to arise, and are directly ascribable to the Western diet.

The consultation

The initial consultation will last about one hour, during which a detailed case history will be taken, including past and present health history, medication, lifestyle, social interactions and diet. There will also be an assessment of physiological functions. Some, mainly non-invasive, laboratory tests may be ordered, such as hair mineral analysis or hormone panel tests.

An account of what the patient is willing to undertake must be made, and recommendations are given. These may range from taking supplements to dietary manipulation or fasting (at the correct times of year) and changes in lifestyle. Many nutritional therapists now work in conjunction with family doctors.

Conditions that may respond to nutritional therapy

Specific conditions that may respond to a nutritional approach include the following:
- Bowel problems
- Depression and anxiety states
- Digestive problems
- Food sensitivities
- Lack of energy
- Most chronic inflammatory conditions (rheumatic and skin).

It must not be forgotten that prevention is more valuable than cure, and dietary advice sought before a problem is evident is a wise precaution. This can be especially relevant preconceptually, during pregnancy and breastfeeding.

Osteopathy

Osteopathy is an extremely popular system of complementary medicine that focuses on the musculoskeletal system (the bones, joints, muscles, ligaments and connecting tissue), and attempts to establish the optimum potential for health by restoring function and mobility to this system. Osteopaths view the person as a unit in which structure, function, mind and spirit need to be in balance for the maintenance of good health.

Osteopaths are trained to diagnose and treat faults or imbalances that occur due to injury, physical stress, accident, disease or protracted emotional stress. The aim of treatment is to allow the body to restore normal function, with each patient being treated as an individual.

Historical perspectives

Osteopathy was originally established as a system of medicine in the second half of the nineteenth century by an American doctor, Andrew Taylor Still (1828–1917). Still originally worked as a surgeon during the American Civil War (1861–5), but later became disenchanted with conventional medicine, which attempted to fight disease by using treatments that often had side effects that were more severe than the symptoms of the disease itself. Still became interested in developing a system of medicine that could stimulate the body's own self-regulating mechanisms, and he combined his medical knowledge of anatomy with an early study of engineering to develop the therapeutic basis of osteopathy.

Although Still's ideas initially met with great opposition from the conventional medical profession in the USA, osteopathy has now gained full recognition, and osteopaths have full medical practice rights in all states. Much of the research that has been carried out into the effectiveness of osteopathy has been conducted in the USA, reflecting the way in which this therapy has been accepted within the mainstream of medical care.

Osteopathy reached the UK at the turn of the century. The British School of Osteopathy was set up in 1917 in London by Dr Martin Littlejohn, who had previously studied under Still. Today the profession of osteopathy is rapidly expanding, and there are several training institutions offering honours courses in osteopathy. Training is demanding and lengthy, and student osteopaths study anatomy, physiology, pathology, biomechanics and clinical diagnostic methods. In addition to the skills of osteopathic manual diagnosis and treatment students also learn about the interpretation of clinical tests, and the relevant areas of physiology and sociology.

Osteopaths are taught to take clinical responsibil-

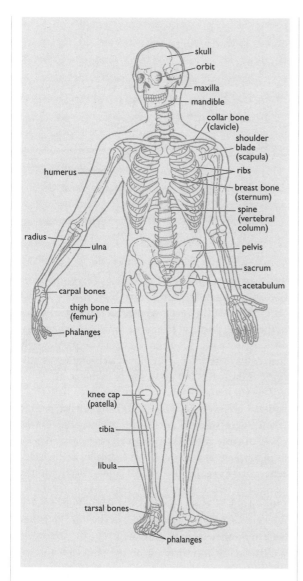

skull
orbit
maxilla
mandible
collar bone (clavicle)
shoulder blade (scapula)
ribs
breast bone (sternum)
spine (vertebral column)
humerus
pelvis
sacrum
acetabulum
radius
ulna
carpal bones
thigh bone (femur)
phalanges
knee cap (patella)
tibia
libula
tarsal bones
phalanges

ity for their patients and are able to identify conditions for which osteopathic treatment may not be appropriate. They are trained in the skills of clinical diagnosis, and are thus able to determine a suitable treatment approach and recognize the presence of serious conditions that might require referral to a conventional medical practitioner.

Basic background

Over the years, a number of approaches have come to constitute the basis of osteopathy. Some are largely theoretical, others more practical; some have been emphasized more than others, and some have been played down, but taken together, they repre-

sent a fair picture of how osteopathy is understood by its practitioners on a global basis..

• **The holistic approach.** The body is regarded as being an integrated unit made up of systems that are dependent upon each other for harmonious functioning. In this way, the osteopathic approach has much in common with other holistic systems of healing. From the holistic perspective, which is taken by osteopaths, the functions of mind, emotions, spirit and body are seen as being mutually supportive and interdependent, meaning that good health comes from a balanced relationship between the various parts and systems of the body as a whole.

• **Emphasis on the intimate relationship between structure and function of the human body.** Osteopathic practitioners generally acknowledge the links between problems in the skeletal and muscular structure and problems with the functioning of specific organs. Therefore, neck pain or tension can be related to chronic headaches, while poor circulation can also lead to general states of fatigue or lethargy. Alternatively, symptoms suggesting that specific organs are not functioning well can also indicate problems with the skeletal or muscular framework.

• **A basic conviction that the body possesses the ability to regulate and heal itself.**
Osteopaths attempt to enhance and support the self-healing mechanisms of the body either through constructive manipulation of the joints and soft tissues, or by suggesting positive changes in daily routine. These may include the adoption of dietary improvements, taking appropriate exercise or adjusting conventional medication.

• **The importance of treating the individual patient.** During osteopathic treatment the patient will quickly become aware that the therapy is attempting to restore their whole system to health, rather than concentrating on the piecemeal removal of symptoms. The osteopath tailors his therapeutic approach to each individual patient in order to speed progress towards recovery. Therefore, two patients may consult an osteopath for treatment of the same condition (such as migraines), but the treatment and advice given to one may be subtly different from those given to the other.

• **The intimate link between mind and body.** The crucial relationship between physical problems and the state of the mind has been established by the developing field of psychoneuroimmunology. The latter is a discipline that has drawn attention to the negative impact that stress can have on the body, leaving it open to repeated infection and resulting in compromised ability to defend itself against serious illness. Osteopaths are especially well placed to work within this field, since they are often able to relieve chronic states of muscular pain and tension that are the result of emotional stress, anxiety or depression. Osteopathic manipulative treatment has also been demonstrated to have effects well beyond the rectifying of structural imbalance in the skeletal system since improved blood-pressure levels, urine output, bowel movements and respiratory function have been attributed to appropriate osteopathic manipulation.

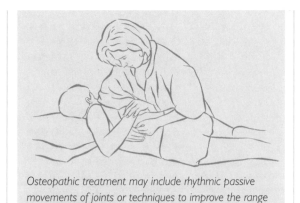

Osteopathic treatment may include rhythmic passive movements of joints or techniques to improve the range of movement of specific joints.

The consultation

When you visit an osteopath for the first time, a full medical history will be taken. The practitioner will ask questions about current symptoms, when they began, what makes them more or less troublesome and how they affect your general experience of health. In addition, details of your past medical history will be taken, together with information regarding any medication or other treatments that you are currently receiving.

The next stage of the consultation will be a thorough physical examination so that the mobility of your body can be evaluated and any areas of weakness, strain or injury can be identified. You may also be asked to perform a simple series of movements, so that assessment of musculoskeletal function can be considered alongside aspects of lifestyle such as work and leisure activities. Putting together this information enables your osteopath to make a full diagnosis, so that a suitable treatment plan can be decided upon.

Osteopaths use their hands both to discover the underlying cause of painful and debilitating problems and to carry out treatment. Osteopathic treatment may include the use of gentle stretching of soft tissues, rhythmic passive movements of joints or special techniques to improve the range of movement of particular joints. Gentle techniques are often used, particularly when treating children or elderly patients. Many osteopaths use what are termed 'cranial' osteopathic techniques, in which the osteopath's highly trained sense of touch is used to identify and correct disturbances and limitations of tissue mobility around the head and neck, as well as throughout the whole body.

Osteopathy is a safe and natural approach to health care. A survey revealed that it is used by a wide variety of patients, including a large proportion of people who suffer from back trouble. Most back pains are the result of mechanical disturbances in the spine, postural strains or injuries to the spinal discs. Osteopathy has been shown to be particularly successful in treating painful and debilitating conditions in the spine and other joints in the body.

The survey also showed that just over half of all patients are women. This is perhaps not surprising when many women are working mothers, leading stressful daily lives that can give rise to a variety of musculoskeletal disorders. For example, many headaches originate from stiffness and tension in the neck, which osteopathic treatment can often relieve. Osteopathy is also beneficial during and after pregnancy, which puts considerable strains on the lower back and other related structures.

Osteopaths also treat a wide age range of patients. Increasingly, parents are seeking osteopathic treatment for their children suffering from conditions such as colic, fretfulness and glue ear. Sportspeople, often in their teens and early twenties, find that osteopathic treatment can not only help them overcome injury, but also help them to keep their bodies in the peak of physical condition.

Many of the problems that osteopaths see are caused by working conditions, perhaps from sitting for long hours at computer terminals or carrying out heavy manual jobs. All of these can give rise to abnormal tension in the neck, arms and hands. Osteopaths treat many conditions relating to the workplace, and can give remedial advice and preventative exercises.

Nearly a quarter of patients seen by osteopaths

are in their forties, as this is a time when many people give up regular exercise and their tissues start to lose some of their elasticity. These factors make our bodies more prone to injury and osteopaths are able to assess posture, strength and flexibility of muscles, tensions and ligaments. Treatment is then formulated to alleviate current problems and to help prevent recurrences.

Many elderly patients also seek an alternative to painkillers for the aches and pains often associated with growing older. For more permanent relief it is necessary to eliminate the underlying cause of the pain, a job which the osteopath's highly developed sense of touch is specifically trained to do. Osteopathy can also help in reducing pain and stiffness in the less acute stages of arthritis, and help patients maintain their mobility and independence.

Conditions that may respond to osteopathy
Patients suffering from any of the following may benefit from consultation with an osteopath:
- Asthma
- Backache
- Bronchitis
- Constipation
- Ear infections
- Headaches
- Lumbago
- Muscular tension
- Neck pain
- Neuralgia
- Osteoarthritis
- Sciatica
- Sports injuries such as sprains and strains
- Stress-related disorders.
  Cranial osteopaths may be able to help with conditions that specifically affect the head such as:
- Disorders in infants and children that can be traced back to birth trauma or injury
- Dizziness and giddiness
- Sinusitis

Reflexology

Reflexology is an increasingly popular form of complementary therapy that involves applying gentle pressure to points on the feet or hands. The application of regulated pressure to certain parts of the feet (called reflexes) has a therapeutic influence on those organs, glands or parts of the body that correspond to the reflex being stimulated.

The feet are regarded as a mirror image of the body: the right foot represents the right half of the body and the left foot the left. Isolated parts of the foot are seen as being connected to certain organs and body parts such as the lungs, kidneys, bladder and reproductive organs.

Although pressure applied to appropriate parts of the feet has an effect on specific body parts, reflexologists maintain that their therapy has a beneficial effect on the whole system by encouraging the release of stress and tension, encouraging the body's own self-healing mechanisms, enhancing a general sense of well-being and stimulating increased energy and vitality.

Historical perspectives
Although the roots of reflexology can be traced back to ancient India, China and Egypt, the development of the system now in popular use owes a great deal to the work of American physician Dr William Fitzgerald. Working at the turn of the last century, Fitzgerald developed a form of treatment called zone therapy. By applying pressure to certain parts of the body it was discovered that a pain-relieving effect could be produced in other areas. Fitzgerald was so impressed with these results that he is recorded as having conducted minor surgical procedures using this technique of analgesia.

The basis of zone therapy rested upon the theory that the body could be divided into ten zones made up of vertical sections running through the body extending from the toes to the top of the head, and down again to the hands. These zones were regarded as being linked by a flow of energy (resembling the meridian theory of acupuncture, see page 41) so that pressure applied to one part of the body could have an effect elsewhere in the same zone.

The practice of modern reflexology also owes much to the work of American physiotherapist

Eunice Ingham (1889–1974) who developed the theoretical basis of foot reflexology. She mapped out areas of the feet that were likely to have a therapeutic effect when stimulated by pressure. Ingham's work was continued and developed by her nephew, who was responsible for setting up the IIR (International Institute of Reflexology).

This popular therapy is now practised on a global basis, with particular interest being shown in European countries (it has been estimated that over 6000 European doctors, physiotherapists and nurses make use of it). Reflexology was introduced to the UK in the 1960s by a pupil of Eunice Ingham, Doreen Bayly, who set up her practice and offered courses for clinical training. It is a growing therapy in the USA.

The consultation

Reflexology has a wide appeal because of its direct, 'hands-on' nature and the pleasant sensations it causes. Appointments should last approximately one hour. Treatment may be given on a weekly basis, or appointments may be needed twice or three times a week for more pressing problems. However, in some straightforward cases, three or four visits may be all that is needed in order to improve the situation substantially.

An initial assessment involves asking general questions about the client's state of health and medical background, and investigating specific problem areas in detail, before the practitioner conducts an examination of the feet (sometimes the hand may also be included).

Once treatment is under way, your reflexologist will ask you to lie in a comfortable reclining position with your feet raised and shoes, socks, tights or stockings off. Your reflexologist will begin to move his or her thumbs and fingers gradually over your foot, using small, precise movements. By working systematically over the foot the therapist can locate the parts that are tender or sensitive and thereby determine the areas of your body in which all is not well. At the beginning of the treatment, your therapist will make note of any areas on the sole of the foot that may be subject to developing corns, calluses or diseases of the skin such as eczema or athlete's foot. These are relevant because they may suggest to your reflexologist that there is a poor blood supply to these areas, or a possible nutritional problem may exist.

The feet are treated by applying pressure to sensitive areas in order to break up tiny adhesions (crystal-like deposits), improve blood supply, unblock nerve impulses, free the energy flow and enhance the self-healing mechanism of the body. The correct amount of pressure applied to sensitive areas is thought to break down tiny crystal-like deposits that may develop around nerve endings as a result of accumulated waste materials. By working on these deposits, a reflexologist encourages the body to rid itself of toxic waste through the bloodstream, thus improving the overall circulation and general blood supply to the rest of the body.

Reflexology may also be beneficial for people who do not yet suffer from a specific health problem, but feel that their health is slightly under par and that they may be heading for potential illness. In this situation a reflexologist can provide preventative treatment in support of the self-healing mechanism of the body, while pointing out to their client areas of weakness in the body. Since reflexology enhances the functioning of all body systems, it can also help sportspeople to maintain optimum health and fitness.

Reactions to treatment may often involve a profound sense of relaxation and well-being, and there should be no dramatic, unpleasant reactions. However, occasionally a 'healing crisis' may occur as toxic waste is being removed from the system. This may be experienced as loose bowel movements, a nasal discharge, skin eruption or a temporary worsening of existing conditions.

Conditions that may respond to reflexology

Reflexologists may be called upon to treat a variety of problems including any of the following:
- Arthritic problems
- Asthma
- Chronic pain
- Circulatory disorders
- Constipation and irritable bowel syndrome
- General stress-related problems
- Headaches
- High blood pressure
- Migraines
- Painful periods
- Sinus problems
- Urinary problems

Conditions where reflexology may need to be used

with caution, or may be unsuitable include the following:

- Arthritis of the feet
- Cancer
- Diabetes
- Epilepsy
- Heart trouble
- Osteoporosis
- Phlebitis
- Thrombosis

Reflexology should not be used during the first trimester of pregnancy, but thereafter it can be extremely beneficial. This therapy can also be of great practical value during childbirth, since it offers an alternative form of pain relief to conventional drugs. It is important always to follow a practitioner's advice before embarking on self-help reflexology when pregnant or suffering from any of the conditions mentioned above.

It is also possible for patients to benefit from this therapy when recovering from surgery such as a hip- or knee-replacement operation. By having reflexology treatment before and after an operation it may be possible to ease pain and encourage speedy healing of traumatized tissue. It is also possible that the general relaxation-inducing effect of reflexology as a therapy could be of immense benefit to those who have undergone the physical and psychological stress of surgery.

Although self-help reflexology techniques may be used for limited, acute problems, it is best to consult a trained practitioner when suffering from a well-established, chronic health problem.

Shiatsu

This dynamic form of body treatment uses a variety of different kinds of pressure and stretches to stimulate the flow of energy along pathways (or meridians, see page 41) that are understood to traverse the surface of the body. Shiatsu may be regarded as a parallel therapy to acupuncture in that it seeks to rebalance and harmonize the flow of essential energy or qi (see page 36) throughout the system as a whole.

By stimulating and establishing the optimum flow of qi through the use of shiatsu, acupuncture or qi gong, the body's own capacity for self-healing can be enhanced, so that the whole system becomes more resilient and able to regulate itself more effectively. In this way, mental, emotional and physical health should be improved.

Historical perspectives

Although traditional massage in the Far East has a well-established history, the descriptive term shiatsu (a combination of two words meaning 'finger' and 'pressure') is relatively new. It is related to the pressure techniques incorporated in the do-in-ankyo system, which embraces a range of therapeutic aspects, including diet, meditation, manipulation, massage and exercise. It is a traditional Chinese massage which found its way to Japan by the eighth century. Shiatsu, however, was not developed into a coherent and comprehensive therapy until the early part of the twentieth century by Tokujiro Namikoshi.

Basic background

Shiatsu is rapidly gaining popularity in the West both as a preventative therapy and a treatment for a wide range of health problems. It is regarded as a safe and effective system of healing that can improve specific physical problems of restricted movement of joints, pain, stiffness and tension, while also being capable of affecting the whole system, stimulating a general sense of emotional uplift or relaxation.

The consultation

As with other forms of bodywork such as chiropractic and osteopathy, it will be necessary for your practitioner to make a diagnosis before embarking on an appropriate course of treatment. He will take a full case history, including details of treatment given in the past. Examination will also involve a combination of observation, pulse-taking and palpation of affected areas in order to evaluate their condition.

Once an assessment has been made, and your practitioner has decided that your case is one that may benefit from shiatsu, treatment will begin. Each session may last anything from thirty minutes to an hour and requires no special preparation before-hand, other than avoiding eating a large meal or drinking alcohol. Since you can expect to remain clothed during the course of treatment, whatever garments are worn should be comfortable, and loose enough to allow for a wide range of movement without any sense of restriction or discomfort.

A shiatsu session may involve instruction on ener-gizing exercises in order to stimulate the flow of qi. Once treatment is under way you will be asked to lie on the floor on a firm, supportive surface such as a futon while your practitioner applies regulated pressure to the parts of your body that require treat-ment. Pressure may come from the practitioner's hands, elbows, feet or knees and the degree of stim-ulation used may vary from very firm to light, and may feel like a rubbing movement, kneading or holding the pressure at one specific point for a period of time. For the latter, pressure is applied for a few seconds at a time, and may be repeated up to three or four times at the same spot. The practi-tioner is aided by the basic force of gravity when applying static, leaning pressure to his client. His own relaxed body weight is used in a controlled manner, so that the client feels no discomfort.

Possible techniques that may be used during a shiatsu treatment may include sustained, steady pressure, supporting pressure that permits the prac-titioner to maintain a balanced distribution of body weight without causing undue strain to the client, and vertical pressure. These techniques may be used while the client is lying on the belly, back or either side, or when sitting.

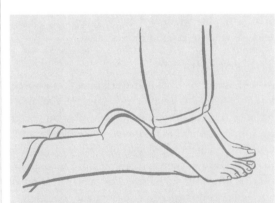

Techniques used during a Shiatsu treatment may include sustained, steady pressure, supporting pressure or vertical pressure.

It is considered helpful to rest for approximately fifteen minutes after treatment in order to give the body a chance to recover and reorient itself. This can be important because, although a sensation of euphoria can occur, a shiatsu session can also induce a feeling of drowsiness or sleepiness.

SHIATSU IN PRACTICE

The more vigorous shiatsu techniques may not be suitable where a high fever is present, if the patient has inflammation, a slipped disc, fractures, infec-tious disease, heart disease or cancer, or where steroids or cortisone are being taken.

Direct pressure should never be applied over any area where there is a bruise, injury, scar tissue, swelling, or a cut or graze. On the other hand, using less dynamic, gentle shiatsu technique is an appro-priate complement to other supportive treatments for treating patients suffering from some forms of cancer or heart disease.

Depending on the severity or established nature of the problem, weekly sessions may be necessary initially, gradually letting the gaps widen between appointments to fortnightly intervals or more. Shiatsu can be part of a health maintenance programme, when treatments may be spaced less frequently.

Conditions that may respond to shiatsu

Although practitioners of shiatsu regard this therapy as very patient-centred rather than oriented towards the relief of certain specific, limited conditions, patients suffering from any of the following may benefit from shiatsu treatment:

• Back pain
• Constipation
• Convalescence from illness
• Depression
• Diarrhoea
• General digestive problems
• General symptoms of stress and tension
• Headaches
• Insomnia
• Menstrual problems
• Migraines
• Pain that is related to postural problems
• Sluggish immune-system reaction, leading to recurrent or persistent infections

PRACTICALITIES

How to use this book

Once you have established the nature of the problem — say, recurrent headaches, or a skin disorder, turn to the 'Treatment Guide' section of this book. Here you will find an initial description of common conditions, with primary symptoms frequently given in bullet-point form. At this stage you will have a chance to confirm the details of your problem.

It is important to establish at the outset whether you are suffering from an acute or chronic condition, since the former tend to respond to alternative self-help prescribing, while the latter are more likely to need help from a trained practitioner. See pages 74-75 for information on how to identify which category your problem belongs to.

If symptoms are mild or intermittent in nature they may respond to information contained in the 'Preventative measures' section alone. These are straightforward modifications to general lifestyle, diet or exercise that may do a great deal to improve the situation in the long run. This approach can be of value if you are unsure about alternative self-prescribing, but feel that you want to take positive steps in improving your situation, rather than experiencing the frustration of adopting a passive role with regard to illness.

Always pay special attention to the sections headed 'Seek professional help', since this is where firm guidance is given about symptoms suggesting a condition that must be referred to a conventional medical practitioner. Professional medical help is

necessary in two important sets of circumstances:
• Acute problems treated by self-help measures at home that begin to show signs of deteriorating into a more serious condition demanding conventional medical help, ideally accompanied or followed by non-conventional treatment.
• Problems that should from the outset be dealt with by a trained alternative or conventional medical practitioner in order to improve. This section will give pointers on how to identify symptoms relating to such conditions.

If you feel confident about using an appropriate alternative self-help technique, move on to the advice headed 'Alternative treatments'. In most cases you will find that this is divided into two sections, with the first listing alternative treatments that can be used externally in the form of creams, ointments, aromatic baths, scented massage oils or as poultices or compresses. These measures may be especially appropriate for helping skin conditions, inflamed or slightly burnt skin, muscular strains, sports injuries or general muscular tension associated with stress. Exploring these options initially if you are a newcomer to alternative measures may be an excellent way of building up your confidence in using alternative medicines.

The first section often also includes advice on home remedies, and gives valuable hints on using everyday ingredients to soothe the pain, discomfort and irritation of illness. This is an excellent way of gaining confidence in using self-help techniques to deal with straightforward acute health problems, without yet entering the realms of self-prescribing alternative medicines that may be taken internally.

The second section, entitled 'Medicines intended for internal use' will give an overview of the possible options of medicines that may be taken in tablet, tincture, tea or decoction form. Medicines included in this section are likely to include herbal, biochemical, homoeopathic or anthroposophical approaches. Generally speaking, it is best to choose one of these approaches at a time rather than using a combination of two or three, since it can otherwise be extremely difficult to work out the reaction to any one therapy. Deciding on which approach to use first may depend upon the practical issue of availability: for example, it is likely to be easier to obtain biochemic tissue salts or homoeopathic medicines from a high-street chemist than to buy an anthroposophical preparation. If more time is available, anthroposophical or herbal preparations may be readily found in health-food shops.

Do bear in mind that you can use a cream, ointment, essential oil or compress at the same time as an alternative medicine that is taken internally in order to speed up a general positive reaction.

Remember that when selecting biochemic tissue salts, homoeopathic medicines, or flower remedies the medicine chosen needs to match the symptoms experienced by the patient as closely as possible. In this way it should be possible to make a reasonably firm choice between one medicine and another. For further information on selecting the appropriate medicine, see the information given within each therapy section in this chapter.

As a rule, it should not be necessary to take alternative medicines over an extended period of time in order to maintain an improvement. In this way, alternative medicines tend to differ from orthodox drugs. For example, inhaled steroids for asthma or beta blockers for high blood pressure must be taken long term to improve symptoms. Alternative medicines, used wisely and competently, should gently steer the body as a whole towards a state of improved health. Once this has occurred, the need for alternative medical support should become unnecessary as the body regains its sense of equilibrium and well-being.

In short-term, acute problems that respond well to home prescribing, alternative medicines should, ideally, not be necessary for more than a few days before improvement sets in. In more pressing circumstances, where symptoms are more marked, improvement should be apparent within hours rather than days. If it becomes necessary to take alternative medicines over an extended period, professional alternative medical help should be consulted to help you manage the situation more effectively.

For instructions on how to take the selected alternative medicine, as well as the dosage, see the relevant section under the individual therapy heading in this chapter, from pages 79–90.

Do not abandon alternative self-help if the first approach you select does not improve the situation. It does not necessarily mean that alternative medicine is not effective or appropriate for you, since you may simply need to modify the dosage or change to a more appropriate therapy. However, do not delay in seeking professional conventional or alternative medical advice if symptoms show signs of deterioration or intensification.

Differentiating between acute and chronic conditions

ACUTE CONDITIONS

An acute medical condition arises suddenly and lasts for a limited time. It may or may not be serious. The following acute problems are likely to respond to alternative self-help treatment:
- Bites
- Bruises
- Chickenpox
- Colds
- Colic
- A brief episode of constipation
- Coughs
- Croup
- Cuts and grazes
- Diarrhoea
- Earache
- Food poisoning
- Hangovers
- Heartburn
- Indigestion
- Influenza
- Measles
- Minor burns and scalds
- Mouth ulcers
- Mumps
- Muscle strain
- Nappy rash
- Nosebleeds
- Shingles
- Short-lived anticipatory anxiety
- Sore throats

- Sprains
- Stings
- Teething
- Travel sickness
- Whooping cough

CHRONIC CONDITIONS

A chronic medical condition is one that develops slowly, or lasts for a long time, or recurs periodically. It may or may not be serious. The following chronic problems require alternative or conventional professional medical advice and treatment:

- Acne
- Anxiety
- Arthritis (osteo or rheumatoid)
- Asthma
- Cold sores
- Cystitis
- Depression
- Eczema
- Hay fever
- Hiatus hernia
- Hot flushes
- Insomnia
- Irritable bowel syndrome
- Migraines and tension headaches
- Osteoporosis
- Painful periods
- Post-natal depression
- Pre-menstrual syndrome
- Psoriasis
- Sciatica
- Sinusitis
- Thrush

The following conditions should receive swift, emergency medical treatment due to their potentially serious nature:

- Accidents involving injury to the head
- Childhood infectious illnesses that occur in babies under six months
- Collapse or breathing difficulties that are accompanied by blue-tinged lips, fingernails or fingertips
- Distressing or severe abdominal pains that last for more than an hour
- Inhalation of a foreign body
- Multiple fractures
- Rapidly advancing swelling around the face, lips, or throat (signs of anaphylactic shock)
- Second- or third-degree burns and scalds

- Severe bleeding
- Shock
- Sunstroke
- Suspected meningitis
- The sudden appearance of rashes
- Traces of blood in vomit or stools
- Unexplained drowsiness or confusion
- Vomiting and diarrhoea in babies or the elderly (because of the strong risk of dehydration)

When to consult a therapist

Throughout this book situations that require prompt conventional medical help have been clearly outlined. However, there are other situations needing alternative or complementary medical advice. These may include any of the following:

- Chronic conditions (see left-hand column for a list of problems that fall into this category). These are usually recurrent episodes of illness that tend not to clear up of their own accord, even if optimum conditions for recovery are present and a great deal of time goes by. Symptoms will often get progressively worse as the condition becomes more established. However, describing a problem as 'chronic' need not mean that symptoms are exceptionally severe, since an acute problem can sometimes give rise to more intense symptoms. On the other hand, acute illnesses tend to be characterized by a short lifespan and usually clear up of their own accord, provided optimum conditions are present for recovery.
- Acute conditions that begin to recur frequently or show signs of increasing in intensity or severity also require help from a trained practitioner, since this suggests that the self-help prescriber is getting out of his depth.
- Acute conditions that initially respond to home prescribing but cease to continue improving, show signs of gradually getting worse or changing symptoms.
- It is important to remember that most alternative medicines are not intended to be taken over an extended period. If you become dependent on an alternative medicine to keep symptoms at bay, it is best to consult an alternative practitioner to have the benefit of more deep-seated, extended treatment that is more likely to have a long-lasting effect.
- If you suffer any symptoms listed in the 'Seek professional help' sections in this book, obtain appropriate help without delay, since these are an indication that you may have a potentially serious

problem. Depending on your problem, you may need to go to the accident and emergency department of your local hospital, or call on the services of your family doctor. In less pressing circumstances, existing patients of an alternative therapist may choose to contact their practitioner instead.

Obtaining remedies

Herbal treatments can be bought as pre-mixed manufactured preparations or as single or mixed dried herbs. The manufactured medicines are usually combinations of various herbs, roots and barks and are available as tablets, capsules, mixtures, tinctures, ointments and creams and are available from health-food shops and high-street pharmacies. However, the dried herbs themselves are only available from specialist suppliers, as are Chinese or ayurvedic herbs or preparations.

The thirty-eight flower remedies are also available from many health-food shops and a few pharmacies, or direct from the manufacturers by mail order.

The needs of the newcomer who is self-prescribing homoeopathic, anthroposophical, biochemic or herbal medicines should be more than adequately met by using over-the-counter retail outlets such as health-food shops and high-street pharmacies. As homoeopathy, in particular, has grown in popularity and profile in the past decade, homoeopathic remedies have become widely available. Health-food shops and high-street pharmacies keep a wide range of homoeopathic remedies, often in both 6c and 30c (see page 87), while specialist homoeopathic pharmacies stock an excellent range of remedies in a wide variety of potencies from very low to the highest. A specialist pharmacy, where the staff can be an extremely helpful source of advice and guidance about home prescribing, is likely to be more appropriate for the experienced homoeopathic home prescriber or practitioner. This is also the case for the complete range of biochemic tissue salts.

Anthroposophical medicines however, are a different proposition. Although there is a selection of over-the-counter preparations available through most health-food shops and a number of high-street pharmacies, the majority of anthroposophical medicines are only available as pharmacy only or through a prescription from the doctor. This is because the complex nature of this system of medicine does not lend itself readily to self-diagnosis and self-prescription.

If you need to order a remedy from a homoeopathic pharmacy, it is usually because the potency falls outside the lower end of the spectrum or when a lesser-known remedy is required.

Using and storing medicines

Under each therapy heading in this chapter (pages 79–90) there are specific recommendations that should be observed in storing alternative medicines. Natural medicines appear to have an almost indefinite shelf-life when stored in optimum conditions, and there are certain rules that should be followed that apply to their storage. They include the following:

• Keep medicines in a cool, dust-free, well-ventilated space where they are unlikely to become contaminated by excess humidity or moisture. Extremes of temperature can also be a problem, so, if possible, keep them where the temperature is fairly stable.
• Dark glass jars are usually best for those preparations that may react adversely to sunlight, such as aromatherapy oils, fresh herbal remedies or homoeopathic medicines.
• Always keep caps of jars and bottles tightly closed in order to avoid the risk of evaporation.
• Some preparations may be adversely affected by strong aromatic odours, such as camphor, eucalyptus or peppermint, so it is important to keep them in as odour-free an environment as possible. For this reason it is best to keep essential oils and aromatic herbs separate from biochemic, anthroposophical and homoeopathic preparations.
• It is generally better to use glass containers rather than plastic jars or bottles, since the latter can result in chemicals leaching from the container into the contents.
• If you want to keep a close track of the freshness

of your medicines, label each container carefully with the date of purchase.

• If medicines spill out of their containers, throw them away rather than attempting to put them back.

• Exposure to X-rays at airports may also interfere with the medicinal effectiveness of homoeopathic remedies. This problem may be avoided by requesting that remedies are examined by staff, rather than leaving them in bags or suitcases that pass through security scanners.

Putting together an alternative first-aid kit

A tremendous amount of flexibility is possible when choosing the contents of an alternative first-aid kit, since different approaches can be dictated by personal preference, family requirements and available budget.

Once you have obtained a basic range of alternative medicines it becomes very easy to decide what should be added to expand your repertoire of remedies. This is often the best way of setting about building up a practical alternative first-aid kit, since buying remedies becomes an organic process that expands naturally to meet your individual requirements. This approach avoids too great a financial outlay, and it also helps avoid making mistakes at the outset when remedies may be bought that are theoretically useful, but not needed in practice.

Basic first-aid supplies – such as the following – will be needed in addition to the alternative remedies suggested:

• Sterile absorbent gauze

• A pair of sharp scissors

• Sterile lint

• Bandages

• Waterproof self-adhesive plasters of varying sizes and shapes

• Arnica

• Tweezers

BEGINNER'S KIT

• Aloe vera (in gel form or fresh plant)
• Arnica (homoeopathic medicine)
• Arnica cream or ointment (herbal cream)
• Calendula cream or ointment (herbal cream)
• Calendula tincture (herbal tincture)
• Lavender (Lavendula angustifolia, essential oil)
• Rescue Remedy (flower remedy)
• Tea tree (Melaleuca alternifolia, essential oil)

ACCIDENT AND EMERGENCY KIT (PLUS SPORTS INJURY KIT)

• Apis (homoeopathic medicine)
• Balsamicum ointment (anthroposophical medicine)
• Bryonia (homoeopathic medicine)
• Calendula and hypericum tincture (herbal tincture)
• Cantharis (homoeopathic medicine)
• Carbo veg (homoeopathic medicine)
• Combudoron ointment and lotion (anthroposophical medicine)
• Eucalyptus globulus (essential oil) **NB** Not to be used on children under three years old
• Geranium (Pelargonium asperium, essential oil)
• Lavender (Lavendula angustifolia, essential oil)
• Ledum (homoeopathic medicine)
• Nervone (mineral tissue salts)
• Rescue Remedy (flower remedy)
• Rhus tox (homoeopathic medicine)
• Symphytum (homoeopathic medicine)
• Tea tree (Melaleuca alternifolia, essential oil)
• Urtica urens (homoeopathic medicine)
• Urtica urens tincture (herbal tincture)
• Zief (mineral tissue salts)

COMPREHENSIVE KIT

• Aconite (homoeopathic medicine)
• Aloe vera (in gel or plant form)
• Arnica (homoeopathic medicine)
• Arnica cream, ointment or tincture (herbal tincture)
• Arsenicum album (homoeopathic medicine)
• Belladonna (homoeopathic medicine)
• Bryonia (homoeopathic medicine)
• Calendula cream, ointment or tincture (herbal tincture)
• Chamomile (dried flower heads or herbal tea)
• Combudoron ointment and lotion (anthroposophical medicine)
• Comfrey ointment (herbal ointment)
• Echinacea tincture (herbal tincture)

- Eucalyptus globulus (essential oil) **NB** Not to be used for children under three years old
- Gelsemium (homoeopathic medicine)
- Hypericum cream, ointment or tincture (herbal tincture)
- Ignatia (homoeopathic medicine)
- Lavender (Lavendula angustifolia, essential oil)
- Nervone (mineral tissue salts)
- Nux vomica (homoeopathic medicine)
- Peppermint (dried or fresh herb)
- Pulsatilla (homoeopathic medicine)
- Rescue cream and drops (flower remedy)
- Slippery elm powder (herbal)
- Tea tree (Melaleuca alternifolia, essential oil)
- Witch hazel (herbal)
- Yarrow (dried or fresh herb)

PARENT AND BABY KIT

- Arnica (homoeopathic medicine)
- Calendula tincture and cream or ointment (herbal tincture and cream)
- Chamomile (Chamaemelum nobile, essential oil)
- Chamomilla (homoeopathic medicine)
- Colocynthis (homoeopathic medicine)
- Combination E (mineral tissue salt)
- Combination R (mineral tissue salt)
- Ferrum phos (homoeopathic medicine)
- Kreosotum (homoeopathic medicine)
- Lavender (Lavendula angustifolia, essential oil)
- Mag phos (homoeopathic medicine)
- Rescue Remedy cream and drops (flower remedy)
- Ravensar (Ravensara aromatica, essential oil)
- Rosewood (Aniba roseaodora, essential oil)
  NB Ointments may contain lanolin.

Guidelines to consumers: how to find a qualified practitioner

In many ways, the best way of finding an alternative practitioner is by word of mouth, since an enthusiastic recommendation from a friend, colleague or family member whose opinion you trust may be of much more help than information about the qualifications of the therapist in question alone. The positive verbal recommendation also means you can ask straightforward questions of the existing patient such as: How are consultations conducted? What is expected of the patient? What is the average fee? What is the professional manner of the therapist like?

When you have contacted the therapist, questions you might like to ask in an initial conversation before or during the consultation may include any of the following:
- How long have you been in practice?
- Where did you train, and for how long?
- Are you registered with a professional body that has an established code of conduct, code of ethics and complaints procedure?
- If you are registered with a professional body, are you covered by a professional indemnity insurance policy?
- How experienced are you in treating patients who suffer from a similar condition to mine?
- On what basis are fees charged, and how long is treatment likely to be needed for?
- Are you happy to advise over the telephone for any acute problems that may occur during the course of my treatment? Is there an extra charge for this service?
- Are you happy to work alongside any conventional medication that is being given at the time of the consultation?
- What is your view of conventional treatment?
- Would you be happy to communicate with my family doctor if necessary?

If you cannot get a personal recommendation, the next best step is to obtain a list of registered practitioners in your area, if possible. They should have been trained to a level acceptable to an established professional body in order to be included on the register. It is quite appropriate to ask each professional organization how long it has been established, the requirements and qualification it demands of the therapists included on the register, and if it adheres to a code of ethics and professional conduct. On pages 353–6 you will find a list of organizations that will help you find a practitioner in your area. In the absence of a register word of mouth can be very helpful.

Health-food shops can also provide helpful advice and guidance about local practitioners, and public libraries should list information about local training centres or colleges running courses in specific alternative therapies. College staff can be especially helpful in providing lists of trained practitioners in your area and may also have important links with other therapists in different, but related alternative therapies.

Once you have located a practitioner, you may want to speak briefly on the telephone to ask some of the questions mentioned above. Most practitioners will be happy to have a short conversation with prospective patients, although others may use their receptionists to deal with patients' enquiries. You can also ask if it is possible to visit his or her consulting rooms in advance. This should not usually be necessary, but it can be helpful to visit clinics where acupuncture, shiatsu, massage or reflexology are being carried out to check that the rooms are comfortable and warm. This can also be an appropriate moment to check that standards of safety and hygiene are being met, for example, in the case of sterilization of acupuncture needles.

Aromatherapy oils

Aromatherapy is the use of essential oils to improve physical and emotional wellbeing through massage, baths and inhalations. It is especially effective in the treatment of stress-related problems and many chronic conditions.

The following guidelines should apply at all times:
• All essential oils must be mixed with a carrier oil before use.
• Always do a patch test for allergic reaction. A

good place is the inside forearm.
• Do not use essential oils on children under five without first consulting a qualified aromatherapist.
• Some essential oils affect the action of homoeopathic remedies – always check first.
• Always keep essential oils away from eyes and never put drops into the ears.
• Be especially careful when using a bath-oil blend of essential oils and carriers, as it will make the surface of the bath greasy.

Selecting and purchasing essential oils
It is important to buy the best quality oils available when putting together a basic aromatherapy kit. Look for oils that are 100 per cent pure essential oil rather than a product labelled as an 'aromatherapy oil' – the latter is already diluted in a carrier oil.

Flower oils are incredibly expensive, costing over £100 per one teaspoon of essence. However, any professional aromatherapist will mix up a blend containing a few drops of the precious oils in a carrier at a much more affordable price.

Storing essential oils
If aromatic essences are stored properly, they should remain in good condition for several years. However, once a bottle has been opened, its chances of degeneration increase due to the potential process of oxidation, which occurs when the essential oil comes into contact with oxygen, altering its original structure.

However, your essential oils will have the best chance of survival if the following tips are followed:
• Essential oils should always be stored in a cool, dark place, well away from the rays of direct sunlight.
• Always keep the cap or stopper firmly in place between use in order to avoid the extreme evaporation that can take place if oils are exposed to the air.
• Always keep your essential oils stored away from the reach of children.
• Avoid essential oils coming into contact with synthetic material such as rubber, as some oils can cause such substances to perish or dissolve. Highly polished or varnished surfaces can also be damaged by direct contact with aromatic essences.

Putting together a beginner's kit
Although the range of essential oils available may seem bewildering, it is best to start in a fairly restricted way to gain familiarity with the oils. It can

be helpful when choosing a basic selection to make sure you do not overlook the importance of following your own preferences and dislikes. This is very important, since a great deal of the pleasure of becoming familiar with aromatherapy is bound up with the sensuous pleasure of enjoying the aroma of the oils that you use.

However, it is also helpful to be aware that pure essential oils are unlikely to smell like any perfume you have come across before, due to their very concentrated, aromatic nature. As a result, be careful not to dismiss an essential oil at first sniff just because it is an unfamiliar smell. On the other hand, if it continues to smell uninviting it is probably best to concentrate on using other oils that smell much more attractive. Remember also that 'neat' aromatic essences do not tend to smell as attractive as diluted oils, and that an essential oil can take on a new personality when blended with other complementary aromatic essences.

Selecting essential oils for treatment

To establish the appropriate essential oils for treating an individual condition, turn to the 'Treatment guide' section dealing with the medical problem. Once the general advice has been consulted, turn to the section on aromatherapy oils which should be found under the heading 'Alternative treatments: Topical preparations'. Here you will find suggestions of essential oils that may be used to relieve the condition and their methods of external application.

Methods of application

Although many of us may associate aromatherapy treatments with having a scented massage, it is important to appreciate that this is a healing system that can have a much broader and more flexible application. Essential oils may be used in any of the following ways:

Inhalation

This is a simple way of enjoying the therapeutic benefits of aromatherapy and especially helpful in clearing the head and nasal passages and calming the mind. The most straightforward way to inhale your selected essential oil involves decanting two to three drops of oil onto a clean handkerchief and inhaling as often as needed. This method can be especially useful for clearing congested nasal passages during a heavy cold. Steam inhalations may also be useful in easing the discomfort of colds. Simply add two to four drops of essential oil to approximately 500ml (18fl oz) boiling water. Cover your head with a towel and gently inhale and exhale the fragrant steam. However, do not continue for more than five minutes, and avoid steam inhalations of any kind if you are asthmatic.

Scented baths

A very small amount of essential oil can be added to a warm bath to induce relaxation, ease muscular aches and pains, uplift the spirits or soothe sensitive skin. It is very important to add the essential oil *after* the taps have stopped running, otherwise a high proportion of the essential oil will evaporate before you have had a chance to soak in the water. Use between four and eight drops of oil, dispersing it well by agitating the bath water. Avoid bathing in very hot water since it can have an adverse effect on skin tone and result in a feeling of enervation. **NB** Never put essential oils in baths meant for babies or small children – infants have a habit of rubbing their eyes if splashed and there is a possibility of some essential oil getting into their eyes.

Aromatic compresses

Warm or cold compresses can be an extremely effective aid in easing muscular aching, swelling, inflammation or bruised tissue. When preparing a cold compress, add six drops of essential oil to a bowl containing 500ml (18fl oz) cold water. Agitate the water to disperse the oil and soak a clean piece of cloth or towelling in the liquid. Once it has been saturated, wring out well and place the damp cloth over the affected area. Secure in place and replace it with a fresh cool compress once it has begun to get warm. To make a warm compress follow the same instructions, using warm instead of cold water.

Warm compresses are most suitable for treating muscle aches and pains, the localized discomfort of cystitis, toothache, painful periods, pains that date from long-standing injury or boils and abscesses. Cool compresses, on the other hand, are more appropriate for soothing the pain of recent falls or injury, general swelling and inflammation, headaches, the inflammation of high temperature and the early phase of sprains and strains.

Vaporization

This is an exceptionally useful way of enjoying the

benefits of essential oils when direct contact between the oils and the skin (for example, in a massage blend or aromatic bath) is not appropriate. Vaporization is particularly good for pregnant women, babies and infants and anyone who has an extremely sensitive skin. An oil burner or vaporizer consists of a glass, porcelain or earthenware container that has space for a small candle to be placed inside. The small reservoir over the candle may be filled with water and a few drops of essential oil floated on the surface. As the flame gently warms the liquid, the water will evaporate, permeating the room with the scent of essential oil. Alternatively, an electric diffuser can be purchased, which has a filter or ceramic surface that can be kept at a consistent temperature for the burning of essential oils with, or without, the addition of water. Steam diffusers, on the other hand, utilize a cold-air pump that blows tiny amounts of essential oil into the atmosphere.

When using essential oils for massage it is vital to know that they should be diluted in a carrier or base oil before they are applied to the skin.

Creams and gels

Essential oils may be added to a bland, unperfumed cream base or gel base in order to create your own individual brand of salve to be used on unbroken skin to heal bruises, abrasions, minor burns, chilblains and bites and stings. Avoid open wounds – simply apply the salve around the edges of the wound. Up to twenty drops of essential oil may be added to every 30g (approximately 1oz) of cream/gel base. Place the cream or gel in a small, clean glass container and stir in the oils. Replace the lid firmly and store in cool, dark surroundings. If kept under favourable conditions the preparation should remain in good condition for up to six months.

By mouth

Essential oils should not be taken internally.

Undiluted applications of essential oils

Certain conditions can be treated by the application of one drop only of neat essential oil on a cotton bud and used as directed.

Suitable proportions for preparing a massage oil

Generally speaking, one drop of oil should be used for every teaspoon of carrier oil. For a facial massage no more than a couple of teaspoonfuls of blended massage oil may be needed, while a full body massage will use approximately six teaspoonfuls of massage oil.

The following are suitable as base oils for aromatic massage:
- **Sweet almond oil** (cold pressed)
Good for most skin types and suitable for body massage blends. Contains vitamins and minerals.
- **Apricot kernel**
Good for mature, sensitive and dry skins.
- **Avocado pulp** (refined)
Useful for treating mature skin. Contains protein, vitamins A and D, lecithin and essential fatty acids.
- **Hazelnut** (virgin cold pressed)
Suits oily or combination skins.
- **Jojoba** (natural)
Rich in vitamin E.
- **Peach kernel** (virgin cold pressed)
Contains useful levels of essential fatty acids and vitamin E.
- **Rosa rubiginosa**
Excellent for skin care, particularly on old and new scars.
- **Walnut** (virgin cold pressed)
High in unsaturated fatty acids.
- **Wheatgerm** (virgin cold pressed)
A rich source of vitamin E.

Other carriers include hydrolat, linalol, thujanol and gel base. Hydrolat (or flower water) is a by-product of the distillation process, and should not be confused with lavender water, which is a toiletry. The water-soluble molecules from the essential oil delicately fragrance the distillation water, so that there is a 'shadow' of the essential oil.

Safety first

Aromatic essences can have powerful therapeutic effects and need to be treated with a healthy mixture of respect and caution. By being aware of the rules of safety governing the use of essential oils we are more likely to feel confident and positive as we explore the practical and exhilarating art of aromatherapy.

Situations that require caution

Sensitive skin

Although it is comparatively rare for someone to develop a marked allergic reaction to an essential oil (unless they have an intolerance of a wide range of innocuous substances), sensitivity may develop if the same essential oil is used for too long. Those who are particularly at risk are likely to suffer from any of the following: sensitivity to house dust mite or animal fur or hair, hay fever, allergic rhinitis, asthma, eczema or overreactivity to certain foods such as wheat, sugar or dairy products made from cows' milk.

If a sensitivity exists, it may manifest itself as wheezing, swollen eyelids, itching skin or irritated eyes. If any doubt exists as to whether you may be sensitive to an essential oil, it is always worthwhile testing it initially on a small patch of skin before using it more liberally. *Never* use the oil 'neat', but take care to dilute it first in a carrier oil by adding one drop of essential oil to a teaspoon of bland base oil. Apply it to the areas of skin that are most likely to react if there is a problem, such as the inner part of the wrist, crook of the arm or behind the ears. Leave the oil undisturbed for at least twenty-four hours, checking to see if there are any signs of redness or irritation of the skin. If no reaction occurs, there is a good chance that the oil is fine to use. However, if you are still suspicious, try the test again to make sure before using the oil on a larger area.

For those who are especially concerned about an oversensitivity, skin-test base oils on their own to check they do not provoke an adverse reaction.

Sunlight and essential oils (phytosensitivity)

Some essential oils can lead to skin pigmentation if they are applied immediately before exposing the skin to sunlight or a sunbed. The following oils should always be avoided in this context: bergamot, angelica root, citrus oils such as grapefruit, lemon, lime, mandarin, orange and tagetes.

Essential oils in pregnancy and during breastfeeding

It is advisable to avoid the use of essential oils on the skin during pregnancy, although you can use favourite aromatic essences in a vaporizer or diffuser. Although essential oils should be avoided in massage blends during this time, there is no problem associated with using a carrier oil.

Because plant essences can be absorbed via the skin and lungs into the bloodstream, they can also travel into breast milk. As a result, the therapeutic qualities of aromatic oils may be transferred to a breastfeeding baby. Consequently, it is best to avoid

the use of strongly aromatic essences when breast-feeding, always making sure that any residue of essential oil has been removed from your skin before feeding begins.

Children and essential oils

The topical use of essential oils should also be avoided, or used only in extremely low concentrations, on babies and children under the age of three, or preferably, five years old. Simply use a carrier oil when massaging your baby, vaporizing essential oils to scent the air.

Flower remedies

Although a therapist familiar with the flower remedies may be more likely to have the necessary objectivity to choose a remedy appropriate for your mental and emotional state, it is also possible to use this form of medication within a self-help context. Rescue Remedy can be used for any situations that involve shock or trauma; otherwise select any of the flower remedies whose characteristics seem strikingly familiar. Remember that it is possible to make up a treatment bottle from more than one flower remedy, so that if more than one seems appropriate, this need not cause a problem.

Taking flower remedies

• Once the appropriate remedy or combination of remedies has been selected, a stock bottle of the relevant concentrate may be obtained from a health-food shop or pharmacy.

• Fill a sterilized 28g (1oz) dropper bottle with spring water, and add two drops of flower remedy. Add a teaspoon of brandy to the treatment bottle in order to preserve the solution if it is likely to be

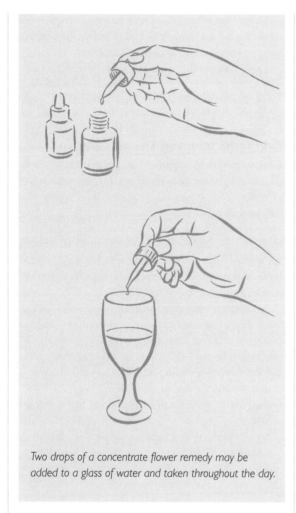

Two drops of a concentrate flower remedy may be added to a glass of water and taken throughout the day.

stored in a warm environment.
• Four drops should be taken in a small glass of water four times a day. The liquid should be held in the mouth for a moment or two before swallowing to achieve the maximum beneficial effect. Make sure that the cap is firmly replaced on the treatment bottle each time after opening.
• In severe situations, doses may be given more frequently (every hour or at half-hourly intervals) until symptoms improve.
• If making up a treatment bottle is inconvenient, two drops of concentrate may be added to a glass of water and sipped at intervals throughout the day.

Rescue Remedy
This combination formula is made up of the following flower remedies:
• Impatiens
• Clematis
• Rock rose
• Cherry plum
• Star of Bethlehem.

Rescue Remedy is especially valued for its calming and stabilizing effect on the mind and body during or after experiencing any form of shock or trauma. Rescue Remedy is available in liquid or cream form and may be used alone or in combination with any other flower remedies.

It also appears to play a useful role as an adjunctive treatment when receiving massage, chiropractic treatment or dental work. Rescue Remedy is non-toxic, non-addictive and free from any known side effects. It is not a substitute for essential emergency treatment in the event of a serious accident but there are substantial numbers of personal accounts suggesting that Rescue Remedy can help ease the panic, fear and severe mental stress that are likely to occur as a result of an accident, so it can be a useful tool in easing stress symptoms while waiting for emergency help to arrive.

Additional situations that might call for Rescue Remedy include bereavement, anticipatory anxiety, hysteria, job interviews and anxiety about public speaking.

How to use Rescue Remedy
Internally
• Add four drops of Rescue Remedy concentrate to a quarter of a glass of water.
• Sip at regular intervals for as long as it is necessary, holding the liquid for a second or two in the mouth before swallowing.
• If water is not readily to hand, take Rescue Remedy directly from the bottle, placing four drops under the tongue. Make sure that the glass dropper does not come into contact with the mouth, or you may risk bacterial contamination occurring in the concentrate.
• If the patient cannot swallow, or it is inadvisable to give anything by mouth, Rescue Remedy concentrate may be applied directly to the lips, wrists or behind the ears.
• Once signs of improvement appear, there is little need for repetition of the remedy unless and until symptoms recur, when the directions given above should be followed once again.
Externally
• Rescue Remedy cream may be applied to bruises,

cuts, grazes, scratches, sprains, minor burns, bites, haemorrhoids and any area of minor inflammation.
• Once you are sure the wound or affected area is clean, smooth the cream gently into the problem area, or apply to a sterile piece of clean gauze or lint, and bandage securely over the wound.
• Rescue Remedy cream may be applied as often as required, and may be continued for a while after superficial healing has taken place.
• If shock and trauma have occurred as a result of a minor injury, Rescue Remedy concentrate may be given by mouth as well as using the cream as a topical application. In this way, the emotional impact of an accident may be eased while the cream soothes the external wound.
• Rescue Remedy may also be given to animals and plants which show signs of stress or trauma. Add ten drops to a bucket of water for large animals, while the same dilution can be used in a watering can or spray for plants.

Biochemic tissue salts

The twelve single biochemic tissue salts are sold in the 6x potency (strength) and are numbered from one to twelve in alphabetical order by Latin name. In addition to the single tissue salts, combination formulas are also available, aimed at treating specific ailments. Once you have read about your ailment in the 'Treatment Guide' section of this book, and you find that more than one tissue salt is indicated, using a combination formula can be much more straightforward than taking a number of single tissue salts at one go.

There are eighteen combination formulas in total. Each container of tablets will be labelled with a letter from A to S and the conditions that may be treated by that specific combination. These formulas are prepared according to the same principles as the single tissue salts, and dosage instructions are identical.

Single and combination formulas of mineral tissue salts can be easily obtained from most health-food shops, high-street chemists, or homoeopathic pharmacies.

Taking biochemic tissue salts

Tablets should be dissolved in the mouth or under the tongue, rather than swallowed whole with a glass of water. This means the tablets make contact with the mucous membranes in the mouth, which encourages absorption into the bloodstream as quickly as possible. The tablets should not need to be chewed because of their soft, melting consistency, an especially important property when administering tissue salts to children.

In certain limited situations tissue salts can be made into a paste for external application. Crush ten to twenty tablets into a fine powder between two teaspoons, or sandwich them in a fold of clean paper and crush with a rolling pin. Add a small amount of boiled, cooled water to the fine powder to make a smooth paste, which can be applied to bites, wounds or stings.

Small children and babies may need to take their tissue salts in liquid form. This can be easily done by crushing the appropriate tissue salt as suggested above and dissolving it in water or a bottled feed.

Dosage

There is no hard and fast rule that must be followed routinely when using biochemic tissue salts. The most important principle is the need to match the optimum dosage to the severity of the symptoms experienced. In other words, frequency and size of dosage should be increased for abrupt, severe symptoms, while conditions that build slowly, or remain at a low level of intensity may require less frequent repetition over a longer period of time.

An average example of dosage for an adult is four tablets three times a day until the situation shows signs of improvement, when tablets should be gradually phased out. On the other hand, very severe symptoms would require an increased dosage of four tablets taken at hourly intervals until improvement of the condition sets in.

Once the condition shows definite signs of easing,

the dosage may be reduced to three tablets taken three times a day, or four tablets taken twice a day. Once symptoms have cleared, the appropriate tissue salt should be taken for an extra two or three days in reduced dosage in order to guard against a return of symptoms as the body adjusts to the tissue salt being withdrawn.

For long-standing conditions of insidious development, it may be necessary to pace dosage at a different level. A well-established, low-grade problem may respond best to a regime of low dosage that is continued for a few weeks. This allows for an increase in the dosage if symptoms begin to escalate.

A mild or low-grade condition may respond best to two tablets taken twice a day to keep symptoms at bay. If symptoms intensify the dosage may be increased to three or five times a day, and reduced again as soon as signs of improvement become apparent.

Biochemic tissue salts are believed to be free of side effects, and overdosing is thought to be impossible. However, it is always important to bear in mind that for the maximum benefit to be obtained, it is important to find the optimum dosage for each individual. This makes complete sense if we consider the fact that each of us has a unique metabolism and that we are likely to experience illness in our own individual way.

Since there are no recorded side effects, biochemic tissue salts are regarded as being safe to take in pregnancy. However, if you feel uneasy about using any form of medication in pregnancy, avoid the use of tissue salts in the first trimester.

Dosage for babies and children is also straightforward. One tablet crushed and included with a feed six times a day is suitable for babies, while toddlers should have two or three tablets three times a day. Nursery-age children may be given four tablets three times a day, while children over six years of age may require five tablets three times a day. These are flexible guidelines for dosage, so remember that the frequency of dosage in children should be matched to the severity of the condition experienced.

Storage

Although biochemic tissue salts have a relatively long shelf-life, the container of tablets should not be kept for more than three years once opened. They should be stored in dry conditions out of direct sunlight.

Homoeopathic remedies

While homoeopathic remedies can be used very successfully at home, they are not suitable in all situations. The conditions that respond best to homoeopathic self-help are acute conditions (see 'Differentiating between chronic and acute conditions', pages 74–76), such as colds, food poisoning, cuts and bruises, and immediate symptoms of emotional distress following bad news or shock. Chronic conditions are not suitable for self-help because they arise from a fundamental weakness in the system, which is best identified and treated by a trained practitioner.

For the most successful results the home prescriber should have a clear idea of the information needed from the patient at the outset, so avoiding a host of prescribing pitfalls and confusion at a later stage.

Getting essential information from the patient

• It is extremely helpful to identify any factors that may have made the patient more vulnerable to the onset of illness. These potential triggers can be very wide-ranging and may include anything from being exposed to a severe chill to suffering an emotional trauma. These may be tolerated perfectly well at other times, but if they occur when someone is at a low personal or physical ebb they can be the trigger that tilts the balance towards a state of ill health.

• Write down the primary symptoms of illness, bearing in mind that you are interested in any emotional and physical changes that have occurred since the onset of ill health. For instance, if the patient normally has a flushed complexion or if they are irritable as a rule, these are not relevant symptoms when prescribing for an acute illness. On the other hand, if the patient looks unusually pale, or has become uncharacteristically tearful and emotional since feeling unwell, these are important symptoms. Do not neglect the exploration of any emotional changes that have developed since illness began.

• When there are strong leading symptoms such as nausea, pain or feverishness, detailed questions should be asked of the patient. For example, if a headache is the main problem, ask what sort of pain it is, and what gives relief or makes it feel more intense.

• Once as much information as possible has been obtained about the main problem, ask further questions about any other changes. Simple questions might include the following: Are the eyes sensitive to light or has there been any nausea since illness began? Ask questions that seem relevant, always keeping at the forefront of your mind that you are trying to pick up any changes that have occurred as a result of the illness.

• Make sure that you also do not overlook asking general questions about sensations that affect the whole system. In other words, has the patient become more chilly, heated, restless, or lethargic since illness began? At this point explore factors that are responsible for making the patient feel a sense of relief from or aggravation of symptoms. These can be extremely broad in nature and may include cool air, movement, rest, heat, eating or company.

Selecting the appropriate remedy

• Consider the information you have obtained from the patient, initially trying to identify the trigger or strong contributing factor that encouraged illness to develop. This could be anything from stress or trauma, working too hard for too long or becoming extremely cold or damp.

• Organize the rest of the symptoms you have, listing them in order of importance or intensity. You could underline the most intense or marked symptoms with three lines, those that are less characteristic or milder in nature with two lines, and those that are much less intense but still present with one line. These may be regarded as 'General features'.

• Make a special note of any symptoms that fall into the category of strange, rare or peculiar features. These are symptoms that may have contradictory qualities, such as nausea that is relieved by eating or dry mouth with lack of thirst. Symptoms such as these are of particular importance, since they can

often be the clinching factor in deciding which remedy is most appropriate.

• In addition, highlight the factors that make the patient feel better or worse, remembering that these must be influences that make a general difference to the patient, as well as being factors that make a difference to specific symptoms. For example, head pains may be eased by contact with fresh, cool air while the patient may generally be more comfortable for being kept warm. This information may be placed under headings of 'Better from' and 'Worse for'.

The remedy tables

• When using the relevant table in this book, try to match the information included on your own list under the heading of 'General features' with the information listed in the matching column in the book. There need not be a complete match between these two, provided that the most striking or characteristic symptoms (those that have been underlined twice or three times) are mentioned. In other words, the most severe or marked symptoms of the condition must match with the central information in this column.

• Once you are satisfied that there is a comfortable match between the characteristic symptoms of illness and the information listed in the first two columns of the remedy table, check with the information included in the 'Worse' and 'Better' columns to establish that these broadly match the information gathered from the patient. If there is a general correspondence between the information listed under these column headings and the symptoms elicited from the patient, there is a very good chance that the remedy mentioned in the 'Remedy name' column will be the most appropriate for the patient.

• The tables in the book do not have to be used in a rigid or regimented way, but can be employed to creative advantage. If we take the example of someone suffering the miseries of cold symptoms and a cough, or experiencing vomiting and diarrhoea that occur simultaneously, it is possible to amalgamate the information given in more than one table to establish whether one remedy embraces the leading features of both conditions.

• Once you are familiar with using the remedy tables, it will become apparent that a number of homoeopathic remedies appear frequently under different headings. For instance, Belladonna can be appropriately used in treating a wide range of possible conditions that include the following: fever, earache, sore throats, chickenpox, cystitis and sunburn, while Arsenicum album may be helpful in cases of anxiety, vomiting, diarrhoea, flu, coughs, colds, insomnia, heartburn and indigestion.

Choosing the appropriate strength (potency) of remedy

Homoeopathic remedies are available in three strengths, 6c, 12c and 30c: 'c' stands for centessimal dilution – in other words, one drop of the remedy has been diluted in ninety-nine drops of water and alcohol. High-street pharmacies and health-food shops sell 6c potency remedies, and, often, 30c. You will need to order a 12c from a homoeopathic pharmacy, where the staff are often extremely helpful in giving advice and guidance about home prescribing.

Low-potency remedies are most suitable for slow-developing, low-grade symptoms of illness, and should be administered twice or three times a day until symptoms improve. Rapidly developing symptoms need a higher-potency remedy, repeated more frequently – for example, every thirty or forty minutes – at the outset and less frequently as the patient improves.

If you think that symptoms are severe enough to need a high-potency remedy, but you can only buy a 6c, do not worry – just use the 6c more frequently.

Administering the appropriate remedy

• Once you have selected your remedy, tip a single dose (one tablet) onto the cap of the remedy bottle or a clean teaspoon and transfer it swiftly into the mouth. This precaution is important since it allows for minimum contact with the tablets, helping to avoid the possibility of contamination.

• Do not swallow tablets whole with water, but chew or suck them. This allows them to be rapidly absorbed by the mucous membranes of the mouth. Do not take homoeopathic remedies when there are any strong flavours in the mouth that may interfere with the medicinal action of the remedy. These include strong tea, coffee, mints (including spearmint or peppermint sweets or chewing gums), eucalyptus or strongly-flavoured mouthwashes. Additional substances that might interfere with the effectiveness of homoeopathic remedies include some aromatic oils such as Olbas Oil, inhalations, and some essential oils

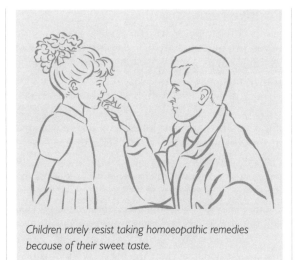

Children rarely resist taking homoeopathic remedies because of their sweet taste.

such as rosemary, lavender or eucalyptus.

• If too many granules or tablets are accidentally spilt out of the remedy bottle, they should be thrown away rather than replaced since they may have become contaminated. As a result, their medicinal potential may have become compromised.

Children and babies

• Granules or powders are better for small children or babies rather than tablets. Although not readily available from retail outlets, these can be easily obtained from a homoeopathic pharmacy by mail order (see page 358).

• If you don't have powders or granules, you can crush tablets into a fine powder to give to a baby. Put a tablet onto a clean teaspoon and crush it by pressing hard with the back of another teaspoon, or place a tablet in a fold of clean paper and grind it using a heavy object such as a rolling pin.

• Put a pinch of granules or powder inside your child's cheek, or rub it along the area where the gums join the cheek.

Assessing the response

After giving the first dose, wait for roughly half an hour, taking note of any changes that are visible in the patient's condition. These changes might include any of the following:

• Reduction in discomfort or pain
• Lessening of feverishness
• Increased or renewed appetite
• Lifting of restlessness, anxiety, despondency and general distress
• Improved energy levels and sense of well-being

Positive responses

• A positive response may simply be a general sense of improvement or relief, despite the fact that specific symptoms are present. For instance, a patient may experience a sense of improved energy, vitality or well-being after taking a well-chosen remedy, even though their symptoms of stomach upset, headache or cough have not yet shown signs of improvement. When this occurs, the degree of distress associated with the symptoms may lift before the symptoms themselves are reduced and disappear. It is important to let this development continue under its own steam, so do not give an additional dose of the remedy unless and until a setback occurs. Again, this relapse could either involve a reappearance of the initial symptoms or a reduction in the sense of well-being or vitality.

Negative responses

• In treating acute or severe symptoms, it may be necessary to repeat the dose of your selected remedy if there has been no substantial improvement within the first half hour. This is especially worthwhile if you are convinced that your choice of remedy is correct, or if there has been a brief improvement that has ceased.
• If there is no improvement after repeating a remedy three times (every half or three quarters of an hour in rapidly developing or severe symptoms), return to the relevant remedy table in case you need to make a more suitable choice.
• Stop the patient taking the remedy if symptoms become more intense after a few doses. This means that the patient's system has become overstimulated. This reaction is easy to spot, in contrast to a situation in which a general deterioration of the original condition occurs. If the patient has become overstimulated, the intensification of symptoms should be rapidly followed by a steady improvement once the remedy has been stopped and the body as a whole is given the chance to regain its equilibrium. In most cases, this problem can be avoided by never repeating a homoeopathic remedy routinely once an improvement is under way.
• If a well-selected remedy has initially had a positive effect, but the symptoms change their nature or focus, reconsult the remedy table. For example, once a remedy has been given, an initially dry, irritating cough may turn into a loose, productive one, or a clear, burning, scanty nasal discharge may become thick, bland and yellowish-green in appearance. If this occurs, it is extremely important that the newly emerging symptoms should be matched by a change of remedy.
• When there is an initial improvement in response to a few doses of a low-potency remedy (such as a 6c), but a relapse occurs, giving a higher potency should be the next step (such as a 12c or 30c). On the other hand, always remember that high potencies have a more powerful action and should not require as frequent repetition as low-potency remedies.

How to store homoeopathic remedies

Generally speaking, provided they are kept in optimum conditions, homoeopathic remedies appear to have an almost indefinite shelf-life. To maintain optimum conditions follow these guidelines:
• Bright sunlight may damage homoeopathic remedies, so it is best to store them in a dark place.
• Continued exposure to air may also cause problems, so make sure you replace the tops of remedy bottles securely after use.
• Contact with extreme heat or cold can be problematic, so remedies are best kept in stable, moderate temperatures.
• Exposure to X-rays at airports may interfere with the medicinal effectiveness of homoeopathic remedies, so ask for remedies to be examined by staff, rather than leaving them in luggage that passes through security scanners.
• Aromatic substances such as Olbas Oil, some essential oils, inhalants or camphorated products can also damage homoeopathic remedies.

Herbal remedies

Herbal preparations

Herbal remedies can be prepared in any of the following ways for use at home.

Poultices and compresses

These are used as external treatments to ease pain, inflammation or stiffness. To make a herbal compress soak a clean piece of soft cloth in a warm or comfortably hot decoction (see below). Wring it out slightly until it is comfortably moist, and apply it as

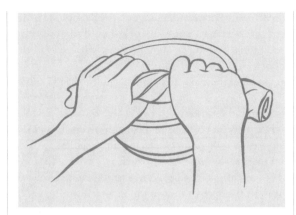

warm as possible to the problem area. Once it begins to cool, replace it with a fresh, warm compress.

Poultices may be made by mixing the required herbs to a warm paste by adding hot water or cider vinegar. Wrap the hot mixture in a clean piece of soft cloth or gauze and apply to the affected area. As with the hot compress, always reapply a fresh hot poultice once the original one has cooled down.

Decoctions

Decoctions make the active ingredients of hard or woody herbs soluble and readily assimilated. Decoctions may be made from roots, bark, nuts or wood that should be ground down, cut or chopped into small pieces. Measure the appropriate amount of herb into an enamel pan and add cold water, bring to the boil, cover and simmer for ten to fifteen minutes. Strain and use while hot.

Tinctures

Tinctures must be used in small amounts because of their concentrated nature. The proportion of herb to liquid should be one to five (i.e. 100g (3½oz) of herb to 500ml (18fl oz) of liquid). Once the herbs have been selected, measure the appropriate amount into a dark-glass, securely stoppered jar or bottle and cover them with alcohol (a spirit such as vodka is most suitable for this purpose). The mixture should be kept securely covered in a warm, dark place and shaken thoroughly twice a day. After a couple of weeks, strain the tincture through muslin, squeezing well to obtain as much of the liquid as possible. Store the strained liquid in tightly closed, clean, dark-glass bottles. If you do not want to use alcohol, or if it is not available, cider vinegar can be used. Tinctures may be used to make compresses, added to base

creams and ointments, taken diluted in water or teas as a medicinal treatment, or applied to wounds, minor burns or grazes as a healing agent.

Infusions

You can make an infusion from plants that are plentiful in aromatic oils or from leaves or petals of flowers. When preparing an infusion add the measured amounts of herbs to a warmed teapot (ideally made from porcelain or glass) and add boiling water. Keep covered for roughly ten to fifteen minutes, and strain before drinking warm. Remember when using dried herbs that smaller quantities need to be used than

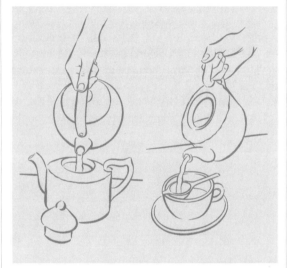

when using the same herbs in a fresh form (one part of a dried herb is roughly equivalent to three parts of the same fresh herb).

Gathering, preparing and storing fresh herbs

• It is important to gather plants at the optimum time to enjoy their maximum medicinal potential. Ideally, leaves are best gathered when flowers are in bud and leaves are green and fresh.

• Flowers should be gathered at the same time of day as leaves (ideally early in the day), soon after they fully open. Any foreign bodies or insects should be carefully removed from flower heads before they are used.

• Roots are best gathered as the growing season draws to an end, which ensures that they will provide their maximum nutritional content. Discard any damaged specimens, and wash the remainder thoroughly in cold water to remove residual dirt and soil.

• Herbs should be dried as soon as possible after gathering in order to avoid loss of essential oils or bleaching of the leaves. Pick out any foreign bodies and damaged or discoloured leaves. Remove flower heads and chop roots or bark into small pieces about 2.5cm (1in) thick.

• The ideal place for drying large quantities of herbs in bunches is a warm spare room or shed. Smaller quantities can be dried in an airing cupboard (provided it has reasonable circulation of air) or cool oven. Small quantities of herbs may be dried by spreading them on trays and turning them at regular intervals.

• When drying herbs, steady, slow heat tends to produce the most favourable results. The room should be warmed to a stable temperature (32–34°C/90–93°F) before the herbs are brought in. After two or three days reduce the temperature to 25–27°C (77–81°F) to conclude the process.

• As a general rule, herbs take an average of five to seven days to dry. When leaves are ready they should break easily between the fingers, petals should rustle but not fall apart, roots or bark should snap readily, and stems and stalks should break with very little effort.

• Once herbs have been successfully dried, some may be stored whole (such as tarragon, thyme, marjoram, chamomile flowers or mullein), while others may be reduced to a rough powder by crushing with a rolling pin or placing in a grinder.

• Once herbs have been dried and reduced, store them in dark, airtight glass jars as soon as possible to prevent the herbs absorbing moisture from the air. If clear glass is used, make sure that the herbs are stored in a dark, cool place so that there is less chance of their essential oils being damaged by contact with sunlight. Avoid plastic containers at all costs because they may cause herbs to 'sweat'; instead use earthenware pots or airtight wooden boxes.

• Once the herbs are ready for storage, label each jar or box straight away with the date and name of the herb to avoid confusion later on.

FIRST AID

This section gives complementary health advice only for common, minor accidents and emergencies. Since the main focus of this book is on natural medicine, it was decided that it was not appropriate to include orthodox first aid measures such as cardiopulmonary resuscitation and the recovery position, or the treatment of major accidents such as fractures or deep cuts and burns. Such emergencies are best treated by summoning professional help and consulting a standard first aid reference text.

Bites and stings

Bites and stings are likely to come from any of the following sources:

Bites
• Fleas
• Animals such as cats or dogs
• Snakes
• Spiders
• Midges
• Mosquitoes

Stings
• Wasps or bees
• Hornets
• Jellyfish
• Nettles
• Scorpions

Common symptoms that occur as a result of a bite or sting include the following:
• Redness, heat, and inflammation of the area immediately surrounding the sting or bite.
• Itching, stinging or burning of the affected area.
• Swelling or puffiness of the skin.
  Depending on the severity of the reaction, the above symptoms can range from mild irritation and discomfort, to very distressing itching and swelling.

Practical self-help
• See general first aid suggestions for cuts and grazes (pages 99-100).
• Clean and bathe the affected area with a soothing, antiseptic lotion or diluted tincture (details are given in the table on page 93).
• If a sting has been left behind, as in the case of a bee sting, scrape it gently until it comes out, ensuring that it is not pushed further in, and the venom sac is not ruptured.

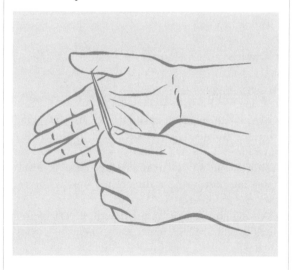

• If cool bathing with a diluted tincture is soothing, continue to do this as often as is needed, until the discomfort has eased.
• Try not to scratch, as this will release histamine and increase irritation.

Preventative measures
• Use a natural insect repellent, such as garlic. Although the idea of using copious quantities of garlic oil on the skin is unacceptable to most people, eating garlic regularly and in plentiful quan-

tities is often enough to keep insects at bay. Fresh elder leaves rubbed on the skin produce a similar effect.

• If you have a history of attracting midges or mosquitoes, make sure you wear light clothing at night that covers your arms and legs. In order to remain as cool as possible, ensure that these items of clothing are made from natural fibres such as linen or cotton.

• Avoid wearing scented toiletries out of doors.

• Try to keep calm if you come in contact with a bee or wasp. They are not aggressive by nature, and are more likely to sting if they meet with a panicked response.

SEEK PROFESSIONAL HELP

If the person who has been stung has a history of a severe allergic response to wasp or bee stings (see anaphylactic shock, below). They may be wearing a Medic Alert necklace or bracelet carrying this information, in case they become unconscious. Additional symptoms of anaphylactic shock may include:
• Shallow, rapid pulse
• Pallor
• Clammy skin
• Faintness

Arrange for emergency medical treatment if:
• A dog bite has been sustained.
• Signs of redness or inflammation are extending from the wounded area, especially if the possibility of tetanus is suspected. Symptoms of tetanus include rapidly advancing rigidity of the affected area, developing into distressing spasms of the muscles of the back and abdomen.
• A sting has occurred in the mouth, especially in a small child. While emergency help is being obtained, give ice cubes to the patient to suck.
• A poisonous bite has been sustained from a snake, scorpion or spider. Some people may experience a very severe reaction to poison ivy, or a sting from some jellyfish occurring in tropical waters.

ANAPHYLACTIC SHOCK

Anaphylactic shock is a very severe allergic reaction that can be caused by insect stings, certain foods (e.g. peanuts, seafood) and some drugs, such as penicillin. Symptoms include:
• Swelling of the lips, throat and face
• Wheezing and shortness of breath
• A sudden rash
• Abdominal pain, vomiting or diarrhoea
• Lowered blood pressure, dizziness, unconsciousness

Anyone suffering from anaphylactic shock needs *immediate* medical attention, which will include oxygen and an injection of adrenalin, otherwise they may die. Your priority is to call for emergency medical treatment.

It is worth noting that with bites and stings, it is perfectly appropriate to take the relevant remedy internally, while also applying a topical preparation to the skin.

Topical preparations

These are lotions, tinctures or creams that are applied to the skin to soothe and heal. Choose from any of the following, but bear in mind that none of the substances mentioned for application to the skin should be taken by mouth.

Anthroposophical medicines

• Combudoron lotion or ointment may be applied to insect bites or wasp stings. Always dilute the lotion (one part tincture to ten parts of boiled, cooled water) before applying to the affected area. Those with sensitive or reactive skins should note that the ointment contains lanolin.

Aromatherapy oils

• After a bite or sting, apply a drop of lavender oil to the affected area every hour until irritation eases.

• After a bite or sting, wash with lavender hydrosol and apply a drop of lavender oil on a cotton bud to the affected area three times during the day of the bite.

Herbal preparations

• For stinging, inflamed, itchy bites, use diluted Urtica urens tincture. Dilute one part of tincture to ten parts of boiled, cooled water, and apply to the affected area as often as needed.

• After a bee sting has been removed, bathe the wound in diluted Hypericum and Calendula tincture, apply calendula cream or ointment to speed up the healing process and cover with a clean dressing.

• Diluted feverfew tincture may be used as an insect repellent.

Home remedies

• For a bee sting, apply a mixture of bicarbonate of soda and water to the inflamed area once the sting

has been carefully removed. Parsley juice or honey may also ease irritation of the skin.
• For wasp stings or flea bites, a solution of vinegar or lemon juice and water may be applied to the skin.
• Irritation and distress caused by nettle stings can be eased by rubbing dock leaves or plantain on the affected area.

Medicines intended for internal use

These ease pain, reduce inflammation and encourage a speedy resolution of the problem.

Biochemic tissue salts

Stings from insects may be treated with tissue salt No. 9. If symptoms are severe, tablets may be taken hourly until relief is obtained.

HOMOEOPATHIC MEDICINES

Type	General features	Worse	Better	Remedy
Bee or wasp stings that are puffy, pink and raised	Affected area looks very swollen and waterlogged. Pains are stinging, burning, and extremely sensitive to warmth. Apis is useful for hives that follow being stung by a bee or wasp	Heat in any form, e.g. overheated rooms, warm compresses or bathing Touch	Cool applications to the painful area	Apis
Bites and stings of any variety that feel cold to the touch	Although the affected area feels cool, it is much relieved by contact with cool air, bathing or compresses. The site of the sting or bite looks very red and swollen. Pains are pricking and stinging	Warmth	Cool air, bathing or cold compresses to the painful area	Ledum
Bee stings with extreme burning around the site of the sting	Pains are stitch-like, burning and itchy. Unlike apis and ledum, stings that require Urtica urens are made worse by contact with cool air or water. Urtica urens is useful for itching and hives that follow a bee sting	Touch Contact with water Cool air		Urtica urens
Midge bites that are extremely itchy and sensitive	Pains from bites are stinging and sharp, causing extreme mental and physical irritability. The least touch is resented because of the discomfort it provokes. Staphysagria is very helpful as an insect repellent for those who are habitually bitten by midges	Least contact	Warmth Initial scratching	Staphysagria
Shock following a bite or sting	Restlessness, fearfulness and panic. Over-sensitivity to pain with a terror of being touched. Affected area is swollen, and burning to the touch	Being approached Warm surroundings Open air	Resting	Aconite

Blisters

A blister forms when the skin is damaged by heat or friction, or in response to an allergic reaction. Some infections such as shingles, impetigo, cold sores or chickenpox can also result in the production of blisters. These pockets of watery fluid give a chance for new skin to grow underneath, while the liquid in the blister is gradually absorbed. Once this has occurred, the top layer of skin gradually dries until it becomes naturally detached.

It is very important to avoid pricking a blister or removing its top layer of skin, since the fluid forms a protective covering that discourages infection setting in. If the covering of a blister is removed prematurely, the skin may be left feeling sore and raw, and open to the risk of infection.

Blisters that are likely to be subject to friction may be protected by a sterile, padded adhesive dressing. On the other hand, a blister that has accidentally or spontaneously burst may be left uncovered, provided there is no risk of infection or friction from rubbing.

Practical self-help
See the burns and scalds section (pages 96-98).

Alternative treatments
Treat as for burns and scalds (pages 96-98).

Bruises

Bruises usually occur as the result of a traumatic incident such as a fall or accident, or they can be caused by a blow. The severity of these injuries can vary enormously: some cause little distress or pain, while the victim of a serious accident may require hospital treatment in order to deal with internal bruising, or damage to the head, spine or vital organs.

A bruise occurs when blood seeps into the tissues beneath the skin. The characteristic appearance of a bruise is initially purple, changing to a greenish shade as the bruise gradually disappears. The surface of the skin is tender to touch in the early stages of bruising, becoming less painful as the bruise fades away.

Practical self-help
• Apply cold compresses or ice packs to the bruised area at ten-minute intervals. This will alleviate swelling and pain. Do not use ice-cold compresses if the surface of the skin has been broken.

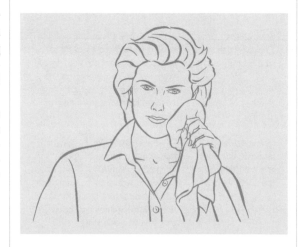

• If a limb has been badly bruised, move it as much as possible. In the case of a bruised leg, resting while keeping the limb raised on pillows above heart level.

HOMOEOPATHIC MEDICINES

Type	General features	Worse	Better	Remedy
Any bruise sustained as a result of accident or injury	Arnica is the first remedy to give after a fall or accident. It is strongly recommended for the emotional and physical shock that follows injury. Arnica also eases pain and promotes rapid healing of bruises by encouraging speedy re-absorption of blood	Touch Being approached Movement Effort	Lying with the head lower than the body	Arnica montana
Black eyes that are soothed by cool bathing	Injured area feels cold and numb. Bruised tissue is extremely sensitive and very swollen. Pains are stabbing or tearing	Warmth Movement	Cool bathing Exposure to cool air Resting	Ledum
Bruised shin bones or any other area with a very thin covering of skin	Ruta is recommended for deep bruising that has damaged the periosteum (the membranous sheath that covers bones). This can result in pains that persist long after surface bruising has healed	Resting Lying on the painful area Walking out of doors Touch	Warmth Moving about indoors	Ruta
Deep bruising of tissues	Bellis perennis is recommended for the bruising and after-effects of a heavy blow that damages deep-seated tissue, e.g. a fall or blow to the breasts. The deep bruising that follows surgery may also call for this remedy	Hot bathing Touch	Cold locally applied Movement	Bellis perennis
Injury or bruising to the eyeball	Symphytum may be needed after a blow to the eyeball from a blunt object, e.g. a tennis ball. To be considered if Arnica has helped with initial swelling around site of injury, but pain persists	Touch		Symphytum

specialist will need to check the retina for damage.

Alternative treatments

It is worth noting that when bruising occurs, it is perfectly appropriate to take the relevant remedy internally, while also applying a topical preparation to the skin.

Topical preparations

These are lotions, tinctures or creams that can be applied to the skin to soothe and heal. None of the preparations listed should be taken by mouth.

Aromatherapy oils

Wash the area with helichrysum hydrosol and seek professional advice: ask for a blend with helichrysum in a gel base.

Herbal preparations

• Arnica may be applied to the bruised area in the form of lotion, massage balm or ointment. Arnica is extremely effective at soothing painful, sensitive,

bruised skin. The lotion may be applied to the bruised area on a compress, or a tablespoonful can be added to a warm bath if there is generalized aching or soreness. However, never apply Arnica to any area where the skin is broken; instead choose Calendula or Hypericum skin preparations, which are more suited to application on grazed or cut skin.
• Comfrey ointment may be applied to bruised, painful skin to ease discomfort.
• Mullein oil may be applied gently to bruised tissue in order to soothe the sensitive area.

Flower remedies
Rescue Remedy cream may be applied to the bruised area.

Home remedies
• Applying poultices to the injured area can be an effective and soothing way of healing bruised tissue. A simple one may be made from marigold petals sandwiched between two layers of gauze, and applied, warmed, to the bruised skin. This is especially soothing if bruising has occurred where there is little skin covering the area, e.g. bruised shins or black eyes.
• Another easy (but rather sticky) poultice may be made from a teaspoonful of dried marjoram, a little vinegar and enough honey to turn the mixture into a thick paste. Alternatively, rolled oats will make a soothing poultice when boiled with water into a thick paste and applied (cooled) onto a cloth, before bandaging in place over the bruise.
• Witch hazel is a soothing and cooling liquid when applied to inflamed or bruised skin. However, take care that its action is not too astringent for sensitive skins.
• Onion juice (rub an onion cut in half on a bruise), lavender or thyme vinegar may speed up the healing of bruises when applied to tender skin.

Medicines intended for internal use
These are used to ease pain, reduce inflammation and encourage a speedy resolution of the problem.
Anthroposophical medicines
Arnica montana tablets may be taken for generalized symptoms of shock and trauma following physical injury. It is also specifically helpful in promoting re-absorption of blood from bruised tissues.
Flower remedies
Rescue Remedy may be taken as often as required in order to help with the shock that accompanies an accident.

Burns and scalds

Burns and scalds frequently happen as the result of accidents at home, and children and the elderly are especially at risk. The range of severity can vary enormously from minor scalds and burns to extremely traumatic skin damage that requires specialized emergency medical treatment. Advice given here relates to minor burns only.

Burns can be caused by any of the following:
• Contact with kitchen equipment such as very hot oven shelves, doors or ceramic rings on the top of a cooker.
• Falling against central-heating radiators that are kept at too high a temperature.
• Over-exposure to strong, direct sunlight.
• Chemical burns from contact with corrosive chemicals.
• Electrical burns.

Scalds may happen as a result of:
• Contact with steam from a boiling kettle or saucepan that holds very hot liquid.
• Spilled hot drinks.
• Very hot bath water: children and the elderly are especially at risk.

The measures below relate only to first- and second-degree burns.

Practical self-help
• If any burnt clothing is stuck to the skin, do not attempt to remove it, but immerse the clothed, damaged area in cool water (provided the surface of the skin has not been broken). Take off clothing and jewellery that can be moved safely from burnt areas, since this may become difficult to remove once swelling begins.
• Once you have cooled the burnt area, apply clean, non-fluffy dressings in an effort to prevent infection. Make sure that you avoid any dressings that use cotton wool, lint or adhesive tapes. If clothing is

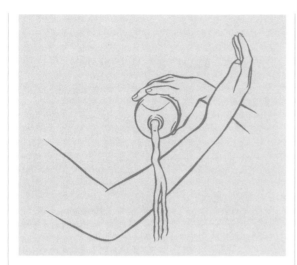

stuck to the burn, do not remove it, but cover lightly with a clean piece of cloth.
• Make sure that blisters are not broken, since these form a protective covering over the burnt area. If they are ruptured, the risk of infection increases greatly. It is best to avoid handling burnt skin in an effort to protect the damaged area as much as possible.

Chemical burns
• Chemicals used in home cleaning products can be very destructive if they come in direct contact with the skin. When dealing with a chemical burn, great care should be taken to ensure that the caustic agent does not come in contact with the skin of the person who is helping the casualty.
• Rinse the burnt area under cool, running water and treat as suggested above.

Preventative measures
There are a variety of practical steps that may be taken to minimize the risk of burns and scalds at home. These include:
• Ensuring that flexes of kettles, handles of saucepans, mugs of very hot liquids, and calor gas, or electric fires are kept well out of the way of small children.
• Checking the temperature of bathwater, and keeping central-heating radiators at a moderate level of heat.
• Making sure that small children are out of the kitchen when meals are being prepared.
• Keeping household cleaning products locked away, or on very high shelves that a toddler or small child cannot reach. Also making sure that cleaning agents are not transferred to other containers, e.g. soft-

drink bottles. This can lead to confusion that may have fatal consequences.
• If you are elderly, making bright lighting a priority in order to protect against shadowy, poorly lit conditions where falls, burns and accidents can take place more readily.
• Keeping matches and cigarette lighters out of the reach of small children.
• Never smoking in bed.
• Installing home fire extinguishers and smoke alarms where appropriate.
• Not keeping inflammable materials such as petrol in the house.

SEEK PROFESSIONAL HELP
• If the casualty has severe burns that cover an area larger than 2.5cm (1in) in diameter. In these cases emergency medical attention is necessary.
• If burns are on the face or over a joint.
• If burns are deep.
• If burns are in the mouth.
• If there are indications of infection around a burn. These may include:
• Excessive or persistent inflammation or redness
• Swelling
• Pus formation
• If an electrical burn has occurred.
• If a person with sunburn develops symptoms of severe heatstroke (page 104).

Alternative treatments

Topical preparations
These are lotions, tinctures or creams that can be applied to the skin to soothe and heal. Choose from any of the following if dealing with a minor burn but bear in mind that none of the substances mentioned for application to the skin should be taken by mouth.
Anthroposophical medicines
Combudoron lotion or ointment is extremely soothing when applied to minor scalds or sunburnt skin. Dilute one measure of the lotion to ten parts of boiled, cooled water and bathe the injured area, or soak a clean compress with the solution and cover the inflamed skin. The ointment may be all that is needed in situations where the burn or scald is very minor. However, bear in mind that caution may be needed if the user is sensitive to the lanolin base of the ointment.

HOMOEOPATHIC MEDICINES

Type	General features	Worse	Better	Remedy
Minor first-degree burns	Red, burning, itchy burns or scalds. Stinging sensations may also be marked with general sensitivity to touch. The homoeopathic remedy may be taken internally, while the diluted tincture may be applied to the skin	Touch and contact		Urtica urens
Minor second-degree burns and scalds	Stinging, inflamed skin with blister formation. Use diluted hypericum tincture on the skin, switching to diluted calendula tincture if the blister breaks	Touch and contact		Urtica urens

Aromatherapy oils

Dilute ten drops of lavender oil in a teaspoonful of gel base and apply to the inflamed area.

Herbal preparations

• Diluted Urtica urens tincture makes a very soothing and calming solution when applied to minor burns and scalds. One part of tincture should be added to ten parts of boiled, cooled water.

• If blisters have broken on a minor burn or scald, diluted marigold tincture should be used to bathe the affected area. Dilute according to proportion suggested above for nettle tincture. After bathing, Calendula cream or ointment may be applied to the damaged area in order to inhibit infection, and speed up healing. Bear in mind that some skins may react to the lanolin base of the ointment.

• Provided the skin has not been broken, the injured area may be immersed in cool water for about ten minutes. In order to soothe and provide pain relief, ten drops each of Calendula and Hypericum tincture may be added to the water.

• Comfrey ointment may be applied to minor burns and scalds.

• Vitamin E oil may be applied to minor burns and scalds in an effort to soothe, heal and discourage scarring.

Home remedies

• For minor burns and scalds that can be treated at home, slit open an aloe vera leaf and apply the juice to the inflamed area.

• Apply a gauze compress that has been soaked in distilled witch hazel to minor burns and scalds and fix it gently in place.

• Cabbage leaves make a soothing compress when applied to minor burns. Prepare them by removing the central rib, dipping them in boiling water, and crushing with a clean rolling pin. Place over the inflamed area and bandage gently in position.

• Minor sunburn without complications may be treated at home with the juice of an aloe vera plant, or a soothing compress may be made from cucumber juice or infusion of marigold flowers. If none of these is readily available, a solution of bicarbonate of soda, or natural, unflavoured yoghurt may be very soothing when applied to sunburnt skin.

Medicines intended for internal use

These ease pain, reduce inflammation and encourage a speedy resolution of the problem.

Flower remedies

Rescue Remedy may be given as often as required in order to minimize any residual shock that can occur as a result of a burn or scald.

Biochemic tissue salts

No. 5 (kali mur) may help aid recovery after a minor burn or scald has occurred. Other possibilities include Combination D or Combination M.

Depending on the severity of the symptoms, tablets may be taken hourly until relief is obtained. Take three doses daily in less pressing circumstances.

Cuts and grazes

Cuts (lacerations) and grazes (abrasions) can vary from a slight scratch or graze, which can be easily treated at home, to a large gash that requires hospital treatment. Advice given here relates only to minor cuts. Any wound that breaks the skin carries with it the risk of infection, so thorough cleaning of the injured area is essential.

Practical self-help
• Bathe the wound with an antiseptic solution in order to remove any debris or dirt that may have entered the graze or cut. Soaking the injured area in an antiseptic solution is helpful in encouraging the removal of any debris.
• Once the wound looks clean, apply an antiseptic cream to a sterile gauze dressing and cover the injured area.

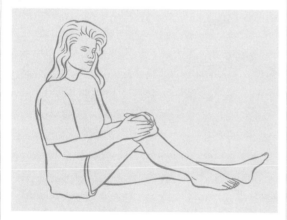

SEEK PROFESSIONAL HELP
If the casualty is suffering from any of the following, make sure you get professional medical help:
• Wide or deep cuts that cannot be held together with dressings or bandages. Cuts that require stitches are often long, jagged, deep, or involving areas of skin that cover joints.
• Profuse or severe bleeding accompanying an injury or wound.
• Numbness, tingling, or loss of strength in an injured limb.
• Deeply embedded debris or dirt that cannot be removed by cleaning or bathing.
• Severe cuts to the face, chest or abdomen.
• Signs of infection surrounding a graze or cut. These may include heat, redness or inflammation, any suggestion of swelling or pus developing in or around the injured area, a high temperature (40°C/102°F), red streaks radiating from the wound along the injured limb.
• Severe cuts to the palm of the hand, or the sides of the fingers which can become easily and rapidly infected.
• Bleeding from the nose or ear following a fall or blow to the head. While you are waiting for the emergency services, let the patient lie on the side that is bleeding with a pad loosely covering the ear or nose.

If the patient has not been immunized against tetanus, professional advice should be consulted.

Alternative treatments
See the section on bites and stings (page 92) for an explanation of the use of topical treatments and medicines that can be taken internally.

Topical preparations
These are lotions, tinctures or creams that can be applied to the skin to soothe and heal. Choose from any of the following, but bear in mind that none of the preparations listed below should be taken by mouth.

Anthroposophical medicines
Marigold (Calendula) ointment may be applied directly onto the cut or graze, or onto a dry, sterile dressing. Before applying the ointment, calendula lotion may be used to bathe or soak the wound. One teaspoon of lotion should be diluted in a glass of boiled, cooled water. Calendula is an excellent choice of ointment or lotion to treat wounds and grazes because it slows down bleeding, encourages healing of damaged tissue, and acts as a natural antiseptic. However, because of its efficacy in promoting speedy healing of tissue, it is essential to check that all debris that could promote infection has been removed from deep cuts. Otherwise there is a risk that surface healing could take place, sealing in infection at a deeper level. Those with sensitive or reactive skins should note that the ointment contains lanolin.

Aromatherapy oils
Wash the affected area with lavender/thymus linalol hydrosol.
Biochemic tissue salts
A couple of tablets of tissue salt No. 4 may be crushed into a powder and applied to small cuts. When this remedy is used topically, it slows down bleeding and encourages rapid healing.
Herbal preparations
• Bathe a minor wound with diluted tincture of marigold (Calendula). If the cut is deep, Hypericum diluted tincture may be used to bathe the wound in order to ease pain and speed up the healing process.
• A mixture of Calendula and Hypericum may be obtained in tincture, cream, or ointment. Use the diluted tincture for bathing wounds (one part tincture to ten parts boiled, cooled water), and the cream for cuts and lacerations. The ointment is more suited to grazed, roughened skin.
• Distilled witch hazel on cotton wool may be used to bathe cuts and grazes. It helps stop bleeding and encourages healing to take place.
• Vitamin E oil may be applied to scar tissue in an effort to promote speedy healing.
Home remedies
• If none of the above is available, warm soapy water may be used to bathe or swab wounds. Alternatively, a teaspoon of common salt, or a few drops of lemon juice may be added to boiled, cooled water as a makeshift antiseptic solution.
• A mixture of garlic and honey is reputed to promote the healing of wounds showing signs of potential infection.
• A wet compress may be made from sage or marigold flowers. An infusion of thyme leaves in boiled, cooled water is also suitable for bathing cuts, grazes and other small wounds such as scratches.

Medicines intended for internal use
These ease pain, reduce inflammation and encourage a speedy resolution of the problem.
Flower remedies
Rescue Remedy may be taken as often as required in order to help with the shock that accompanies an accident.

HOMOEOPATHIC MEDICINES

Type	General features	Worse	Better	Remedy
Cuts and bruises that occur together	Generalized state of shock that accompanies an accident.	Touch Being approached Movement	Resting with the head lower than the body	Arnica Arnica slows down, and promotes re-absorption of blood. Although appropriate for internal use **never** apply Arnica to lacerated skin
Wounds that involve crushing of areas rich in nerves, e.g. fingers	Pains may be intermittent with a tendency to shoot along the injured limb. Affected areas are sore and very sensitive to touch	Touch Movement Contact with cold air	Keeping the injured part as still as possible	Hypericum Hypericum is suitable for deep cuts or those that are near areas rich in nerve supply.
Incised wounds, e.g. as a result of surgery	Pains are stinging and sharp in nature with maddening sensitivity to touch.	Touch Making a mental effort Becoming stressed or upset	Warmth Resting	Staphysagria Staphysagria is especially recommended for wounds that are accompanied by a sense of violation, e.g. hysterectomy, or Caesarean section

Eye injuries

Although many of us are squeamish about eye injuries, there are practical steps that may be taken to deal with a minor eye injury, and simple pointers that can be used to identify when expert medical help is needed.

Damage may be sustained to the eye and the surrounding tissues from the following:
• Foreign bodies such as gravel or dirt entering the eye.
• Corrosive chemicals accidentally squirted into the eye.
• A scratch to the eyeball.
• A blow from a blunt object, resulting in damage to the eyeball or bruising of the soft tissues covering the eye socket.

Practical self-help
• If a foreign body has entered the eye, never attempt to remove anything that has penetrated the eyeball (the white part of the eye). Ensure that no foreign body is removed from the pupil.
• Make sure that the patient is not tempted to rub the eye in an effort to dislodge the object. There is a risk that this may do further damage to the eye.
• If a foreign object is floating freely on the white of the eye, the casualty should sit down with their head tilted backwards. The lower eyelid should be gently pulled down as the casualty looks up. If nothing is visible, let the lid return to its original position and lift the upper eyelid. A foreign body may be removed gently on a clean piece of cloth or tissue.
• Alternatively, the eyelid may be gently pressed down with a firm object (such as a matchstick) in an effort to get the foreign body to adhere to the inside of the eyelid. It can then be very gently removed once the eyelid is gently pulled backwards. However, never use this method if you suspect that an object is even slightly embedded in the eye.
• If a floating object has been initially obvious, but has disappeared under the top lid, carefully pulling the upper eyelid down, and letting it gently slide back into place may be sufficient to remove the foreign body.
• If the object cannot be removed, place a clean pad over the affected eye, securing it lightly in place with a bandage. In addition, seek professional medical help as quickly as possible.
• Black eyes (bruising to the soft tissues surrounding the eyes) may be treated by applying a clean, cool, damp cloth to the affected area in order to reduce swelling. Do not apply ice packs to this area if the skin has been broken.

SEEK PROFESSIONAL HELP
Prompt medical help is needed if:
• A foreign object is situated on the iris or pupil of the eye.
• A foreign body is embedded in the white of the eyeball.
• A foreign body cannot be located or removed.
• The eye is damaged through contact with corrosive chemicals.
• The casualty has blurred vision following a black eye.
• Severe pain or light sensitivity are present.

Alternative treatments
It is worth noting that with very minor eye injuries, it is perfectly appropriate to take the relevant remedy internally, while also applying a topical preparation locally to the affected area. However, eye injuries as a rule require professional medical help, rather than being suitable for self-help treatment. If in doubt about the severity of an eye injury, always seek professional medical advice.

Topical preparations
These are lotions, tinctures or creams that can be applied to the skin to soothe and heal. Choose from any of the following, but bear in mind that none of the substances mentioned for application to the skin should be taken by mouth.

Aromatherapy oils
As a general rule, essential oils should never be applied to the eyes, regardless of how much they have been diluted. This is because of the risk of irritation or inflammation of the delicate tissues of the eye.

Herbal preparations
• After a foreign body has been safely removed, bathe the affected eye in a diluted solution of

HOMOEOPATHIC MEDICINES

Type	General features	Worse	Better	Remedy
Irritation of the eye following entry of a foreign body	Remaining soreness or numbness after foreign body has been removed. Injured area feels enlarged or swollen.	Light Cold draughts Touch Shock	Resting Moderate temperatures	Aconite Aconite is often referred to as 'the Arnica of the eye', and is recommended for shock and fear that follow injury
Injury to the eyeball from a blow with a blunt object		Touch		Symphytum Symphytum is often needed after Arnica has dealt with the initial bruising and swelling
Black eyes that feel numb and cold	Sensitive, swollen tissue around the site of bruising, with tearing, stabbing pains. Tenderness is eased by cool bathing	Movement Warm compresses Warm bathing	Exposure to cool air Cool bathing Cool compresses	Ledum
General bruising, shock and trauma following an accident	General bruising, tenderness and sensitivity.	Movement Touch Being approached	Resting with the head lower than the body	Arnica Arnica eases pain and encourages re-absorption of blood. Eases the physical and emotional trauma that accompany injury
Black eyes that are terribly sensitive and painful	Pains are excessive in proportion to the severity of the injury and persist for a long time. Long-lasting discomfort after a foreign body has been removed	Touch Movement Cold, damp air	Bending the head back Keeping still	Hypericum

Euphrasia or Calendula tincture. Dilute four drops of tincture in 150ml (5fl oz) of boiled, cooled water.
• Mountain daisy tincture may be used to bathe black eyes according to the proportions given above. Do not use mountain daisy cream or tincture if the skin is broken, and only use it on the soft tissues surrounding the eye socket, never directly on the eyeball. Diluted mountain daisy tincture may be used to bathe the swollen area, or it may be applied to a clean cloth, which can be held to the affected area as a cold compress. It will ease pain, reduce swelling and encourage bruises to heal faster by promoting re-absorption of blood.

Home remedies
• If eyes are sore or irritated after a foreign body has been removed, a soothing eyewash may be made from

a weak saline solution. Two level teaspoonfuls of sea salt should be dissolved in a pint of boiled water. Once the saline solution has cooled, pour it into a sterilized bottle. Use as needed to bathe the eyes, ensuring that the eyebath is kept scrupulously clean.
• Soothing compresses may be made from cotton wool pads saturated with the following solution. Add two drops of Euphrasia tincture to two tablespoons of rose water and one tablespoon of boiled, cooled water.
• A comforting compress for black eyes may be made from cotton wool soaked in witch hazel. However, make sure that the liquid does not seep between the eyelids, as it may make the eyes smart.
• A cooled infusion made from herbal teas such as elderflower, chamomile or fennel may be extremely

soothing when used to bathe the eyes, or as cool compresses when added to cotton wool pads.

Medicines intended for internal use

These ease pain, reduce inflammation and encourage a speedy resolution of the problem.

Anthroposophical medicines

Arnica is specifically indicated where severe bruising has occurred (e.g. affecting the soft tissues surrounding the eye), but it may also be helpful in easing the symptoms of general shock and trauma that follow injuries and accidents.

Flower remedies

Rescue Remedy may be taken as often as required in order to help with the distress that may accompany an eye injury. Dissolve a few drops in a small glass of water, and sip frequently. Alternatively, drops may be applied directly to the tongue if water is not available.

Fainting

A faint is a brief loss of consciousness that occurs due to a shortage of blood to the brain, usually caused by a drop in blood pressure. A variety of triggers can cause us to experience this disorienting problem: these may include standing up too quickly, or experiencing extreme pain or shock. Severe fatigue can also leave us open to the possibility of fainting, since this can result in a slow heart rate that can adversely affect the circulation of oxygen to the brain.

Other potential factors can include a history of heart disease or diabetes, or inadequate oxygen in the blood. The latter may be associated with rapid breathing (hyperventilation), an overactive thyroid gland or anaemia, or drinking an excessive amount of strong tea, coffee or alcohol. Such stimulants can result in rapid breathing (hyperventilation), which adversely affects oxygen levels in the blood.

Practical self-help

• If a faint has occurred, lie the patient flat with the legs in a slightly elevated position. This is important because it helps restore the blood supply to the brain.

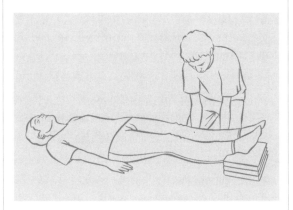

• Loosen any tight clothing around the neck and waist, and check that there is nothing in the mouth that might be swallowed.
• If there are any signs of distress, including difficulty in breathing, lie the patient on their side and send for emergency medical help immediately.

Preventative measures

• Try to make a point of never rising too quickly from a crouching position with your head lowered. Always lift your head slowly at first, gradually raising yourself to an upright position.
• When standing in one place for an extended period of time, raise your heels, flex your toes or contract and relax your calf muscles at regular intervals.
• Avoid standing up too quickly after lying down or reclining in a chair. Instead, sit up straight and perch on the edge of the chair for a little while before standing.
• Avoid going for too long without food, since low blood sugar can also contribute to dizziness and faintness. Instead, try to eat a little at regular intervals if you have a tendency to feel faint.
• Drink plenty of non-alcoholic fluids.
• If the first signs of a faint occur (dizziness, light-headedness, weakness in the legs or pallor and coldness of the skin), make sure that you rest for a short time in order to recover. Once you feel recovered, don't get up too quickly or spend too long in a standing position afterwards. If lying down with the

feet slightly higher than the body is not possible, sitting with your head between your knees for a few minutes may do a great deal to make you feel better.

SEEK PROFESSIONAL HELP

Emergency medical help should be obtained if consciousness is lost as a result of an injury, or if a faint occurs for no obvious reason.

Loss of consciousness that lasts for more than a minute or two requires medical help.

If any of the following occur after gaining consciousness, lose no time in getting professional medical help:
- Blurred vision
- Tingling or numbness in any part of the body
- Protracted disorientation and confusion
- Inability to speak
- Reduced movement or strength in the arms or legs

If fainting occurs on a repeated basis it should be investigated by your family doctor in order to establish the likely underlying cause.

Alternative treatments
Home remedies
- Beetroot juice has a reputation for reducing a tendency to giddiness and dizziness.
- A mixture of lemon juice and honey may ease fatigue and disorientation if blood-sugar levels have dropped as a result of not eating at regular intervals.
- If a faint has occurred, give the patient a mixture of one dessertspoon of honey and a pinch of cinnamon dissolved in a cup of water. This soothing mixture has a reputation as an excellent restorative after the disorientation and distress of a faint.

Medicines intended for internal use
These relieve giddiness and faintness.
Flower remedies
Rescue Remedy can be extremely helpful in easing the shock and trauma of a faint. A few drops may be placed directly on the tongue as soon as the patient shows signs of returning to consciousness, or a few drops may be dissolved in a small glass of water and sipped at regular intervals. In addition, a drop or two of Rescue Remedy may be added to a hot cup of sweet tea in order to ease shock as the patient is recovering.

Heat/sunstroke and heat exhaustion

Heatstroke, also known as sunstroke, is a potentially serious problem that can develop with alarming rapidity in very hot, sunny or humid conditions. As with many conditions, those especially at risk include the very young and the elderly, since they can become dehydrated very rapidly.

Symptoms occur after excessive exposure to direct sunlight and may include any of the following:
- Dizziness and nausea
- High temperature (40°C/102°F)
- Dry skin
- Restlessness and irritability
- Semi-consciousness or severe drowsiness
- Rapid pulse
- Rapid or irregular breathing

Heatstroke may be preceded by heat exhaustion, which is often triggered by drinking too little in hot or humid conditions. As a result, too much fluid and salt are lost through perspiring and the following symptoms may occur:
- Weakness, prostration, faintness and exhaustion
- Dizziness
- Nausea
- Rapid pulse
- Headache
- Muscle cramps

If this condition is neglected, it can develop into heatstroke. Mild cases of heat/sunstroke may respond to self-help measures very well, but it must be stressed that severe episodes of this condition constitute a medical emergency requiring rapid medical help. See the advice in the 'Seek professional help' section for a listing of symptoms indicating that emergency medical aid is needed.

Practical self-help
Heat exhaustion
• Encourage the casualty to rest in cool, peaceful surroundings with the feet raised a little higher than the body.
• Loosen clothing around the neck and waist and ensure that the patient does not feel hemmed in, or lacking fresh air.
• Give water to drink in order to prevent dehydration.

Heat/sunstroke
The first objective is to cool the patient down as quickly as possible without causing shock. Loosen or remove clothing and sponge the body down with cool water. Alternatively, a sheet may be soaked in cool water, wrung out thoroughly, and wrapped around the body. If a fan is available, direct the cool air in the direction of the casualty.

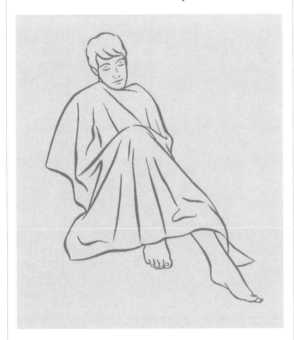

The patient should be placed in a comfortable, semi-reclining position in the coolest, airiest surroundings possible. If a headache is distressing, make sure that exposure to light and noise is kept to a minimum. Monitor the patient's temperature at regular intervals in order to check that it is not becoming dangerously high (above 40°C/102°F).

If the skin has become inflamed and burnt, see the alternative treatments suggested below for information on soothing preparations that may be applied to the skin.

After the patient has recovered, make sure that he or she is not exposed to severe extremes of temperature, since they may become vulnerable to a recurrence of the problem.

Preventative measures
• Avoid exposure to the sun when its rays are strongest. This is the period between 11am and 3pm.
• Build up gradual tolerance to the heat of the sun, always staying out of direct sunlight during the time of day suggested above.
• Ensure that a good quality sunblock is worn at all time, always remembering to re-apply it after swimming.
• The vulnerable areas of the head and back of the neck should always be shaded by a hat in hot, sunny climates.
• If the first symptoms of sunstroke appear, go indoors as quickly as possible and begin self-help measures. Be especially vigilant with children, who may show signs of irritability and restlessness as an early response to excessive exposure to sunlight.

SEEK PROFESSIONAL HELP
• If sunburnt skin has become blistered, always seek a medical opinion.
• If a dangerously high temperature develops (40°C/102°F or above), medical help should be sought at once.
• Severe drowsiness may be the precursor of unconsciousness. If this happens, or the casualty lapses in and out of consciousness, emergency medical attention is essential.
• A severe headache also indicates that medical attention is needed.
• Since heatstroke constitutes a potentially life-threatening problem, if there is any cause for concern about the casualty's condition, always seek medical help and advice. This is especially important if the patient is very young or eldely.

Alternative treatments
If the patient has heatstroke complicated by sunburn, topical preparations are mainly of use *after* the initial emergency has been dealt with by medical help.

Topical preparations

These are lotions, tinctures or creams that can be applied to the skin to soothe and heal. Choose from any of the following, bearing in mind that none of the substances mentioned for application to the skin should be taken by mouth.

Aromatherapy oils

• A soothing topical application on hot skin is lavender hydrosol – using a spray is very effective.
• Five drops of lavender in two teaspoons of gel base will help ease sunburn.
• Ten drops of lavender oil in a cool bath helps

HOMOEOPATHIC MEDICINES

Type	General features	Worse	Better	Remedy
Sunstroke with severe headache that is aggravated by bending the head back	Sudden onset of symptoms with throbbing headache that is relieved by contact with cool air, but may be made worse by ice-packs applied to the head. Skin is flushed and itchy. Explosive pains move up the body	Bending the head backwards Heat to the head Jarring Movement	Cool conditions Fresh, open air Uncovering Elevating head	Glonoin
Sudden onset of violent symptoms that are relieved by bending the head backwards	Burning heat, dryness and bright redness of skin with terrible restlessness. Throbbing headache with severe pains in temples. Pulsating pains radiate in a downward direction from the head	Cold draughts Checked perspiration Light Noise Jarring movements Looking at bright objects	Light bedclothes Bending the head backwards Resting propped up in bed	Belladonna
Heat exhaustion with sudden fainting and chilliness	Although burning sensations are present, patient also feels icy cold. Skin is bluish and clammy, with a tendency to muscle spasms and cramps. Severe headache with nausea, pallor and secretion of an increased amount of urine	Cold drinks Touch Pressure	Dressing Lying down	Veratrum album
Severe cramps with heat exhaustion	Faintness, chilliness and pale clammy skin with chilliness. Very weak and prostrated with heavy, cold sweats. Jerking, cramping and twitching of muscles of the toes, fingers and calves with risk of convulsions	Raising arms Movement Touch	Cool drinks	Cuprum met
Collapse with craving for fresh, cool air	Exhaustion from dehydration with cold body and hot head. Faintness and collapse come on suddenly with bluish-tinged, clammy skin. 'Air hunger' with strong need to be fanned	Warmth Chill Pressure of clothes Lack of fluid	Cool, fresh air Being fanned Elevating feet Cold drinks	Carbo veg

diminish inflammation and the discomfort of sun-burnt skin.

• For children, always seek professional advice.

Herbal preparations

• Aloe vera juice can be immensely soothing when applied to sunburnt skin. If the plant is not readily available (the leaves may be crushed and the juice applied directly to the skin), commercially produced formulations are available in gel form.

• Urtica urens reduces inflammation and stinging sensations. Alternatively, a few drops of Urtica urens tincture may be applied to cool bathwater.

Home remedies

• Compresses may be made from fresh cucumber juice, or an infusion of marigold.

• Cold sage tea, Indian tea, or elderflower infusions are very soothing when applied to inflamed skin.

• The liquid that is strained from infused quince seeds can be used to ease the discomfort of sunburnt skin.

• Bicarbonate of soda or baking soda may be made into a paste with water and applied to painful areas. Alternatively, two tablespoons of the powder may be added to cool bathwater.

• Live, plain yoghurt makes a cooling balm when applied to sunburnt areas straight from the fridge. Avoid flavoured or sweetened varieties.

• Calamine lotion is often used as a soothing lotion where the skin is itchy or inflamed. However, although it may initially ease the heat and sensitivity of sunburnt skin, it will encourage dryness and peeling.

Medicines intended for internal use

These are given in order to reduce a high tempera-ture, and encourage a speedy resolution of the problem.

Flower remedies

Rescue Remedy may be taken as often as required while medical help is on its way in order to relieve the symptoms of shock and trauma that accompany a severe condition such as heat – or sunstroke.

Nosebleeds

The lining of the nose is very sensitive, and even blowing the nose heavily can rupture a tiny blood vessel and cause bleeding.

Nosebleeds are not usually serious unless they are profuse.

Practical self-help

• If a spontaneous nosebleed has occurred, instruct the patient to lean well forward and suggest they should breathe through the mouth while the soft part of the nose is pinched firmly. Make sure that any blood that enters the mouth is spat out in order to avoid vomiting. If nosebleeds are associated with any injuries, seek prompt medical help.

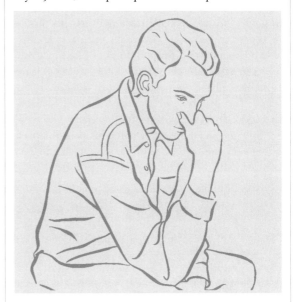

• If there are any signs of loss of consciousness, get medical help immediately. If the casualty seems drowsy, give them nothing to eat or drink.

• Check that the casualty's breathing rate and pulse are not erratic or accelerated.

• Do not drink alcohol or hot drinks for twenty four hours.

SEEK PROFESSIONAL HELP

Prompt medical help is needed if:

• A foreign body visibly remains in a puncture wound. See section on puncture wounds (page 109) for additional information.

• There is bleeding from the nose after a head or chest injury.

• The casualty suffers from haemophilia, a blood disorder, affecting men only, that prevents the natu-ral blood-clotting mechanism that effectively seals a wound. Similar problems may occur with patients

taking anticoagulant or antithrombotic drugs.
• If nosebleeds are recurrent – this can be a sign of high blood pressure or a blood disorder.

Alternative treatments

Topical preparations

These are lotions, tinctures or creams that can be applied to the skin to soothe and heal. None of the preparations listed below should be taken by mouth.

Home remedies

• Crush a leaf of yarrow and rub it gently inside the nostrils. However, make sure that you do not push it inside the nostrils to a point where it may be inhaled or cannot be retrieved. Alternatively, make an infusion by steeping two teaspoonfuls of crushed yarrow leaves in a cup of boiling water. After straining, leave to cool, and soak a pad of cotton wool with the liquid. This may be used to plug the nose, ensuring that it does not enter the nostrils too far.
• Apply a cold compress of witch hazel to the back of the neck and the bridge of the nose in an effort to slow down bleeding.
• Soak a wad of cotton wool with distilled witch hazel or lemon juice and pat the nasal passages externally with it.

Medicines intended for internal use

These ease pain, reduce inflammation and encourage a speedy resolution of the problem.

Flower remedies

Rescue Remedy may be taken as often as required in order to help with the shock that accompanies blood loss.

A tendency to recurrent nosebleeds may benefit from alternative medical help from a practitioner working in any of the following therapies:
• Anthroposophical medicine
• Ayurvedic medicine
• Traditional Chinese medicine
• Homoeopathy
• Naturopathy
• Western medical herbalism

HOMOEOPATHIC MEDICINES

Type	General features	Worse	Better	Remedy
Bright red, spurting or gushing bleeding	Terrible nausea and cold sweat with blood loss. Nausea is made very much worse by movement of any kind. If bleeding is severe it may be accompanied by breathlessness or weak pulse	Movement Warmth Lying down	Fresh, cool air Sitting still	Ipecac
Bleeding associated with a fall or accident	General state of shock and trauma with blood loss.	Being approached Touch	Lying down	Arnica If other indications are not present, Arnica is the first homoeopathic remedy that should be given as soon as possible after an accident
Steady, oozing blood loss with faintness	Bleeding results in collapse. Blue-tinged skin that is very cold and clammy to the touch. Craving for fresh, open air with internal burning sensations	Warmth Stuffy surroundings Movement	Being fanned Fresh, cool air	Carbo veg
Nosebleeds or minor wounds that bleed excessively	Frequent nosebleeds provoked by overly violent blowing of the nose. Severe anxiety and need for reassurance with blood loss	Cold air or surroundings Physical effort	Reassurance Massage	Phosphorus

Puncture wounds

Although puncture wounds can be generally dealt with in a similar way to other cuts and grazes, there are specific problems associated with this type of injury that require extra attention: see 'Practical self-help' below. Only very minor puncture wounds are dealt with here.

Puncture wounds may occur when any of the following enter the skin:
• Nails
• Drawing pins
• Glass
• Splinters
• Bites or stings
• Any other object that is sharp enough to become embedded in the skin

Practical self-help

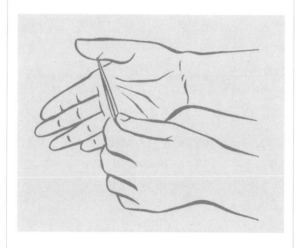

If a small sharp object has entered the skin, it may be removed by gentle, but thorough soaking in an antiseptic solution. This should also help clear out any additional dirt or debris that may have entered the wound.

If a splinter is embedded in the skin, remove it carefully using a sterilized pair of tweezers. Before using the tweezers, bathe the area surrounding the point of entry with an antiseptic solution. Dry the skin by gently wiping in an outward direction from the wound. Once the splinter has been removed, bathe the wound once again with an antiseptic solution, dry and cover with a sterile dressing. If the splinter cannot be removed, seek medical help.

SEEK PROFESSIONAL HELP

Call for medical help if:
• A sharp object is firmly embedded in the wound and cannot be removed with ease.
• The foreign body is preventing loss of blood.
• Dirt or debris is embedded in the skin and cannot be removed by cleaning or bathing the wound.
• The casualty has puncture wounds affecting the hands rather than the fingers.
• The casualty has puncture wounds affecting the joints, since they are likely to become infected more rapidly.
• There is any sign of infection surrounding a puncture wound. This might include heat, inflammation, red streaks radiating from the site of entry or pus formation in the area around the wound.
• A puncture wound remains sensitive and painful for more than forty-eight hours following the accident.
• The casualty has not been immunized against tetanus.

Alternative treatments

It is worth noting that in the case of puncture wounds, it is perfectly appropriate to take the relevant remedy internally, while also applying a topical preparation to the skin.

Topical preparations

These are lotions, tinctures or creams that can be applied to the skin to soothe and heal. Choose from any of the following, but bear in mind that none of the substances mentioned for application to the skin should be taken by mouth.

Anthroposophical medicines

• Marigold (Calendula) ointment is suitable for puncture wounds that have bled steadily. It may be added directly to the wound, or applied on a clean, dry dressing after bathing with diluted hypericum or calendula tincture. It is an excellent choice of ointment or cream because it slows down bleeding, acts as a natural antiseptic and encourages healing of lacerated tissue. However, great care must be taken with deep puncture wounds in order to ensure that all dirt and debris have been removed. Otherwise there is a strong risk that superficial healing may take place speedily, effectively sealing in infection at a deeper level. Those who have sensitive or reactive skins should note that the ointment contains lanolin which may provoke a skin reaction.

• Balsamicum (a combination of Calendula and other ingredients) ointment may be used to soothe and heal minor puncture wounds. Those with sensitive skin should note that the ointment contains lanolin.

Herbal preparations

• The wound should be bathed in a solution of diluted Hypericum tincture. One part tincture should be added to ten parts of boiled, cooled water. If this is unavailable, Calendula tincture is an appropriate second choice. Alternatively, use a mixture of Hypericum and Calendula, combining the healing and pain-relieving properties of both in equal measure.

• After the wound has been bathed thoroughly, Hypericum cream should be applied to the wound on a clean dressing and bandaged in place.

Alternatively, a cream containing a combination of Calendula and Hypericum may be used.

• Distilled witch hazel may be used on cotton wool to swab wounds. It slows bleeding and encourages healing.

• Scar tissue may heal more rapidly if vitamin E oil is applied daily.

Home remedies

• If none of the items mentioned above is at hand, use warm, soapy water to bathe or swab wounds. Alternatively, a few drops of lemon juice or a teaspoonful of common salt may be dissolved in boiled, cooled water.

• Sugar may be added to a cleaned minor wound in order to speed up healing and prevent scarring. The injured area may be covered with granulated white sugar and protected with gauze. Rinse four times daily and repeat the process.

• A wet compress may be made from marigold flowers or St John's wort. A cool infusion of elder-flower is also suitable for bathing wounds.

HOMOEOPATHIC MEDICINES

Type	General features	Worse	Better	Remedy
Puncture wounds that bleed freely (initial stage)	Needed immediately after accident has occurred. Bruising and extreme tenderness around site of wound.	Touch Being approached Jarring movement	Lying with head lower than the body	Arnica Arnica helps physical and emotional trauma that accompany accidents and blood loss
Raised, puffy, puncture wounds with rosy-pink swelling	Severe inflammation and swelling around the wound with stinging pains. Terrible sensitivity to heat that makes discomfort much worse	Warm compresses Warm air Resting Touch	Cool air Cool compresses Movement	Apis
Puncture wounds with hyper-sensitivity to pain	Lacerating, sharp pains with terrible sensitivity to touch. Darting, intermittent pains shoot up the injured limb	Touch Jarring movement	Keeping still	Hypericum
Puncture wounds from bites and stings that are relieved by cold	Affected area feels cold and numb and is soothed by contact with cold	Warm bathing Warm air Movement	Cool bathing Cool air Resting	Ledum Follows Arnica well if there is marked residual bruising and swelling around the wound.

Medicines intended for internal use

These ease pain, inhibit infection and encourage a speedy resolution of the problem.

Flower remedies

Rescue Remedy may be taken as often as required in order to help with the shock that often accompanies an accident. Drops may be placed directly on the tongue, or dissolved in a small glass of water and sipped as needed.

Splinters

See the section on puncture wounds (page 109).

Sprains and strains

SPRAINS

A sprain is an injury that commonly affects the joints of the ankle, knees, wrists and fingers. The pain and discomfort occur because of torn ligaments (the fibrous tissues that hold a joint in place). The damage usually occurs because of excessive stress or demands being put upon a joint, often as the result of a fall or an injury sustained during exercise. The pain that ensues can vary from mild to very severe, depending on the extent of the damage that has been done to the ligament.

Although mild sprains are very common and generally not regarded as a serious problem, they can lead to an underlying weakness in the affected joint, which is then more vulnerable to repeated sprains in the future. However, sensible first aid measures taken at the time of injury, followed by careful use of the damaged joint in the future should minimize future problems.

Symptoms of sprains are likely to include the following:

- Swelling around the injured joint.
- Distortion of joints in severe sprains.
- Discoloration of the skin around the site of injury.

Practical self-help for sprains

- If a minor sprain has occurred, apply an ice pack or cold compress to the injured area. However, do not use ice-cold applications if the skin has been broken.
- Support the affected joint with a crêpe bandage and rest it initially as much as possible.

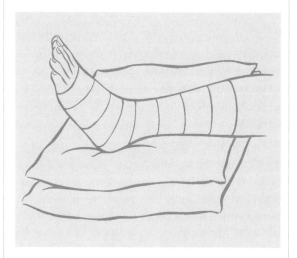

- After forty-eight hours of rest and support, begin to exercise the joint gently, avoiding putting any weight on it.
- When resting, keep the foot raised on a stool or chair so that the swelling is encouraged to drain away.

SEEK PROFESSIONAL HELP

If you suspect a SPRAIN, call for medical help if:
- The joint is distorted, accompanied by extreme pain, suggesting that a severe sprain has occurred.
- A joint remains unusable twelve to twenty-four hours after the accident.
- The joint cannot be straightened.
- The affected limb looks blue, or the injured area feels cold or numb.
- The casualty suffers from osteoporosis (porous, or brittle bones). In such a situation it may be difficult to differentiate between the symptoms of a severe sprain and a fracture.
- A child appears to have sprained his or her wrist.

If a child falls on their wrist, fractures affecting the wrist joint may be mistaken for a sprain.

If you suspect a STRAIN, call for medical help if:
- The injured area is very swollen.
- Pain is very severe or persistent.

STRAINS

Strains are the result of muscles becoming over-stretched, usually as a consequence of too vigorous exercise by those who are unaccustomed to it. Other possible causes include violent sports activities, or exercising muscles that have not had a chance to warm up. When muscle fibres are damaged, the damaged tissue contracts and may become swollen as a result of internal bleeding. Very rarely, the injured muscle may be so severely ruptured that it is completely torn through. However, this is an unusual occurrence, with most people experiencing much more minor damage as a result of physical exercise.

If a slight strain has occurred, there should be a fairly rapid, complete recovery without complications. However, the healing process is likely to take longer in the elderly. If a muscle is ruptured, the consequences may be serious unless medical help is obtained. Minor strains can be successfully treated at home, while a ruptured muscle may require surgery.

Practical self-help for strains
- Ensure that rest is taken while pain persists.
- Bandaging the damaged area firmly will help support the muscle, but make sure that the strapping is not too tight. Overenthusiastic binding can be hazardous because the circulation in the damaged area may become obstructed.
- Once the pain has eased, it is very important to move the injured limb in order to keep joints flexible.
- If a muscle strain is preventing ease of movement, use of crutches may be recommended for a leg injury, or a supportive sling for a damaged arm. Physiotherapy may also be recommended, depending on the severity of the damage to the affected muscle.

Alternative treatments

It is worth mentioning that with sprains and strains, it is perfectly appropriate to take the relevant remedy internally, while also applying a topical preparation to the skin.

Topical preparations

These are lotions, tinctures or creams that can be applied to the skin to soothe and heal. Choose from any of the following, but bear in mind that none of the substances mentioned for application to the skin should be taken by mouth.

Aromatherapy oils
Cold compresses using chamomile are very soothing when applied to a strain or sprain.

Anthroposophical medicines
Provided the skin has not been broken, arnica ointment can be rubbed into the painful area twice daily in order to ease pain and reduce swelling.

Herbal preparations
- Cool compresses may be made from witch hazel, daisy or Arnica. An ice-cold compress can be made from witch hazel by freezing it in an ice cube tray. The cubes can be wrapped in a cloth and held to the painful area. Half a teaspoonful of Arnica tincture can be dissolved in a pint of cool water, which can be used to bathe the injury. Alternatively, a length of cloth or towel can be dipped into a cooled infusion of daisy and wrapped around the painful area as a cold compress.
- If Arnica cream or ointment helps initially, but ceases to be of use after a while, switch to ruta ointment.
- Comfrey ointment may be used in order to relieve the pain of bruises and sprains. Apply morning and evening after bathing the painful area in warm water. However, do not apply it to broken skin, and care should be taken not to continue using it for more than ten days. It is also not recommended for use in pregnancy or during breastfeeding.

Home remedies
- A bag of frozen peas makes an excellent substitute for an ice pack. Hold it to the painful area at regular intervals in order to reduce swelling and ease pain. However, do not use an ice pack if the skin has been broken.
- A simple and soothing compress may be made by applying crushed cabbage leaves to the painful area and binding firmly in place.
- One teaspoonful of turmeric may be mixed with a little honey to form a paste and applied to the painful area twice daily to reduce inflammation and speed up healing.
- An olive oil and garlic liniment may be made by steeping ten cloves of garlic in 250ml (9fl oz) of olive oil. Massage gently around the injured area as required.

HOMOEOPATHIC MEDICINES

Type	General features	Worse	Better	Remedy
Immediate pain and swelling following injury		Movement Touch Exertion	Lying with the head low	Arnica Arnica relieves the trauma and pain of injury, promotes re-absorption of blood and reduces swelling. Also reduces emotional shock that accompanies injury
Established stage of sprains and strains that are much worse when moved	Severe tearing pains that are much relieved by a night's rest, and aggravated by the slightest movement.	Motion Touch Muscular effort Rising from a sitting position	Heat Keeping as still as possible Firm pressure to injured part	Bryonia Bryonia is often needed after Arnica has initially helped with pain and swelling
Established sprains and strains that feel better for continued movement	Pains are especially severe when resting in bed, resulting in extreme restlessness. Injured area is much more comfortable during continued movement.	Cold Damp conditions Lying, sitting or standing still First movement Overexertion	Warmth Warm compresses Continued movement that does not exhaust	Rhus tox Rhus tox is often required if Arnica has helped with the initial trauma and swelling of injury
Established sprains that affect the wrists, knees and ankles	Pain and stiffness with inflammation. Injury from repetitive movement rather than one violent action, e.g. tennis elbow. Pain in one small area: feels as though a nail were sticking in injured joint	Damp, cold Resting Lying on injured part Walking out of doors Touch	Warmth Movement indoors	Ruta
Established sprains and strains that are soothed by cool bathing	Affected joint is swollen and hot to the touch, but not red. Stabbing pains are worse for becoming warm in bed. Pain and stiffness in injured limb is relieved by contact with cold water	Becoming warm Movement Warm bathing	Resting Cool compresses Cool bathing Contact with cool air	Ledum

Medicines intended for internal use

These ease pain, reduce inflammation and encourage a speedy resolution of the problem.

Biochemic tissue salts

The swelling and pain of strains and sprains may be treated with one of the following formulations of tissue salts: Combination I, Combination P or No. 4. Combination I is suitable for the treatment of muscu-lar pain. Combination P for aching legs and feet, while tissue salt No. 4 may be indicated for inflamed, painful muscles. In severe cases, tablets may be taken hourly until relief is obtained. Alternatively, if symptoms are less traumatic, four tablets may be taken three times a day, reducing the dosage as symptoms improve.

TREATMENT GUIDE

EAR CONDITIONS

Earache

See page 284 in the section 'Childhood Problems'.

Infection of the outer ear canal (otitis externa)

This may be a localized infection of the outer ear canal (such as a boil or an abscess) or a general state of infection affecting the lining of this area as a whole. Infections of this kind may often be set off by swimming, because moist skin is very vulnerable to any infection that may be water-borne. Alternatively, localized or generalized infection may occur after scratching the inner ear in an effort to ease itching or remove excess wax.

Symptoms may include any of the following:
• Irritation in the ear followed by pain and discomfort.
• Discharge from the ear.
• Pain on moving the outer part of the ear by gently pulling on the ear lobe.

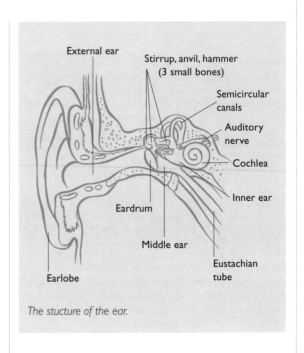

The stucture of the ear.

• Some degree of hearing loss if the outer ear canal becomes blocked by pus formation.

Practical self-help
• Keep the ear as warm and dry as possible by using ear plugs when in contact with water (e.g. when showering), and placing a warm, dry pad over the ear in order to ease pain.
• Thoroughly clean any hearing aid worn in the affected ear.

SEEK PROFESSIONAL HELP
• If pain is severe and does not respond rapidly to self-help measures.
• If there are any signs that the bone underneath the ear is painful, and/or if the skin behind the ear looks red and inflamed.
• If there are any indications of stiffness in the neck, drowsiness or general debility accompanying an ear infection.

Alternative treatments

It is worth noting that with outer ear canal infections, it is quite appropriate to take the relevant remedy internally, while also applying a topical preparation to the inflamed ear.

Topical preparations

These are lotions, tinctures or creams that can be applied to the skin to soothe and heal. Choose from any of the following, bearing in mind that none of the substances mentioned for application to the skin should be taken by mouth.

Aromatherapy oils

Use one drop only of any of the following essential oils on a cotton wool bud, and gently rub over the outside of the ear: tea tree (Melaleuca alternifolia), lavender (Lavendula angustifolia) or Roman chamomile (Chamaemelum nobile). *Never* use essen-tial oils inside the ear. For children, always seek professional advice.

Herbal preparations

Hypericum oil can also be used as above in order to ease irritation and inflammation of the ear.

Home remedies

• Ground ivy oil can also be extremely soothing and healing when used as suggested above. In order to make the oil, several generous handfuls of the crushed, fresh plant should be steeped in a jar containing 600ml (1 pint) of good-quality sunflower or olive oil. The solution should be left to stand in a sunny place for one month. Shake the liquid occasionally and strain the oil through a fine muslin cloth before use.

• Warm compresses soaked in chamomile tea placed around the ear will help in soothing pain and encouraging the body to deal with infection.

HOMOEOPATHIC MEDICINES

Type	General features	Worse	Better	Remedy
Inflammation of the outer ear that sets in after getting chilled	Rapidly developing, severe symptoms that cause great restlessness and anxiety. Extreme sensitivity to, and intolerance of noise and pain that drives patient to a frenzy	Exposure to cold winds / Pressure / Touch / At night / Noise / Bright light	Resting / Moderate temperatures / Sweating	Aconite
Ear infection with sudden swelling of the outer ear	Inflammation and pain of the outer ear with cold sensations in affected area. History of swollen glands and poor-quality bones and teeth. Ear problems set in after getting wet or excessive mental strain	Exposure to cold draughts of air / When teething / At puberty / Movement	Warm, dry conditions / Summer weather / Lying down	Calc phos
Inflammation of the outer ear canal with hearing loss	Stitch-like pains in the ears from laughing, talking or swallowing. Cracking sounds in the ears are made worse by swallowing and blowing the nose. Swollen glands with outer ear infection	Touch / Damp and cold / At night / Cold / Speaking / Laughing / Bending head backwards	Fresh air / Lying down / Eating	Manganum

- Garlic capsules can be an excellent way of obtaining an oil that can be warmed and applied to the ear by piercing the capsule with a pin. Alternatively, vitamin E oil capsules may be used in the same way.
- Lemon, parsley or onion juice may also be squeezed onto a warmed piece of cotton wool and applied to the ear in order to ease infection and irritation.

Medicines intended for internal use

These ease pain, reduce inflammation and encourage a speedy resolution of the problem.

Biochemic tissue salts

Pain and irritation in the ear may be eased by tissue salt No. 1 or No. 7, the latter often being needed by those who are much worse in hot weather. If symptoms are severe, tablets may be taken every hour until relief is obtained.

If problems with an outer ear infection do not rapidly respond to self-help measures, or if symptoms recur, professional medical help should be sought. Any of the following therapies may provide appropriate help with the problem once the initial acute phase has been dealt with:

- Anthroposophical medicine
- Homoeopathic medicine
- Naturopathy
- Traditional Chinese medicine
- Western herbal medicine

Infection of the middle ear (otitis media)

A middle ear infection occurs as a result of a bacterial or viral infection developing in the cavity of the middle ear. The resulting inflammation leads to swelling and blockage of the Eustachian tube (the connecting tube that extends between the cavity of the middle ear and the back of the nose). If a bacterial infection has developed, pus will form in the cavity of the middle ear, which, if left untreated, may lead to rupture of the eardrum. Children are far more likely to get ear infections if there is a smoker in the house. Smoking in another room does not solve the problem because smoke travels.

Middle ear infections often develop as a complication following a virus or infection of the nose and/or throat (e.g. as a result of a cold). Symptoms may include any of the following:

- A sensation of fullness in the ear
- Severe, distressing, stabbing pains
- Diminished hearing
- Feverishness.

If the infection is bacterial, the appearance of a discharge is usually accompanied by a reduction of pain. This is the result of the pressure of pus having built up to the point where the eardrum has been ruptured. Treatment with antibiotics has no influence on whether or not the eardrum ruptures. Antibiotics do reduce the pain, but increase the chances of glue ear (sometimes called chronic secretory otitis media) developing.

If problems with middle ear infections become chronic (long-standing), the characteristic features to look out for are deafness and problems resulting from this, for example, delayed language development or behavioural difficulties in children, or depression and irritability in adults. Chronic bacterial middle ear infection is very rare, and discharge occurs only when the eardrum has been perforated.

A chronic discharge is usually caused either by infection of the outer ear canal (see pages 113–16) or cholesteatoma, which needs specialist treatment as it erodes bone and destroys hearing if left unchecked.

Practical self-help

- If a cold develops, suck medicated pastilles or use a spray decongestant in order to keep your nasal passages as clear as possible. By doing so, there is every chance that the Eustachian tubes are less likely to become swollen and spread infection.
- Use alternative or conventional methods of pain relief (such as a painkiller) in order to ease distress and discomfort.
- Keep the ear as clean and dry as possible, and

place a soft, warm, dry pad over the affected ear in order to avoid the likelihood of further infection.

• Contact with warmth often eases the pain of an ear infection. A simple warm compress can be made by wrapping a warm hot-water bottle in a towel, or wringing out a flannel that has been immersed in warm water. However, if a young child is suffering from ear pain, always ensure that warm water is used (rather than boiling) in order to avoid accidental burns or scalds. If cool compresses provide more relief, soak a flannel in cool water, or use a custom-made cool pack, which can be wrapped in a thin, soft cloth before applying to the painful area.

• Avoid, or greatly reduce the amount of dairy foods in the diet, especially if middle ear infections have become a chronic problem. This is important because dairy foods have a reputation for encouraging mucus production, thus making congestive respiratory problems (such as sinusitis) worse.

SEEK PROFESSIONAL HELP

• When any infection of the middle ear causes severe pain, inflammation and/or pus formation.

• If stiffness in the neck, drowsiness or general debility accompany an ear infection.

• If ear problems in babies are accompanied by signs of dehydration. These may include reduced urine output, dry skin, sunken eyes or sunken fontanelle

HOMOEOPATHIC MEDICINES

Type	General features	Worse	Better	Remedy
Rapidly developing, severe, right-sided ear symptoms	Affected ear looks bright red and feels very hot and dry. Feverishness with ear pain and extremely dry, hot bright red skin. Swollen glands with throbbing pains in throat and ears. Extreme irritability and bad temper with pain	Excitement or stimulation Chill Noise Jarring movement Bright light	Warm compresses Sitting propped up in bed in a dark room	Belladonna
Rapidly developing ear pain that is less violent than symptoms calling for Belladonna	Itching, pulling, drawing pains in the ear. Left-sided, or more severe pain in the right ear than the left. Face may be pale or flushed with ear pain.	Contact with cool air Touch Noise Effort At night	Cool compresses Lying down	Ferrum phos Ferrum phos often needed in the initial stage of ear infection before discharge has developed
Ear infections with thick, yellowish discharge (established stage)	Sharp, splinter-like pains in ears and throat with pussy discharge. General chilliness with extreme sensitivity to contact with draughts of cold air. Uncovering a small part of the body causes disproportionate distress	At night Lying on painful side Chill Being exposed to chill or cold winds	Wrapping up, or covering the head warmly Warm surroundings Rest	Hepar sulph
Persistent, lingering symptoms with yellowish-green discharge	Ear infections develop after getting wet or chilled. Extreme intolerance of stuffy, overheated rooms and craving for cool, fresh air. Weepy and depressed with pain and illness	Rest Stuffy rooms Humidity Lack of attention Evenings	Gentle exercise Cool, fresh air Cool bathing or compresses Cool drinks Having a good cry	Pulsatilla

(the soft spot at the crown of the head in young babies).

Alternative treatments

It is worth noting that with middle ear infections, it is quite appropriate to take the relevant remedy internally, while also applying a topical preparation to the inflamed ear. However, it is important to stress that acute or chronic ear infections should always be investigated by a medical practitioner in order to avoid the potential of long-term damage.

Topical preparations

These are lotions, tinctures or creams that can be applied to the skin to soothe and heal. Choose from any of the following, bearing in mind that none of the substances mentioned for application to the skin should be taken by mouth.

Herbal preparations

• Four or five drops of warm mullein oil can be very soothing when ears are inflamed and painful. Once the warmed oil has been applied to the ear, it should be covered with a warmed, small wad of cotton wool. Mullein oil can be made by placing fresh mullein flowers in a well-washed glass jar with slices of garlic. The contents of the jar should be covered with good-quality olive oil, covered with cheesecloth secured in place by a rubber band and left to infuse in a sunny place for two weeks. The oil should then be strained and kept in clean, small dropper bottles ready for use. Provided it is kept in a cool place, the oil should remain usable for up to two years.

Home remedies

• Warm compresses soaked in chamomile tea placed around the ear will help in soothing pain and encouraging the body to deal with infection.
• Garlic capsules can be an excellent way of obtaining an oil that can be warmed and inserted into the ear by piercing the capsule with a pin. Alternatively, vitamin E oil capsules may be used in the same way.
• Lemon, parsley or onion juice may also be squeezed onto a warmed piece of cotton wool and placed over the ear in order to ease infection and irritation.

Medicines intended for internal use

These ease pain, reduce inflammation and encourage a speedy resolution of the problem.

Biochemic tissue salts

Combination Remedy J or Combination Remedy N

may ease the distress and pain of an ear infection. If symptoms are severe, tablets should be taken every hour until relief is obtained.

If problems with a middle ear infection do not rapidly respond to self-help measures, or if symptoms recur, professional medical help should be sought. Any of the following therapies may provide appropriate help with the problem once the initial acute phase has been dealt with:
• Anthroposophical medicine
• Homoeopathic medicine
• Naturopathy
• Traditional Chinese medicine
• Western medical herbalism

Tinnitus (ringing in the ears)

Tinnitus is experienced as a persistent buzzing or ringing sound that may affect one or both ears. In some cases, the cause may be nothing more complicated than a build-up of wax in the outer ear. However, additional co-factors that may play a part in developing this troublesome condition may include any of the following: loss of hearing, high blood pressure or taking certain drugs such as quinine. Emotional stress that results in anxiety or depression can also aggravate the problem.

Alternative treatments

If tinnitus has become an established problem, professional help may be sought from practitioners working in any of the following therapies:
• Anthroposophical medicine
• Aromatherapy
• Biochemic tissue salts
• Cranial osteopathy
• Homoeopathy
• Naturopathy

- Nutritional therapy
- Relaxation techniques
- Shiatsu
- Traditional Chinese medicine
- Western medical herbalism

EYE CONDITIONS

Blepharitis

Blepharitis occurs as a result of inflammation of the edges of the eyelids. As a result, the margins of the lids look red and scaly and may feel uncomfortable. The condition may be related to eczema of the eyebrows and scalp, and the tendency to flakiness of the affected areas of skin may look rather like dandruff.

If flakiness of the skin on the eyelids becomes severe, particles of skin may enter the eye and set off a bout of conjunctivitis. Alternatively, in a severe case of blepharitis, little ulcers may develop on the margins of the lids and some eyelashes may be lost.

Practical self-help
- If dry, scaly skin on the scalp is a problem, using an anti-dandruff formulation (such as a tea tree oil shampoo) may help.
- Try gently washing the scaly skin around the margins of the lids with a warm, dilute, salt-water solution using a soft, clean cotton wool bud. This should be done each morning and night for a couple of weeks.
- Make a point of washing the hands frequently before and after touching the eyes, and also try to avoid rubbing or scratching the inflamed area.
- If you suspect that blepharitis is occurring repeatedly as a result of being stressed or run down, see the general advice given under 'Preventative measures' in the Boils section (page 219).

SEEK PROFESSIONAL HELP
- If the condition does not respond to self-help measures.
- If there are any signs of infection.

Alternative treatments
It is worth noting that in cases of blepharitis, it is quite appropriate to take the relevant remedy internally, while also applying a topical preparation to the skin. However, blepharitis is a recurrent, rather persistent condition that is likely to require professional help in dealing with the tendency to reappearance of the problem.

Topical preparations
These are lotions, tinctures or creams that may be applied to the skin to soothe and heal. Choose from any of the following, bearing in mind that none of the substances mentioned for application to the skin should be taken by mouth.
Aromatherapy oils
As a general rule, essential oils should never be applied to the eyes, regardless of how much they have been diluted. This is because of the risk of irritation or inflammation of the delicate tissues of the eye.
Herbal preparations
- The inflamed area may be bathed in a solution of diluted Euphrasia tincture. Twenty drops of tincture should be dissolved in four tablespoons of rose water in order to make a soothing lotion. A cotton wool bud should be used in order to bathe the specific areas of skin that are inflamed.
- Diluted Calendula tincture may be used to bathe the inflamed, scaly areas of skin at the lid margins. One part of tincture should be dissolved in ten parts of boiled, cooled water.
- Calendula cream or ointment may be applied to the edges of the eyelids in order to soothe and moisturize the skin, as well as discouraging secondary infection. However, it is important to note that the ointment contains lanolin, which may provoke a reaction in those who have sensitive skin.
Home remedies
- Cold Indian tea can make a soothing, cooling lotion with which to bathe inflamed areas of skin.
- A cold poultice of pulped baked apples may also be of value in reducing inflammation. In order to make the poultice, wrap the softened apples in clean, soft, thin gauze and apply it to the inflamed area as often as feels necessary.

Medicines intended for internal use

These ease discomfort, reduce inflammation and encourage a speedy resolution of the problem.

If blepharitis is severe, or has become an established problem, professional help may be sought from practitioners working in any of the following therapies:

- Anthroposophical medicine
- Biochemic tissue salts
- Homoeopathy
- Naturopathy
- Nutritional therapy
- Traditional Chinese herbalism
- Western medical herbalism

HOMOEOPATHIC MEDICINES

Type	General features	Worse	Better	Remedy
Blepharitis which is worse from cool bathing	Swelling and inflammation of the margins of eyelids with itching, stinging and burning sensations. Eyes water easily and are very sensitive to draughts of cold air	At night Cool draughts of air Bathing with cold water Bright sunlight	Fresh air	Clematis
Blepharitis with a tendency to ingrowing lashes	Red and swollen, or dry, scaly and pale eyelids. Patches of eczema affect the scalp and eyelids with a tendency for the eyelids to become cracked and inflamed. Digestive problems may alternate with disorders of the skin	Cold draughts of air Bright light Scratching During and after a period	After walking in the open air Touch	Graphites
Blepharitis with dry sensation in eyeballs, which feel stuck to eyelids	Inflammation of eyelids with profuse scaly, flaky skin on scalp and eyebrows. Watering eyes from cool compresses. Unhealthy skin in general with a tendency for small boils to develop that do not come to a head	Cool draughts of air to back of head or neck Movement Jarring movements	Fresh air Warmth	Sanicula (aqua)
Blepharitis with dry, crusty eyelids	Eyeballs feel swollen and distended. Shaky vision with a tendency for eyes to water when looking fixedly at an object for any length of time. Patient wants to wipe eyes at regular intervals	Contact with cold air or winds Pressure Touch Looking at one thing for a long time Rubbing	Bending the head backwards Perspiring	Senega

Conjunctivitis

Conjunctivitis develops when the conjunctiva (the transparent membrane that lines the eyelids and the surface of the eye to the edge of the cornea) becomes inflamed. This usually happens as the result of allergic reaction or infection.

The symptoms of infected conjunctivitis may include any of the following:

- Redness, pain and inflammation of the white of the eye.
- Presence of a pussy discharge that may be yellow in colour.
- Crusting and sticking together of the eyelids during sleep.

If conjunctivitis develops as a result of a bacterial infection, both eyes are likely to be affected by a marked discharge. However, if conjunctivitis occurs in response to a viral infection, one eye is usually affected, with a scanty discharge.

The symptoms of allergic conjunctivitis may include any of the following:

- Well-established or recurrent itching and inflammation of the white of the eye.

HOMOEOPATHIC MEDICINES

Type	General features	Worse	Better	Remedy
Rapidly developing conjunctivitis after exposure to cold winds	Dry, gritty eyes with swollen, inflamed lids. Severe light sensitivity with shooting pains in the eyes. Conjunctivitis can set in after a foreign body has been removed from the eye. Patient is extremely anxious and restless with eye symptoms	Cold winds Touch At night Light Sunlight	Resting Moderate temperatures	Aconite
Conjunctivitis that is much worse for warmth	Terribly puffy, swollen eyes with stinging, shooting pains. Tears feel hot. Light sensitivity with marked dislike of having the eyes covered. Rosy-pink, baggy swelling under eyes. Fussy and fidgety with discomfort and pain	Warm bathing Contact with warm air Touch After sleep Warm bathing	Cool bathing Contact with cool air Undressing Movement	Apis
Violent, sudden onset of bright red inflammation of the eyes	Eyes feel hot, dry and burning. Extreme physical and mental sensitivity with pain, and marked intolerance of stimulation and bright light. Eyes feel half closed	Heat of sun Cold draughts or chill Light, noise, jarring Looking at bright or glittering objects	Resting in bed Light covering	Belladonna
Conjunctivitis with established colds	Constantly wants to rub or wipe the eyes because of a sensation that there is something covering the surface of the eye. Burning, profuse, thick, yellowish-green discharge. Tearful and depressed with symptoms	Warmth Evening and night Rest Sunlight	Cool, fresh air Gentle exercise Undressing Rubbing Having a good cry	Pulsatilla

• The conjunctiva may suddenly become puffy during the hay fever season.

Preventative measures

The best way to avoid spreading infective conjunctivitis is to keep your own flannel, towels and cosmetic brushes separate from everyone else's. It is also helpful to observe scrupulous hygiene habits, always washing your hands after touching your eyes.

If conjunctivitis is due to an allergic reaction to pollen, wearing good-quality sunglasses when out of doors may protect the eyes to a certain degree, while bathing the eyes with cool water when indoors may encourage the inflammation to go down.

SEEK PROFESSIONAL HELP

• If a young baby develops symptoms that resemble conjunctivitis.
• If there is any severe redness, pain or inflammation of the eye.
In these cases you should be examined by a medical practitioner or optician as soon as possible.

Alternative treatments

It is worth bearing in mind that in cases of conjunctivitis, it is quite appropriate to take the relevant remedy internally, while also applying a topical preparation to the inflamed area.

Topical preparations

These are lotions, tinctures or creams that can be applied to the skin to soothe and heal. Choose from any of the following, bearing in mind that none of the substances mentioned for external application should be taken by mouth.

Aromatherapy oils

As a general rule, essential oils should never be applied to the eyes, regardless of how much they have been diluted. This is because of the risk of irritation or inflammation of the delicate tissues of the eye.

Herbal preparations

• The soreness and discomfort of conjunctivitis may be greatly eased by bathing the eyes in a diluted solution of Euphrasia or Calendula tincture. Four drops of tincture should be dissolved in 140ml (5fl oz) of boiled, cooled water.
• Cooled infusions made from herbal teas such as chamomile, elderflower or fennel may be very soothing when used to bathe the eyes. Soak cotton wool pads in the appropriate infusion to make cool compresses.
• A weak decoction of golden seal (**NB** do not use during pregnancy) also makes a soothing eyewash. In order to make the decoction, half a teaspoon of the root should be boiled in one and a half cups of water and strained. Cool before applying.

Home remedies

A cool tea bag of Indian tea makes a soothing compress that can be laid over the eyelids.

Medicines intended for internal use

These ease pain, reduce inflammation and encourage a speedy resolution of the problem.

If conjunctivitis is severe, or has become an established problem, professional help may be sought from practitioners working in any of the following therapies:
• Anthroposophical medicine
• Biochemic tissue salts
• Homoeopathic medicine
• Naturopathy
• Traditional Chinese medicine
• Western medical herbalism

Styes

Styes occur when the small glands at the root of the eyelashes become inflamed. Infection sets in, with resulting swelling, inflammation and pus formation. A stye should last an average of seven days, after which the eyelid should return to normal. However, it is possible for more than one to appear at the same time, or for styes to recur after a short interval of time.

Generally speaking, the presence of styes (in common with boils and abscesses) indicates that we may be overstressed and run down.

Practical self-help

• If styes are occurring repeatedly as a result of being stressed or run down, see the general advice given under 'Preventative measures' in the boils section (page 219).

• Check how much sugar is being eaten on a daily basis, since it has been suggested that a high intake of refined sugar (sucrose) in the diet can create an environment that encourages bacterial infection. Common sources of sucrose include biscuits, cakes, carbonated drinks, chocolate and ice cream. Eliminating or drastically reducing the quantity of sugar included in the diet may be helpful in discouraging future episodes of infection.

• Rubbing or scratching the eyes can contribute to further problems, especially in young children. Clipping fingernails quite short can help discourage scratching the delicate area around the eyes. However, care must be taken not to cut fingernails *too* short, as the skin of the nail folds can be damaged, leading to an infection called paronykia.

• Make sure that towels and face flannels are not shared between family members in order to discourage spreading infection.

SEEK PROFESSIONAL HELP

If styes are a recurring problem, especially if associated with boils. Although these may be due to the effect of stress on the immune system, it is important that the person is checked for diabetes.

HOMOEOPATHIC MEDICINES

Type	General features	Worse	Better	Remedy
Rapid onset of symptoms with dry, red eyes	Sensitivity of the delicate area surrounding the eye with pounding, throbbing pains. Extreme intolerance of light with possibly dilated pupils. Bad tempered and irritable with eye problems	Jarring movement Bright light Lying on the affected side Being disturbed	Dark rooms Resting propped up in bed	Belladonna
Large, swollen styes with thick, yellowish pus	Painful, acute sensitivity to draughts of cold air, which cause great distress and irritability. Sharp splinter-like pains with styes. Generally feels relief in warm rooms or when warm compresses are applied	Touch Pressure Draughts of cold air Light Undressing	Warmth	Hepar sulph
Extremely puffy, rosy-pink, swollen, waterlogged styes	Severe swollen styes, with stinging, burning tears. Terrific dislike of warmth and relief from cool bathing or compresses. Generally fidgety and irritable with discomfort	At night After sleep Touch Warmth of room or fire Warm bathing	Cool air Cool bathing Movement	Apis
Styes with greenish-yellow pus that affect the lower lid	Gluey discharge that sticks the eyelids together during sleep. Itchy styes with a constant desire to rub the affected area. Pain and discomfort are made worse by warmth	Warmth Overheated rooms Warm compresses Keeping still	Cool bathing Cool compresses Cool, fresh air Gentle movement in the fresh air	Pulsatilla

Alternative treatments

It is worth noting that with styes, it is perfectly appropriate to take the relevant remedy internally, while also applying a topical preparation to the skin.

Topical preparations

These are lotions, tinctures or creams that can be applied to the skin to soothe and heal.

Aromatherapy oils

As a general rule, essential oils should never be applied to the eyes, regardless of how much they have been diluted. This is because of the risk of irritation or inflammation of the delicate tissues of the eye.

Home remedies

Apply a compress of warmed fresh marigold petals or parsley to the stye. In order to make the compress, soak a soft, clean cloth in a warm decoction or infusion of herbs, and apply it warm to the affected area.

Medicines intended for internal use

These ease pain, reduce inflammation and encourage a speedy resolution of the problem.

Home remedies

Include regular amounts of fresh garlic in the diet, or take a course of powdered garlic tablets. Garlic is reputed to have blood-purifying qualities as well as supporting the body in dealing with bacterial infections.

If styes are severe, or have become an established problem, professional help may be sought from practitioners working in any of the following therapies:

- Anthroposophical medicine
- Homoeopathic medicine
- Naturopathy
- Nutritional therapy
- Traditional Chinese medicine
- Western medical herbalism

CONDITIONS OF THE FACE AND HEAD

Headaches and migraines

An astonishingly wide and varied number of factors need to be taken into consideration if we are trying to identify common triggers for headaches and migraines. They may include any of the following: feverishness, infection, overindulgence, poor posture, lack of sleep, muscular tension, low blood-sugar levels or emotional stress. Although we may feel as though we are looking for a needle in a haystack when we attempt to discover potential triggers for our headaches, isolating the factors that make us vulnerable to developing this unpleasant condition can be invaluable in supporting us in dealing effectively with the problem.

It is also very helpful to establish the category our headaches fall into, so that we are best placed to decide on the most appropriate form of treatment we can employ in order to ease the problem. The following list gives a general idea of the most common types of headache:

- 'Morning after' headaches usually occur after drinking excessive amounts or a mixture of alcohol, such as beer, wine and spirits. This type of headache is regarded as a form of vascular headache because of the relationship between alcohol and widening and relaxation of the blood vessels.
- Vascular headaches are related to dilation (expansion) of the blood vessels that serve the head and neck.

• Tension headaches are often related to muscle tightness and tension in the scalp, face, jaw, neck and shoulders.

• Cluster headaches are one-sided headaches that occur on a sporadic basis. The severity of pain may be very great, to the point of frequently waking the patient from sleep. In addition, the eye and nostril on the side of the pain may exude a water discharge for the duration of the pain. Cluster headaches can last for a few hours, or occur sporadically over a few days and then disappear for a few months.

• Migraines can be a much more intense, broadly based disorder that can have profound effects on the whole system. Possible symptoms include severe headaches, nausea, vomiting, a general sensation of illness, disorientation, numbness or tingling of the face, arms, extremities or one complete side of the body, and visual disturbance.

Practical self-help

If recurrent or severe headaches are a problem it is important to avoid overreliance on painkillers as a way of coping with the situation. Even though taking an occasional painkiller may be appropriate in easing the distress of a severe headache, there are definite disadvantages to reaching for the bottle of painkillers at the first twinge of pain. Possible problems that may result from regular use of analgesics include any of the following: rebound pain when the drug is withdrawn, possible psychological as well as physiological dependence, digestive problems such as nausea and constipation, and dizziness. A great deal of attention has also been drawn to the need for great care in monitoring the use of paracetamol, due to the possibility of liver damage occurring if the recommended dose is exceeded.

Certain foods may contribute to the onset of recurrent headaches or migraines. They include any of the following: alcohol, cheese, strong coffee and chocolate. If we bear in mind that dehydration can also make recurrent headaches worse, it becomes clear that it is also extremely important to ensure that fluid intake is kept up. Avoid tea, coffee or hot chocolate, which can make the problem worse, concentrating instead on fresh fruit juices, soothing herb teas and filtered or mineral water.

Experiencing good-quality, restful sleep is also an essential factor in discouraging tension headaches or migraines that are related to an overly demanding lifestyle. See the general advice on insomnia (page 252) for ways of encouraging a sound night's sleep.

Check that conditions at work are not contributing to the problem, since tension headaches in particular can be made much worse by hunching over a badly lit desk in a poorly ventilated office building. Make a point of ensuring that your chair fits comfortably under your desk so that your feet rest on the floor. Also check that you have adequate

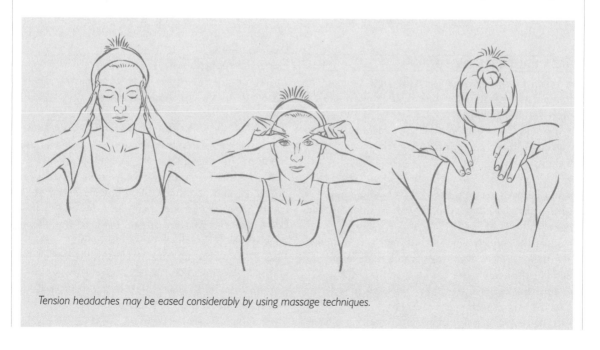

Tension headaches may be eased considerably by using massage techniques.

and firm back support rather than slumping over your desk, or leaning to one side. It is also helpful to be aware that flickering or fluorescent lights can cause particular problems for migraine sufferers, since a flickering light can set off the visual disturbance that is often the first stage of a migraine. The ideal lighting should be bright enough to be able to see clearly and quickly, but not so harsh that it causes eyestrain.

Tension headaches and stress-related migraines can be eased considerably by learning techniques for relaxing and unwinding. These may include learning how to meditate, taking up yoga or having a regular massage. See the general advice included in the section on anxiety (page 237) for helpful hints on ways of stress-proofing your life through breathing techniques and meditation.

It is helpful to bear in mind that eyestrain can also contribute to recurrent headaches. It is a good idea to have a regular eye test in order to eliminate this as a contributing factor. Eyestrain as a cause of headaches can be especially relevant when we reach our forties, since this is a common time for long-sightedness to set in. If you instinctively hold reading material at arm's length in order to read comfortably, it is essential to visit an optician in order to obtain reading glasses.

If postural problems are contributing to recurrent headaches or migraines consulting a teacher of the Alexander Technique may help. Other therapies to consider include acupuncture, chiropractic and osteopathy.

SEEK PROFESSIONAL HELP

• When symptoms occur for the first time, or if they are a new feature (to exclude the possibility of a more serious problem).
• If headaches occur on a daily or recurrent basis, especially if they are present each morning on waking.
• If a headache lasts longer than a day at a time.
• If a headache is accompanied by a high temperature, light sensitivity, vomiting or stiffness in the neck.
• If nausea and drowsiness occur after a head injury.
• If there is severe pain, nausea and/or vomiting on bending the head forwards.
• If painkillers need to be taken regularly in order to ease the pain of recurrent headaches.
• If nausea, blurred vision and vomiting occur, accompanied by severe pain affecting the area within and around one eye.

Alternative treatments

It is worth noting that for headaches and migraines it is quite appropriate to take the relevant internal remedy while also making use of a topical preparation.

Topical preparations

These are essential oils and herbal infusions that can be used to induce relaxation and ease muscular tension. Choose from any of the following, bearing in mind that none of the substances mentioned for external application should be taken by mouth.

Aromatherapy oils

For tension headaches and migraines, use one drop only of peppermint (Mentha piperita) essential oil on a cotton wool bud and rub on top of the forehead at the hairline. For inhalation, use two drops on a handkerchief and, while inhaling keep the handkerchief at least 2.5cm (1in) away from the end of the nose to avoid skin contact.

For menstrual headaches use two drops of clary sage (Salvia sclarea) on a cotton wool bud and gently rub on top of the forehead at the hairline. A lavender (Lavendula angustifolia) and clary sage bath at the end of the day is very relaxing – mix five drops of clary sage with lavender in two teaspoons of sweet almond oil and add to a warm, not hot, bath, agitating the water to disperse the blend. (Use clary sage on the day prior to menstruation and the first day of the period only.)

Herbal preparations

An infusion of rosemary or lavender may be soothing when applied to the affected area. In order to make the infusion, one teaspoon of dried herb should be used for each cup of boiling water. Leave to stand for fifteen to twenty minutes, strain and use warm or cool as required as a local application.

If stress and tension are contributing to tension headaches and migraines, the following herbal soak can be used in a relaxing bath. Mix thoroughly in a bowl: one cup of bran or fine oatmeal, and three cups of dried limeflowers or chamomile flowers. Place the mixture in a muslin bag and soak it in the warm bathwater. Alternatively, make a strong infusion of these herbs (using 50g/2oz of dried herb to every 900ml/1½ pints of water), strain it and add to a warm bath.

Home remedies

• Moistened mint leaves may be very soothing when applied to the temples during a headache.

• Headaches that occur as a result of overexposure to sunshine may respond to the cooling, soothing sensation of slices of raw potato or cucumber placed on the temples and/or the brow of the head.

• Applying vinegar on a cool compress is said to ease the pain and discomfort of a headache.

Medicines intended for internal use

These ease pain and encourage a speedy resolution of the problem.

Home remedies

• Inhaling the fumes of hot malt vinegar has a reputation for clearing the head, while a dash of vinegar may also usefully double up as a substitute for fresh lemon when added to herbal teas.

• An aching head may be eased by chewing fresh basil leaves.

Anthroposophical medicines

Anthroposophical doctors approach the problem of tension headaches and migraines by attempting to correct the fundamental imbalance between the nervous and metabolic systems that is seen to be at the root of the problem, rather than merely patching over the problem by using a short-term painkiller. A preparation called Bidor may be used with a view to rectifying the problem at a fundamental level. Although its use may need to be continued for an extended time for treatment to be effective, this preparation is free of the side effects of conventional medicines used to treat headaches and migraines. As a preventative, one tablet of Bidor 1 per cent may be taken three times daily for up to three months. If an attack occurs, one or two tablets of the 5 per cent may be taken hourly or half-hourly until relief of symptoms is obtained. However, no more than twenty tablets should be taken in any twelve-hour period. Tablets may be swallowed whole with water (this preparation should only be taken under medical supervision due to the nature of the condition).

Flower remedies

Tension headaches that are associated with anticipating a stressful or distressing event, or headaches that follow accident or trauma may respond to Rescue Remedy. Four drops may be added to quarter of a glass of water and sipped as required. If water is not readily available, four drops of Rescue Remedy may be placed on the tongue and repeated as often as necessary.

Biochemic tissue salts

Tension headaches may respond best to Nervone, Combination F or tissue salt No. 6. The latter may be of particular use when an ongoing stressful situation has led to a feeling of physical, mental and emotional burn-out, while Combination F may be of help where migraines have developed in response to nervous tension. Migraines that are connected with biliousness and a tendency to suffer from fluid retention or an irregular urine output in the body may respond to tissue salt No. 11. Low-grade symptoms may be eased by taking three doses a day of the appropriate tissue salt, tailing off the dosage as the situation improves. Problems of a more severe nature or rapid onset may require tablets to be taken at hourly intervals until improvement is obtained.

Herbal preparations

• Feverfew has a reputation for discouraging the onset of migraines. A fresh leaf of the herb can be taken between two slices of bread once a day as a simple preventative treatment.

• An infusion of any of the following may ease tension headaches or migraines: limeflower, valerian, rosemary or vervain. (**NB** The use of rosemary and vervain should be avoided in pregnancy, while valerian should not be used in large doses or over a lengthy period of time, because of its tendency to promote muscular spasms, palpitations and headaches when used incautiously.) In order to make the infusion one cup of boiling water may be added to a teaspoonful of the dried herb. Leave to infuse for fifteen to twenty minutes, strain and sip as a warm drink.

• A cup of meadowsweet tea can soothe the pain of a headache due to the salicylic acid compounds content (related to aspirin) of the flowers and leaves. The tea may be taken three times a day to ease pain and discomfort.

• Headaches and migraines that occur as a result of an accumulation of toxins in the system may be soothed by drinking an infusion of dandelion root. Simmer 25g (1oz) of root in 600ml (1 pint) of water for fifteen minutes. The infusion should be strained and drunk warm.

Professional alternative medical help may be obtained from any of the following:
• Acupressure
• Anthroposophical medicine
• Aromatherapy

HOMOEOPATHIC MEDICINES

Type	General features	Worse	Better	Remedy
Recurrent headaches or migraines brought on by erratic blood-sugar levels	Heavy, throbbing sensation at crown of head with feeling of tightness around brain. Dizziness and disorientation in forehead that is made more intense by bending forward. Needs to eat small amounts regularly in order to keep fatigue and headaches at bay	Excessive physical effort Mid-morning Overheating Sweet foods and sugary drinks Standing for a long time	Walking Movement Fresh air Moderate temperatures	Sulphur
Throbbing headaches that are made much more intense by the slightest movement	Bursting headaches that may be brought on by becoming dehydrated and/or constipated. Dry mouth and skin with marked thirst for cold drinks. Awfully sensitive scalp with pains that are intense from even slight touch. Headache begins above the left eye and shifts to the base of the skull	Becoming too warm The slightest movement Stooping Coughing Eating Touch Physical and mental effort	Peace and quiet Cool surroundings Cool drinks Lying motionless Firm pressure to painful part	Bryonia
Left-sided migraines that come on after sleep	Bursting, constricting pains that extend from the left eye to the side of the nose, or move from left to right side of the head. Dizziness and disorientation are made more intense by closing eyes. Pains may be brought on by overheating or overexposure to sunshine	Overheating On waking In the morning Before or following a period Drinking alcohol Movement	Onset of a discharge (e.g. nose begins to run or a period begins) Cool bathing of affected part Contact with fresh air	Lachesis
Headaches or migraines that are brought about by an excess of alcohol and/or overreliance on prescription drugs	'Morning after' headaches with heavy sensation at the back of the skull. Recurrent sickening headaches with constipation follow too much food, alcohol, smoking and coffee. Awful sensitivity to noise with symptoms at their worst first thing in the morning	On waking Loud noise Becoming chilled Too much coffee Smoking Stress	Warmth Sound, long sleep By the evening and night Peaceful surroundings	Nux vomica
Recurrent cluster headaches associated with puberty, pregnancy or the menopause	Headaches mainly affect the right side with pulsating pains and burning discharge from the eye on the painful side. Dizziness and nausea accompany headaches: both are worse in overheated surroundings. Patient is depressed, fragile and in need of sympathy with headaches	Badly ventilated surroundings Rest In the evening and at night Overly rich, fatty foods Leading up to a period	Cool compresses to painful part Gentle exercise in the fresh air Having a good cry Firm pressure to painful part	Pulsatilla

- Ayurvedic medicine
- Chiropractic
- Homoeopathy
- Naturopathy
- Nutritional therapy
- Osteopathy
- Reflexology
- Shiatsu
- Traditional Chinese medicine
- Western medical herbalism

Neuralgia

The pain and discomfort of neuralgia are caused by inflammation or injury to a nerve. The nerves that can be affected by this problem commonly include those of the face (where the disorder may be called trigeminal neuralgia), or those of the back of the leg (called sciatica, see page 211).

Symptoms may include the following:
- Burning or shooting pains.
- Bouts of tingling and/or numbness in the affected area.

Practical self-help
See practical self-help sections for sciatica (page 212), shingles (page 230) and multiple sclerosis (page 340).
- In addition, it is helpful to make sure that the full range of vitamin B complex is taken because of its role in supporting the nervous system. This may be done by including the following foods in the diet: green leafy vegetables, broccoli, brewer's yeast and mushrooms.
- If life has been particularly stressful, it may be helpful to take a vitamin B complex supplement in order to make sure that levels of this vitamin are boosted.

If symptoms of neuralgia are persistent a professional medical opinion should be sought.

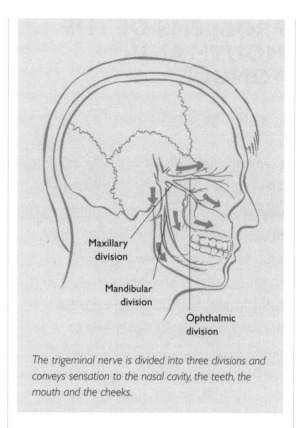

The trigeminal nerve is divided into three divisions and conveys sensation to the nasal cavity, the teeth, the mouth and the cheeks.

Alternative treatments
Since neuralgia can fall into the category of chronic because of its tendency to recur, it is best to seek alternative medical advice from any of the following:
- Anthroposophical medicine
- Aromatherapy
- Biochemic tissue salts
- Chiropractic
- Cranial osteopathy
- Homoeopathy
- Naturopathy
- Osteopathy
- Reflexology
- Shiatsu
- Traditional Chinese medicine
- Western herbal medicine

PROBLEMS OF THE MOUTH AND TONGUE

Cold sores

Cold sores can occur after a cold or other infection, when a person is run down, or after exposure to wind and/or sunshine. The first attack may be symptomless, or may cause ulcers on the mouth and lips, together with an illness resembling influenza. Subsequently the virus lies dormant, and can become active to cause itching, tingling discomfort and painful, crusting blisters.

Once the cold sore has healed, the virus will remain dormant in the system until it is reactivated by stress or the additional factors mentioned above. If reappearance of a cold sore occurs, this heralds the second stage of infection when a blister may form on the lips or beneath the nostrils. When the blister bursts, it develops the encrusted appearance of a cold sore.

Practical self-help

• The *herpes simplex* virus that causes cold sores can be transferred or carried by a toothbrush. Once a blister has appeared, it is important to use a fresh toothbrush in order to prevent spreading infection.
• If you are prone to cold sores, always use an ultra-violet lip block when going out in windy, sunny weather, especially around water or at the seaside, or if you are at altitude or on snow, as these increase your UV exposure due to reflection.
• If you have a cold sore do not kiss anyone who does not have them, and avoid oral sex, even if you only have the tingling that can preclude the onset of blistering.
• Make sure that cold sores are kept as dry and clean as possible in order to minimize the risk of further infection.

• Foods that should be avoided because they may encourage or aggravate cold sores include chocolate, seeds and nuts. Those that help the body fight infection include regular helpings of fresh, raw fruit and vegetables, whole grains, pulses and small portions of fish and dairy products.

SEEK PROFESSIONAL HELP

• If cold sores become a recurrent, or severe problem as a direct result of being run down or in poor health.
• If any symptoms of pain or infection develop in the eyes.

Alternative treatments

It is worth noting that when a cold sore has developed, it is quite appropriate to take the relevant remedy internally, while also applying a topical preparation to the skin.

Topical preparations

These are lotions, tinctures or creams that can be applied to the skin to soothe and heal. Choose from any of the following, bearing in mind that none of the substances mentioned for application to the skin should be taken by mouth.

Aromatherapy oils

Use two drops of ravensar (Ravensara aromatica) on a cotton wool bud and dab on the affected area three to four times a day.

Herbal preparations

Diluted Hypericum tincture may be applied to the affected area in order to speed up the healing process and to ease the discomfort of cold sores. One part of tincture should be added to ten parts of boiled, cooled water.

Flower remedies

Rescue Remedy cream may be applied as often as necessary to the cold sore in order to ease tingling and discomfort and to moisturize the affected area.

Home remedies

• Gel or juice of the aloe vera plant may be very soothing when applied to a cold sore.
• Dabbing a cold sore with witch hazel encourages the blistered area to dry up more speedily.

Medicines intended for internal use

These ease discomfort, reduce inflammation and encourage a speedy resolution of the problem.

HOMOEOPATHIC MEDICINES

Type	General features	Worse	Better	Remedy
Recurrent cold sores affecting the mouth and lips	Cold sores develop after contact with sunlight and windy weather or in response to a viral infection such as a cold. Dry lips with a tendency to crack in the middle. Tingling or numb sensation of lips	Exposure to sunlight Hot weather Salt, sea air Touch	Contact with cool air Bathing with cool water Rubbing	Natrum mur
Cold sores with dry lips that crack in the corners	Crusty, scurfy cold sores around the mouth and lips. Numb, crawling sensations in cold sore, which begins as a blister. Symptoms appear on the left side or move from left to right	Contact with damp, cold air Becoming chilled At rest Jarring movements	Warmth Rubbing Changing position Warm, dry conditions	Rhus tox
Cold sores affecting the lips, lobes of the ears and corners of the mouth	Lower lip becomes dry, cracked and swollen with cold sores. Worn out, exhausted, depressed and run down with symptoms. Tendency to develop warts as well as cold sores	Contact with cold Before a period Pregnancy Touch Rubbing Scratching	Warmth Warm compresses Open air	Sepia
Cold sores that affect the area above the upper lip	Stitch-like, cutting pains in cold sores that may bleed very readily. Lips become dry, cracked and scabby with a sensation of feeling too tight. Easy-bruising skin with a tendency for wounds to heal slowly	On the left side Touch Contact with cold air Eating too much salt	Bathing the face with cool water Rubbing	Phosphorus

Biochemic tissue salts

Cold sores may be encouraged to resolve more speedily by using Combination Remedy D. Four tablets may be taken three times a day, reducing the frequency as symptoms improve. If cold sores cause severe problems, the treatment may be continued for three days after symptoms have cleared up.

If cold sores appear on a recurrent basis, help may be obtained from a practitioner working in any of the following therapies:
- Anthroposophical medicine
- Homoeopathy
- Nutritional therapy
- Naturopathy
- Traditional Chinese medicine
- Western medical herbalism

Gingivitis (inflamed, bleeding gums)

Gingivitis is a commonly experienced condition that leads to the development of red, inflamed, swollen and shiny gums that bleed very readily when they are cleaned. It is a problem that usually develops as a result of food particles lodging at the base of the teeth, leaving the gums vulnerable to swelling and infection. As time goes by, more food deposits occupy the area around the base of the teeth, leading to the formation of a pocket of infection between the gum and the tooth. If the situation is further neglected, a more severe condition may develop, such as destructive gum disease, which can lead to loosening and loss of teeth.

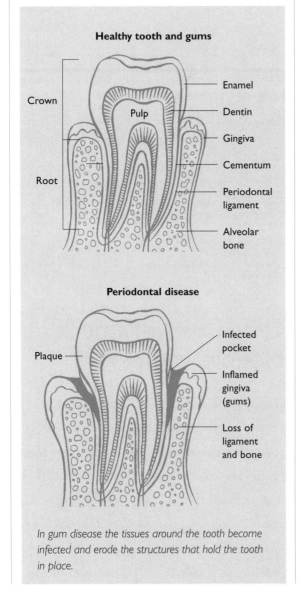

Healthy tooth and gums

Crown

Pulp

Enamel

Dentin

Gingiva

Cementum

Root

Periodontal ligament

Alveolar bone

Periodontal disease

Plaque

Infected pocket

Inflamed gingiva (gums)

Loss of ligament and bone

In gum disease the tissues around the tooth become infected and erode the structures that hold the tooth in place.

Practical self-help

• If there are any indications of sensitivity or bleeding from the gums, make sure that oral hygiene is kept to a very high standard. This may be done by brushing teeth each morning and evening with an anti-plaque toothpaste and using dental floss on a daily basis to remove food particles that may cling to the spaces between the gums and the teeth. Disclosing tablets (which show plaque deposits on the teeth) may be used in order to establish how effectively this is being done.

• Visit your dentist and dental hygienist regularly in order to have your teeth descaled if there are signs of a build-up of calculus (the chalky, hard deposit on the base of your teeth that traps food particles). By flossing and brushing teeth correctly, and taking your dentist's general advice about oral hygiene, it should be possible to discourage the development of serious gum disease.

• Make sure that your diet contains a high proportion of fresh, raw fruit and vegetables, and the minimum of sugary, sticky food and drinks, which can contribute to problems with teeth and gums.

• If you feel that gum inflammation is linked to a general state of poor resistance to infection, increase the amount of vitamin C-rich foods in your diet (such as tomatoes, green peppers, strawberries, citrus fruits and kiwi fruit), or take a course of vitamin C in supplement form.

If you experience swollen, sensitive or bleeding gums that do not respond to the measures suggested above, professional help should be sought from your dentist.

Alternative treatments

It is worth bearing in mind that in the case of gingivitis, it is quite appropriate to take a relevant remedy internally, while also using a local preparation as a rinse or mouthwash.

Topical preparations

These are lotions, tinctures or mouthwashes that can be rinsed around the mouth to encourage healing and discourage the development of infection. Choose from any of the following, bearing in mind that none of the substances mentioned should be swallowed.

Aromatherapy oils

Make a solution using four drops of tea tree oil (Melaleuca alternifolia) in half a glass of spring water

HOMOEOPATHIC MEDICINES

Type	General features	Worse	Better	Remedy
Easy-bleeding, spongy-looking gums	Bad breath with poor-quality teeth and bluish-tinged, inflamed gums. Lips may also look very red and bleed easily	Cold Eating Touch During a period	Warmth Warm food Movement	Kreosotum
Readily bleeding gums on touch or cleaning teeth	Sensitive gums with unpleasant taste in mouth which may be bitter, sour or mouldy. Poor-quality teeth with toothache and swelling of the cheeks. Dry mouth without thirst	Warmth On waking Eating Pressure Before a period	Cool compresses Movement	Lycopodium
Severely infected gums with loose teeth	Well-established gum disease with oozing blood from gums from pressure of cleaning teeth. Unpleasant sour or bitter taste from mouth with bad breath. Chewing causes pain in gums while teeth are sensitive to hot or cold things	Warmth Extreme temperatures Contact with cold air	Fresh air Being fanned	Carbo veg
Easy-bleeding gums with sharp, splintering pains	Swollen sore, flabby gums with loosened teeth that seem spongy and soft. Poor-quality, yellow-tinged teeth with a tendency to cavities. Discoloured, fissured tongue	Touch Jarring movements After eating Contact with cold air	Moderate temperatures	Nit ac

and rinse the mouth by bubbling the mixture around the mouth morning and evening before cleaning the teeth. Do not swallow the solution.

Herbal preparations

• An anti-infective, immunity-boosting mouthwash may be made by dissolving half a teaspoonful of echinacea tincture in half a glass of water. Rinse the mouth twice or three times a day, ensuring that the liquid is distributed into all the crevices of the mouth.

• Propolis tincture may also be used to soothe inflamed, swollen gums. Use the same proportions as those given above for the echinacea mouthwash.

Home remedies

• Local circulation of the gums may be stimulated by brushing the teeth daily with cayenne powder.

• Garlic or vitamin E oil rubbed into the inflamed area will encourage the gums to harden and heal.

Medicines intended for internal use

These ease sensitivity, reduce inflammation and encourage a speedy resolution of the problem.

Home remedies

• Strawberries have a reputation for keeping teeth white and free of plaque, as well as bilberries, blackcurrants and cherries. They should be chewed slowly in order to give ample opportunity for their antiseptic properties to be utilized to the full.

• Sunflower and sesame seeds are also reputed to contain minerals that contribute to developing healthy gums and strong teeth.

Biochemic tissue salts

Tissue salt No. 4 may be helpful in the early stage of inflammation. Four tablets may be taken at the first sign of symptoms, and repeated three times a day until the problem has eased.

Herbal preparations

Drinking rosehip or blackcurrant leaf tea may ease inflammation of the gums that is due to a deficiency of vitamin C or vitamin B.

A recurrent tendency to gingivitis may benefit from professional help from any of the following therapies:
- Anthroposophical medicine
- Ayurvedic medicine
- Naturopathy
- Nutritional therapy
- Traditional Chinese medicine
- Western medical herbalism

Gum disorders

See advice given for gingivitis (page 131) and mouth ulcers (below).

Mouth ulcers

Mouth ulcers occur when the protective lining of the mouth is broken, exposing the sensitive area beneath. Factors that can trigger off ulceration include becoming generally run down or unwell, eating very hot food, rough use of a toothbrush or accidentally biting the tongue or mouth. Occasionally, mouth ulcers may also develop as a consequence of infection such as the herpes simplex virus, which causes cold sores. With herpes simplex, blisters form in the mouth and become ulcers.

We are most likely to become aware of a developing ulcer when we experience the pain, discomfort or smarting that follows eating spicy, salty or acid foods. If we investigate the sensitive area further, we are likely to see a yellow-coloured spot that has a red, inflamed border. Ulcers may occur as large single lesions or in clusters or groups affecting the gums, cheeks or tongue.

Practical self-help

- If an ulcer has occurred as a result of injury from badly fitting dentures, or the broken or rough edge of a tooth, remove the cause of the problem as soon as possible.
- Avoid acid, salty or overly spicy foods to minimize discomfort.
- Soothing, antiseptic mouthwashes and rinses may also ease discomfort and encourage speedy healing of the damaged area.
- If mouth ulcers occur as a result of feeling generally unwell or under the weather, consider taking a good-quality multivitamin and mineral supplement in addition to improving the overall quality of your diet.
- If you suffer from recurrent colds or infections as well as mouth ulcers, take a vitamin C supplement to boost the immune system and discourage further infection. Take 500mg twice a day until the situation has improved. The dose should be reduced if you begin to suffer from digestive problems such as stomach acidity or diarrhoea, or if there is a history of kidney stone formation.

SEEK PROFESSIONAL HELP
- If recurrent ulcers are a problem.
- If an ulcer fails to heal within a three-week period, as this can indicate cancer.

Alternative treatments

It is worth noting that if ulcers have developed, it is quite appropriate to take the relevant remedy internally while also using a local application to speed up the healing process.

Topical preparations

These are tinctures, lotions or mouthwashes that can be applied to the affected area in order to soothe and speed up healing. Choose from any of the following, bearing in mind that none of the substances mentioned for local use should be swallowed.

Aromatherapy oils

Dab ulcers with either tea tree (Melaleuca alternifolia) or ravensar (Ravensara aromatica) essential oil on a cotton wool bud. After ten minutes, rinse the mouth with spring water.

Herbal preparations

• Rinse the mouth with a solution of diluted Hypericum, an effective pain-reliever, and Calendula, an antiseptic, tincture. One part of tincture should be dissolved in ten parts of boiled, cooled water and rinsed around the mouth as often as necessary.

• A soothing infusion may be made from sage or Calendula by adding a cup of boiling water to a teaspoon of dried herb, leaving it to steep and straining off the liquid, which may be used as a mouthwash.

Home remedies

• Lemon juice may be used in warm water as a healing mouthwash.

• Two teaspoons of sea salt can be dissolved in a large glass of warm water and used as a simple

HOMOEOPATHIC MEDICINES

Type	General features	Worse	Better	Remedy
Mouth ulcers with increased saliva	Sweet, metallic taste in the mouth with ulceration and swelling of tongue. Unpleasant taste in the mouth with dribbling of saliva at night. Raw, sore pains in ulcerated areas	At night Becoming heated Extreme heat or cold Contact with anything cold	Moderate temperatures Rest	Mercurius
Recurrent ulcers with offensive breath	Ulceration of the gums and tongue during pregnancy or during a period. Gums look bluish, puffy or spongy and bleed very easily. Burning, pulsating, fiery pains in ulcerated areas	In pregnancy Contact with cold Eating Touch Teething	Firm pressure Movement Warmth Contact with warm food	Kreosotum
Ulceration of mouth and tongue that burns and smarts on contact with food	Mapped appearance to tongue with sores and ulceration. Heavy or tingling sensations in the tongue with a feeling of dryness. Ulceration may follow eating excessive amounts of salt or a period of extreme emotional stress	Heat Contact with acid foods Touch Pressure	Cool liquids Fresh air	Natrum mur
Ulceration of gums and tongue with stitch-like pains	Extremely painful ulcers that are sensitive to touch and strong tastes. Cutting, stinging pains in ulcerated areas. In small children ulcers occur, or may be aggravated, when teething	Touch Cold drinks At night Emotional stress or strain	Warmth Resting	Staphysagria
Spongy, bluish ulcers on gums and tongue	Dryness of mouth with ulceration. Burning pains in ulcers and tongue. Bitter, sour, salty or foul taste in mouth in morning	Cold drinks Contact with cold foods Contact with cold air Eating ice cream, watery fruits, smoking or alcohol	Warmth Sips of warm drinks Distraction	Arsenicum album

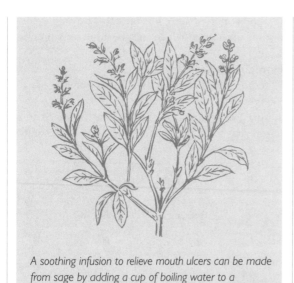

A soothing infusion to relieve mouth ulcers can be made from sage by adding a cup of boiling water to a teaspoon of dried herb.

mouthwash as often as required.
• Vitamin E oil may stimulate healing when applied neat to the ulcerated area.

Medicines intended for internal use

These ease pain, reduce inflammation and encourage a speedy resolution of the problem.

Biochemic tissue salts

Ulcers and sores in the mouth may respond to tissue salt No. 3: take four tablets three times a day until symptoms improve.

A tendency to develop recurrent mouth ulcers may be helped by consulting a professional from any of the following therapies:
• Anthroposophical medicine
• Ayurvedic medicine
• Biochemic tissue salts
• Homoeopathy
• Naturopathy
• Nutritional therapy
• Western herbal medicine

Toothache

Toothache is usually a sign that a tooth is decaying and that prompt dental

treatment is required. Pain and inflammation around the gum may also suggest that an abscess has developed (see 'Boils' on page 219).

If toothache develops that is severe or recurrent, seek dental advice as soon as possible.

Alternative treatments

These suggestions may be helpful in temporarily easing pain. It is quite appropriate to take a relevant remedy internally, while also using a local preparation as a rinse or mouthwash. However, they should not be regarded as a substitute for appropriate dental treatment.

Topical preparations

These are lotions, tinctures or mouthwashes that can be rinsed around the mouth to relieve pain. Choose from any of the following, bearing in mind that none of the substances mentioned should be swallowed.

Aromatherapy oils

Wash the affected part of the face with hydrolat of laurel on a cotton wool bud. Paint a blend of five

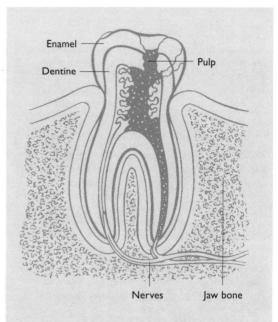

Once the enamel of a tooth has been damaged, bacteria will eat their way through to the pulp chamber, resulting in inflammation and pain.

HOMOEOPATHIC MEDICINES

Type	General features	Worse	Better	Remedy
Early stage of inflammation with marked heat and redness of gum	When used promptly, this remedy can prevent abscess formation. Affected area is bright red and radiates heat. Sharp, piercing pain, throbbing, shooting pains develop rapidly, violently and intensely	Touch Jarring movement	Resting	Belladonna
Toothache with terrific sensitivity to cold draughts of air	Painful area is hypersensitive to cold draughts. Splintering, sharp pains in boils and abscesses.	Cold draughts Undressing Touch Lying on painful part At night	Warmth Wrapping up warmly Humidity	Hepar sulph Hepar sulph encourages 'drawing' process and speedy discharge of pus
Pain in teeth following dental work	Extreme sensitivity to touch and movement. Bruised pains in sensitive area.	Jarring Touch After sleep	Lying with head lower than the body	Arnica Arnica is effective in reducing bruising and swelling after dental work

drops of Roman chamomile (Chamaemelum nobile) mixed with two teaspoons of sweet almond oil or gel base over the inflamed area. Repeat at hourly intervals for four hours. Always seek the advice of a dentist if pain is persistent.

Herbal preparations

Tincture of myrrh may be applied to the inflamed and painful area.

Home remedies

• Cotton wool soaked in onion or garlic juice may be used to temporarily plug a cavity before getting to the dentist.

• Adults may gain relief by soaking a piece of cotton wool in whisky or brandy and plugging the cavity.

• Temporary relief and comfort may be gained by applying a warm flannel to the painful area of the face.

Medicines intended for internal use

These ease sensitivity and provide temporary pain relief.

Biochemic tissue salts

Tissue salt No. 8 may be taken hourly until the pain eases.

RESPIRATORY PROBLEMS

Asthma

Attacks of asthma vary tremendously in severity and seriousness. Some sufferers experience mild tightness of the chest and a slight wheeziness, while others have extreme difficulty breathing and feel as though the chest is encased in a tight band. Although many people with childhood asthma grow out of the problem by their teens, it has been identified as a condition that is affecting a growing proportion of adults and children.

Although attacks of asthma may occur for no obvious

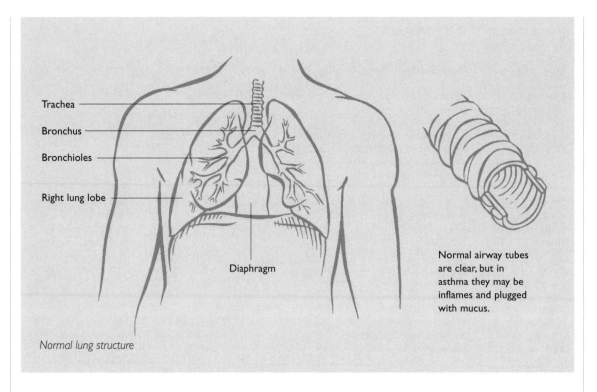

Trachea

Bronchus

Bronchioles

Right lung lobe

Diaphragm

Normal airway tubes are clear, but in asthma they may be inflames and plugged with mucus.

Normal lung structure

reason, there are certain triggers that are readily identified as being responsible for the onset of an attack. These may include any of the following:

• An allergic reaction to house dust mite, animal fur, chemical colourings, additives or preservatives in food, or dairy foods.

• Chest infections.

• Exercise in sharp, cold air.

• Inhalation of chemicals that irritate the air passages.

• Emotional stress, panic or extreme anxiety.
   Symptoms of asthma include:

• Lack of breath with a sensation of painless tightness in the chest.

• Slight or very noisy wheeziness.

• Sweating.

• Increased pulse rate.

• Anxiety.

• In a severe attack, the diminished amount of oxygen circulating in the bloodstream may cause the lips and face to have a bluish tinge.

• Pale, cold, clammy skin.

• Some asthma attacks may be accompanied by a cough because of the accumulation of phlegm in the lungs. Asthma sufferers may also cough in an attempt to relieve the feeling of breathlessness.

• Children may vomit during an asthma attack.

Practical self-help

• Cut down where possible on exposure to potential allergens (triggers that set off an allergic reaction). These may include any of the following: dust, fungal spores (for example, from mould growing in damp housing), pollen, household chemicals, sprays and cleaners, eggs, shellfish, nuts or milk, feathers, pet animals, such as cats and dogs.

   Practical ways of managing contact with possible allergens include dusting and vacuuming each day, avoiding pillows that are stuffed with duck down, choosing fibre-filled pillows instead, and having as limited a contact as possible with airborne pollens. This may be done by staying indoors when the pollen count is high and ensuring that windows and doors are kept shut when the season is well under way.

• If a mild asthma attack is brought on by walking in sharp, cold winds, it may be helpful to sip a warm drink while attempting to relax.

• If wheezing occurs at night, avoid lying flat, as it can make breathing more difficult. Instead, sit propped up on two or three pillows, or try leaning forwards with your elbows supported on the back of a chair. Make a conscious effort to relax your whole body as much as possible while doing this, concentrating on

HOMOEOPATHIC MEDICINES

Type	General features	Worse	Better	Remedy
Nervous asthma with wheezing that is aggravated by lying down	Breathless and wheezy with asthma which is worse for becoming chilled or laughing. Burning sensation in chest with extreme anxiety and restlessness. Coughing bouts may be brought on by cigarette smoke or contact with strong odours	At night Early hours of the morning Chill Physical effort	Warmth Sips of warm drinks Gentle movement Company Fresh air to the head	Arsenicum album
Attacks of asthma that are aggravated by the least movement	Cold sensation of the chest with discomfort during coughing spasms. Difficulty in raising mucus: it can only be brought up with the greatest effort. Sour, unpleasant taste in the mouth	Cold draughts of air Becoming overheated During the winter Stooping Motion Touch	Sitting forward with elbows on the knees During the day Fresh air Warmth	Kali carb
Shortness of breath with a dislike of anything near the mouth	Hiccoughing before an asthma attack. Coughing spasms are eased by cold drinks and aggravated by breathing deeply. Painful tightness of the lower part of the chest	After anger or fright Too much mental or physical stress Touch Movement Raising arms Loss of sleep In hot weather	Cool drinks	Cuprum met
Asthma and breathlessness that are much worse in stuffy, overheated rooms	Smothering feeling when lying down or when lacking contact with fresh, cool air. Has to sit up at night in order to breathe. Asthma gets worse when skin eruptions such as eczema are suppressed by use of topical steroid creams	Overheated rooms Lying flat In the evening At night After eating In pregnancy or puberty	Cool, fresh air Cool drinks or food Undressing Gentle exercise in the fresh air Sitting propped up Having a good cry	Pulsatilla

breathing as evenly and slowly as possible.

• Do not let any pets sleep on the bed, even during the day.

• Dairy products such as milk, cheese, cream and yoghurt should be eliminated from the diet where possible. Dairy foods have a reputation for being potential allergy triggers, and also contribute towards mucus production. As a result, they can aggravate chest problems such as asthma and bronchitis. However, goats' milk appears to be of definite benefit to those who suffer from chest problems, and may be included in the diet in the form of milk,

yoghurt and cheese. Treat convenience foods containing a high proportion of chemical additives and preservatives, peanuts and shellfish with caution.
• If your reactions to stress are contributing to your problems, investigate techniques that can help you cope. These may include meditation, relaxation techniques, hypnotherapy or stress counselling.

SEEK PROFESSIONAL HELP

• If a severe asthma attack occurs and any of the following symptoms are observed:
• Rapid, shallow breathing
• Increased pulse rate, or weak pulse
• Loud wheezing
• Pale, clammy or blue-tinged skin or lips
• Extreme anxiety or panic
• If a severe chest infection develops in an asthmatic.
• If previously mild and infrequent asthma attacks become more frequent and severe.

Asthmatics should always seek professional conventional or alternative treatment for their condition, rather than relying on self-help measures, because of the chronic and, in some cases, potentially life-threatening nature of the condition. This is especially the case if asthma is combined with hay fever and/or eczema.

Alternative treatments
Home remedies
• It has been suggested that a small glass of carrot juice taken each day, or a diet high in vitamin C may reduce the risk of asthma attacks.
• A teaspoon of hot lemon juice taken with or without honey appears to ease chest problems by discouraging mucus production.
• Two cloves of fresh raw garlic should be eaten each day to reduce congestion in the chest.
• Mix one tablespoon of castor oil with one tablespoon of cider vinegar and take daily in order to ease asthma symptoms and catarrh.
Biochemic tissue salts
Temporary relief of minor symptoms may be offered by taking Combination J or tissue salt No. 6. The latter is most useful for attacks of asthma that are brought on by fear or anxiety, while the former is more suitable for seasonal asthma that may be worse in the autumn and winter. If symptoms are severe, tablets may be taken hourly (a medical opinion

should also be sought), or in milder situations tablets may be taken three times daily until improvement has been obtained.
Herbal preparations
• If nervousness or anxiety are contributing to problems with asthma, a warm, soothing cup of lemon verbena tea may help calm the nerves and relax the chest.
• An infusion of equal parts of liquorice (to be avoided in those who have high blood pressure) with chamomile and limeflowers may be helpful in acting as an expectorant and supporting the nervous system. In order to make the infusion, 30g (1oz) of dried herb should be steeped in 600ml (1 pint) of hot water for ten to fifteen minutes before straining.

It is important to stress that the remedies listed above are not mentioned in order to encourage self-help prescribing for asthma. Instead they are suggestions of appropriate remedies that may be helpful in giving short-term relief for mild, acute symptoms. For long-term improvement to be given the best chance to occur, it is essential to seek professional alternative help from practitioners who are trained in any of the following:
• Acupressure
• Anthroposophical medicine
• Aromatherapy
• Chiropractic
• Homoeopathy
• Naturopathy
• Nutritional therapy
• Osteopathy
• Shiatsu
• Traditional Chinese medicine
• Western medical herbalism

Bronchitis

Bronchitis occurs when the mucous lining of the bronchial tubes becomes inflamed. This leads to constant episodes of coughing, as the body attempts to expel the mucus blocking the airways. Bronchitis may occur in acute episodes of limited duration following a cold or sore throat, or may become a chronic problem leading to long-term breathing difficulties. The latter can be a health problem of serious proportions, causing early death in those who suffer severely from the condition.

Symptoms of acute bronchitis may include any of the following:
• Persistent coughing with production of grey, yellow or green phlegm
• Wheezing
• Fever
• Breathlessness
• Pain and discomfort in the upper area of the chest when coughing.

Although anyone may develop acute bronchitis as a complication of a heavy cold or flu, there are certain factors that may predispose us to the problem. These include smoking, suffering from asthma, exposure to atmospheric pollution or persistently damp, cold conditions. However, the main cause of chronic bronchitis is smoking. Infection may cause symptoms to suddenly worsen as additional lung damage destroys the last of the respiratory reserve.

Practical self-help
• Giving up smoking is one of the most important things a bronchitis sufferer can do, since continuing to smoke after attacks of bronchitis have developed will perpetuate the problem. If you are a heavy smoker and have found it difficult to give up in the past, seek as much help and support as possible in order to give up the habit. This may involve using nicotine chewing gum or patches initially, or learning ways of replacing the smoking habit with other activities (such as having a hot drink instead of a cigarette). By consciously becoming aware of the circumstances in which you enjoy smoking, you can adjust yourself to doing other things that may distract you, or may be more pleasurable than smoking. Alternative therapies such as homoeopathy, acupuncture, herbalism and hypnotherapy can also provide a great deal of help and support for those who are trying to come to terms with an addiction to smoking. (See section on addictions on page 236.)
• During an attack of acute bronchitis it is essential to rest as much as possible in surroundings that are neither too hot nor too chilly. Use a humidifier to counteract the dry atmosphere that central heating creates, or place bowls of water near each radiator or fire to moisten the air.
• Avoid smoky atmospheres and coming into contact with people who are known to be in the infectious stage of a cold. The latter is important because those who have long-term problems with bronchitis may find that catching even a slight cold can lead to severe chest problems.
• Avoid mucus-forming dairy foods, opting instead for a largely raw diet that includes a high proportion of raw fruit and vegetables (avoiding dried fruit and bananas as their high sugar content means that they can be mucus-forming). Increase your fluid intake by drinking spring water and fruit juice, which enables you to support your body's detoxifying mechanisms and deal with infection more easily and efficiently.
• See advice given in the coughs section on page 148 for additional ways to help with acute bronchitis.

SEEK PROFESSIONAL HELP
• If symptoms do not improve considerably within 48 hours.
• If body temperature rises above 40°C/102°F.
• If the patient becomes breathless.
• If recurrent chest infections occur after every cold, however mild.

Alternative treatments
It is worth noting that those who suffer from chronic or severe bouts of acute bronchitis should only make use of self-help measures in addition to conventional or alternative professional medical help. This is due to the potential seriousness of severe bronchitis, which requires skilled case management in order to avoid complications.

Topical preparations
These are essential oils, inhalations or rubs that can be applied to the skin to soothe and ease congestion. Choose from any of the following, bearing in mind that none of the substances mentioned for application to the skin should be taken by mouth.
Anthroposophical medicines
Plantago comp ointment (containing plantago and camphor*) may be massaged into the chest morning and night to soothe congestion. However, because of

the inclusion of camphor, this ointment should not be used for children under three years old. (Ingredients marked with a * may interfere with the action of homoeopathic remedies.)

Aromatherapy oils
Make a chest/back rub by blending four drops of any of the following oils in two teaspoons of sweet almond oil, olive oil or one teaspoon of gel base: Eucalyptus globulus (not to be used for small children), sweet green myrtle (Inula graveoleus), ravensar (Ravensara aromatica) or Scots pine (Pinus sylvestris). Use morning and evening. A few drops of essential oil on a tissue to inhale during the day is also useful.

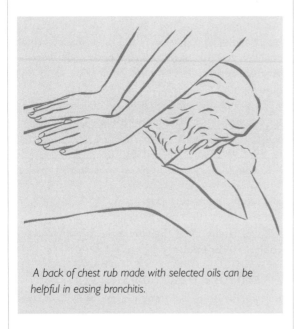
A back of chest rub made with selected oils can be helpful in easing bronchitis.

Herbal preparations
See 'Coughs' on page 151.

Home remedies
A simple inhalant may be made by chopping up several cloves of garlic and adding them to a bowl of boiling water. See 'Home remedies' suggestions in the coughs section (page 149) for additional helpful ideas.

Medicines intended for internal use
These ease coughing spasms, reduce congestion and encourage a speedy resolution of the problem.

Home remedies
• Hot carrot juice has a reputation for easing bronchitis and generally supporting the body in its fight against infection.
• A soothing hot toddy may be made by adding the grated zest of half a thoroughly scrubbed lemon to a glass of hot wine and honey.

Biochemic tissue salts
Combination Remedy J may be used to ease autumn or winter coughs and chestiness. Alternatively, tissue salt No. 4 may be helpful in the first stage of a chesty cough. For mild or infrequent symptoms, take four tablets three times daily, and repeat the dose hourly for more severe chest symptoms.

Home remedies
• If phlegm is greenish in colour, garlic-flavoured honey may be useful in keeping infection at bay. Cover four garlic cloves with 100ml (3oz) of clear honey. Cover, leave the mixture to stand overnight and strain off the juice. Take a teaspoonful of the honey several times a day.
• A mixture of sliced ginger root and a pinch of cayenne may be helpful where phlegm is white and abundant. Add the mixture to an infusion of herbs such as white horehound, coltsfoot, hyssop, yarrow or elderflower. Equal measures of herbs should be infused in 600ml (1 pint) of boiling water before straining for use. However, care should be taken to restrict the use of hyssop to no more than 1–2g to be taken no more than three times daily. See additional information in 'Herbal preparations' in the coughs section (page 00).

A tendency to attacks of severe or recurrent bronchitis may be helped by professional treatment from any of the following therapies:
• Acupressure
• Anthroposophical medicine
• Ayurvedic medicine
• Aromatherapy
• Homoeopathy
• Naturopathy
• Nutritional therapy
• Shiatsu
• Traditional Chinese medicine
• Western herbal medicine

HOMOEOPATHIC MEDICINES

Type	General features	Worse	Better	Remedy
Full-sounding chest with very little mucus raised	Coughing fits and lack of breath are eased by lying on the right side. Suffocating sensations with shortness of breath and rattling, thick mucus. Has to sit up to breathe more easily or cough	Warm rooms Lying down Movement Milky drinks Becoming angry	Bringing up mucus Lying on the right side Sitting upright	Ant tart
Extreme breathlessness and anxiety with bronchitis	Difficulty in breathing and increased wheeziness when lying down. Coughing bouts are increased by laughing, turning over in bed, or contact with strong odours. Alternately dry and loose cough	As the night goes on Early hours of the morning Chill or cold Physical effort	Warmth Sips of warm drinks Gentle movement Sitting propped up in bed Fresh air	Arsenicum album
Very dry, painful cough that is worse for the slightest movement	Hard, dry cough that is brought on by eating or drinking. Sharp pains in chest or at the right shoulder blade. Coughing spasms begin on walking into a warm room. Has to press hands to chest to reduce pain	Movement Stooping Coughing Physical effort Taking a deep breath Eating Drinking Early morning	Firm pressure to painful area Cool, fresh air Sitting up	Bryonia
Violent, incessant coughing bouts with retching in the winter	Gasps between coughing spasms which cause flushed or blue-tinged appearance. Terrible nausea with severe coughing bouts: may vomit once coughing fit is over. Rattling in chest with difficulty raising mucus	Movement Warmth Damp conditions Heat and cold Vomiting Lying down	Fresh air Resting Pressure	Ipecac
Loose, violent coughing spasms with shortness of breath	Chest feels improved by sitting and keeping still. Piercing pain shoots through the left side of the lower chest. Constant problems with chest from catching the least cold. Loose, green phlegm	Contact with warm air Damp weather Pressure Late evening Lying in one position	Fresh air Changing position Lying on the back	Nat sulph

Catarrh

Although a certain amount of fluid mucus is required for the lubrication of the membranes that line the nose, throat and lungs, too much or too little can result in problems. These may appear as a tendency to blocked or congested nostrils, a constantly running nose or an irritating and persistent tendency to clear the throat before speaking. Coughs or earaches can also be an indication of a catarrhal problem.

Practical self-help

• It is best to avoid foods that have a reputation for encouraging mucus production. These include cows' milk and dairy products made from cows' milk, eggs, meat and animal fats, white flour, white sugar and chemical additives.
• Include as many wholefoods as possible in your diet, such as raw fruit, vegetables, salads, whole grain cereals, spring or filtered water and garlic.
• Making a point of taking regular exercise in the

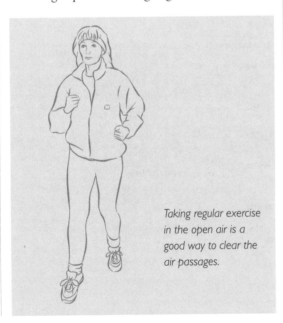

Taking regular exercise in the open air is a good way to clear the air passages.

open air is also recommended as a way of clearing the air passages. Avoid anything that is too strenuous if you are generally unfit, and begin with some brisk walking or short cycle rides.
• Don't smoke, and stop others from smoking in the house.

SEEK PROFESSIONAL HELP

• If general sensations of malaise and high temperature accompany catarrhal problems.
• If nasal discharge is unpleasant-smelling, yellow or green in colour.
• If marked or severe sinus pain occurs that fails to respond to self-help measures within twenty-four hours.
• If catarrhal problems are well established, or occur on a recurrent basis.

Alternative treatments
Topical preparations

These are essential oils or inhalants that can be used externally to ease congestion. None of the preparations listed below should be taken by mouth.

Aromatherapy oils

Put a few drops of Eucalyptus globulus (not to be used for small children), ravensar (Ravensara aromatica) or spike lavender (Lavendula latifolia) on a tissue to inhale during the day. Four drops of any of these essential oils added to two teaspoons of sweet almond oil or a teaspoon of gel base can be used as a chest/back rub morning and evening.

Home remedies

Add the freshly squeezed juice of half a lemon to a cup of warm water. Inhale the warm mixture gently through the nostrils, taking it to the back of the nose.

Medicines intended for internal use

These ease pain, reduce congestion and encourage a speedy resolution of the problem.

Anthroposophical medicines

See suggestions made for anthroposophical treatment of sinusitis on page 159.

Biochemic tissue salts

Tissue salt No. 7 may be useful for mucus secretions that have become thick and yellow. Generally speaking, this is likely to happen in the more established stage of congestion. Combination Q is suitable for catarrhal symptoms that are combined with sinus problems.

Herbal preparations

Golden rod, peppermint, hyssop* or elderflower may be made into an infusion by using one part of each of the herbs mentioned (*only small amounts of this herb should be used: 1–2g, with a maximum dose of twice daily). Lemon juice or honey may be added for flavour in addition to their favourable effect on the mucous membranes. Alternatively, if catarrh is clear and watery, add two slices of fresh ginger to the infusion.

Homoeopathic medicines

See homoeopathic suggestions for sinusitis on page 158. In addition, consider the homoeopathic remedy Natrum mur for catarrhal discharges that are either thin, fluent and clear like uncooked egg white, or thick and obstructive. Those who require Natrum mur may alternate between these two states, while being subject to repeated bouts of uncontrollable sneezing.

A tendency to attacks of severe or recurrent catarrh may be helped by professional treatment from any of the following therapies:

- Anthroposophical medicine
- Aromatherapy
- Ayurvedic medicine
- Homoeopathy
- Naturopathy
- Nutritional therapy
- Shiatsu
- Traditional Chinese medicine
- Western medical herbalism

Colds

The misery of the symptoms of the common cold, although not a serious threat to health, can drastically reduce your quality of life for several days. If additional complications set in, such as sinus problems or persistent catarrh, this can lead to further weeks of discomfort after the original cold has left. You are particularly vulnerable to repeated bouts of infection through the winter if you are suffering from prolonged or severe stress, leaving you with the feeling that you have had one long, permanent cold.

From this rather gloomy perspective, alternative treatments have an enormous amount to offer, since they approach the problem by attempting to boost the body's own healing mechanism, enabling us to feel that we can cope with the symptoms of a cold more easily. Alternative treatments may also speed up the process of a cold, thereby reducing the risk of complications.

The average cold is likely to go through three identifiable stages. Symptoms of the initial stage may include sneezing, soreness or irritation of the throat and a general feeling of unwellness. The second phase is likely to develop into a full-blown head cold, with attendant symptoms of blocked or streaming nose, further irritation in the throat and possible dry cough. At this point mucus discharges should be generally clear in colour. By the last stage, there may be a loose cough, or it may alternate between dry and productive coughing bouts. By this third stage, mucus will probably have taken on a yellowish-green colour, and the nose and ears may feel blocked and congested.

Although these three stages are commonly experienced by cold sufferers, it is possible to experience the first two stages without the third, or to move swiftly through the initial stage without too much trouble, only to find that the last phase seems to go on for ever.

Practical self-help

- Make a deliberate point of resting as much as possible in the early stages of a cold to help your body fight infection effectively. If you keep going, you may end up taking weeks, rather than days to get over the illness. Rest in the early stages of illness will reduce time spent off work overall, and avoids spreading infection to colleagues and friends during the infectious stage (which we are likely to do when we are up and about).
- Keep liquid intake high to flush toxic by-products out of the body as quickly and efficiently as possible. The ideal liquids are water and fresh fruit juice; avoid drinks that have diuretic (fluid-eliminating)

properties, such as tea and coffee. If warm drinks are attractive because they are soothing to the throat, choose refreshing, fruit-based herb teas, or cereal-based coffee substitutes rather than Indian tea or coffee. Also avoid adding milk to hot drinks because dairy products encourage mucus production, which can make chest, sinus, and nasal congestion worse. Avoid alcoholic drinks, as these are dehydrating.

• If your appetite is reduced don't feel obliged to eat, as long as you drink plenty. Foods should be as light and easily digestible as possible, with a strong emphasis on vegetable soups, broths, salads and lightly cooked fish or chicken. Avoid high-fat, indigestible foods such as cheese, red meat and pastries, and do not drink alcohol during the course of the illness. The latter depletes the body of vitamin C, and puts extra strain on the liver, which has to work extra hard to detoxify the body during illness.

• Stay in a stable, moderate temperature, avoiding extreme changes from hot or cold as much as possible. Being exposed to rapid or severe variations in temperature puts extra strain on the body.

• As soon as the first symptoms appear, take a 1000mg vitamin C supplement daily for the duration of the cold. If this causes acidity of the stomach or diarrhoea, reduce the dose (you can also buy 500mg or 250mg tablets) until the digestion settles down once again. Although it is an issue of debate whether vitamin C prevents the development of a cold, there is evidence that using this vitamin in supplement form will shorten the duration of the illness. As a result, it can be helpful to take a limited course of vitamin C as soon as possible after exposure to the cold virus, or as soon as there is any indication that symptoms are developing. Anyone who suffers from kidney stones should avoid using vitamin C supplements for extended periods. Most kidney stones are made of calcium salts, but anyone who suffers from rarer oxalic acid-type kidney stones should be extremely cautious in their use of vitamin C.

• If chest or sinus problems are persistent after developing a cold, take garlic supplements, which are naturally antibacterial and encourage the breakdown of thickened, discoloured mucus.

SEEK PROFESSIONAL HELP

• If severe or persistent cold symptoms develop in the very young or the very old.

• If earache appears as a complication in a young child.

• If feverishness develops in the very young or very elderly that does not improve after using self-help measures.

• If laboured, wheezy or difficult breathing is experienced during a cold, especially by those who have not previously suffered from asthma.

• If a patient who has previously suffered from rheumatic fever develops a sore throat or throat infection.

Alternative treatments

For a cold it is quite appropriate to take the relevant remedy internally, while also using a topical preparation.

Topical preparations

These are lotions, tinctures or oils that can be used externally. Choose from any of the following, bearing in mind that none of the substances mentioned for external use should be taken by mouth.

Aromatherapy oils

A few drops of Eucalyptus globulus (not to be used for small children), ravensar (Ravensara aromatica), spike lavender (Lavendula latifolia) or tea tree (Melaleuca

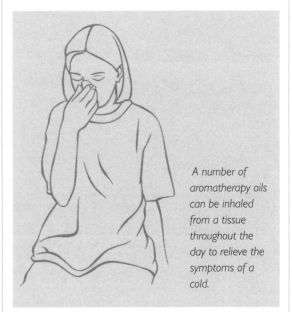

A number of aromatherapy oils can be inhaled from a tissue throughout the day to relieve the symptoms of a cold.

alternifolia) can be inhaled from a tissue during the day. Four drops of any of these oils can be added to two teaspoons of carrier oil or one teaspoonful of gel base for a chest/back rub to be used morning and evening. A few drops of lavender or tea tree can also be added to a bath.

Home remedies

• Warm footbaths have a reputation for easing cold symptoms. One tablespoon of mustard powder should be dissolved in 2 l (3½ pints) hot water, and the feet should be bathed for ten minutes twice a day while symptoms are troublesome.

• Make a strong brew of onions or garlic by simmering in water that has been brought to boiling point.

The steam from the mixture should be inhaled through the nose in order to clear nasal passages.

• Gargling with the following may soothe inflamed or painful throats. One teaspoon of salt and vinegar should be added to a teacup of home-made barley water. However, great care should be taken not to swallow the mixture.

HOMOEOPATHIC MEDICINES

Type	General features	Worse	Better	Remedy
First stage of a cold with earache and sore throat	Swollen, sore throat that is very painful when swallowing. Diminished hearing with ear pains. Becomes alternately pale and flushed in the initial stages of a cold	Chill Jarring Cool drinks Night	Cool compresses Lying down	Ferrum phos
Initial stage of a rapidly developing cold that sets in after exposure to cold winds	Sudden onset of symptoms with feverishness, dry, hot throat and marked thirst. Tonsils feel dry and swollen and make swallowing difficult. Dry nasal passages or hot, scanty nasal discharge. Terribly anxious and restless with high temperature	At night Exposure to cold winds or chill Touch Bright light Noise	Fresh air Rest	Aconite
Violent, abrupt onset of symptoms with high temperature	Skin is generally bright red, hot and dry. Nose and throat are also bright red and inflamed. Severe inflammation of throat makes it difficult to swallow. Irritable and intolerant when ill	Lying flat Jarring Noise Touch Bright light Stimulation	Rest Being lightly covered Resting propped up in bed	Belladonna
Chilly and restless with burning pains that are eased by warmth	Scanty, burning discharges from eyes and nose, with burning discomfort in throat that is eased by warm drinks. Tight, wheezy chest with dry cough: sits propped on pillows in order to breathe. Emotional and physical symptoms get worse at night	At night Lying down Chill Physical or mental effort Being alone	Sitting propped up in bed Warmth Sips of warm drinks Warm applications Company	Arsenicum album
Head colds with streaming clear nasal discharge that runs like a tap	Obstructed breathing from stuffed-up feeling high in the nose. Cold sores with cracked, dry lips and nasal discharge that is either clear, watery and runny, or like uncooked egg white. Severe bouts of sneezing that are made worse by hot sun	Touch Noise Heat Sunlight Making an effort	Fresh, cool air Cool bathing Cool compresses Skipping meals Being left in peace	Natrum mur

Medicines intended for internal use

These ease feverishness, reduce congestion and encourage a speedy resolution of the problem.

Home remedies

Fresh garlic, cayenne pepper, onions and watercress should be included in the diet in order to prevent and treat cold symptoms.

• A basic hot honey and lemon drink may be made even more soothing by adding cinnamon, cloves, ginger or cayenne and a slice of lemon to 600ml (1 pint) of water. Bring the liquid to boiling point, simmer for fifteen minutes and strain. Drink every couple of hours, sweetened with honey to taste.

Biochemic tissue salts

Combination J or tissue salt No. 4 may be effective in reducing feverishness and inflammation in the first stage of a cold. If symptoms are severe, tablets should be taken every hour until relief is obtained. For milder symptoms, take four tablets three times daily until symptoms improve, tailing off the dosage accordingly.

Herbal preparations

• Elderflower or peppermint make soothing herbal teas that settle the queasiness that often accompanies feverishness and the congestion of a head cold. They may be taken with a pinch of mixed spice and a little honey to soothe a painful throat. However, it is important to be aware that peppermint tea may interfere with the beneficial action of homoeopathic remedies.

• Basil tea, made from the fresh or dried herb, may be used to encourage a slight sweat in the early stages of a cold, thus reducing feverishness. A pinch of ground cloves may also be added for flavour and encourage reduction of fever.

Coughs

Persistent, irritating coughing can be one of the most exhausting and enervating symptoms left behind after a heavy cold or bout of influenza. Most conventional medicines such as cough suppressants work by dampening down the coughing reflex, *thus temporarily reducing the severity or frequency of coughing spasms.*

Alternative approaches, however, regard a cough as a necessary mechanism employed by the body in ridding itself of excess mucus or phlegm. When this reflex acts efficiently and effectively, we are able to bring up the phlegm that leads to congestion of the chest, which should make breathing easier. Provided this mechanism works well, we should find that we recover from a cough within a reasonable amount of time with the minimum amount of complications. This is why alternative approaches concentrate on supporting the body in its efforts to loosen and bring up (expectorate) phlegm, rather than discouraging the coughing reflex, which can lead to the problem continuing for longer.

Unproductive, dry coughs may cause bouts of spasmodic coughing that occur at exhaustingly regular intervals. In such a situation, an appropriate alternative remedy can loosen the cough, dislodging mucus. Alternative remedies can also ease the discomfort of the muscular aching in the chest that often accompanies continued, spasmodic coughing bouts.

Practical self-help

• If a cough is especially disturbing at night, avoid taking a milky drink before going to sleep. Dairy products in general appear to contribute to mucus production, resulting in extra chest congestion. Also avoid products made from cows' milk such as cheese, yoghurt and cream.

• Avoid sleeping flat at night, which can aggravate chest problems. Instead, try resting propped up on two or three pillows; this allows the chest to expand and relax more naturally.

• Increase the amount of raw garlic taken in the diet, or take a garlic supplement if the taste is unappealing. Garlic is an important item in the diet because it encourages the breakdown of mucus and phlegm, and because of its antibacterial properties. If it is taken in supplement form, two capsules or tablets should be taken three times a day until improvement occurs. If chestiness is a predictable problem during the winter, discourage problems by taking a course of garlic for the winter months.

• When a cough is dry and croupy, being in a steamy atmosphere can help a great deal, especially if the cough is generally worse for exposure to a dry, cold atmosphere. Try steam inhalations, or spend time in a hot shower or steam-filled bathroom.

• Centrally heated or air-conditioned surroundings can also aggravate a cough. Use a humidifier to counteract the dryness in the atmosphere, or place bowls of water near each fire or radiator. Top up the bowls as the water evaporates.

SEEK PROFESSIONAL HELP

• If a stubborn cough does not respond to self-help measures within a few days.

• If a persistent cough is associated with reduced energy levels or a general decline in well-being.

• If breathing difficulties or distress occur in small children.

• If there is any suspicion that a cough has appeared as a result of a foreign body being inhaled.

• If coughing is accompanied by severe chest pain.

• If severe coughing spasms occur in the elderly or the very young.

• If there are any signs of wheeziness in anyone who does not suffer from asthma.

• If drowsiness or confusion accompany a severe cough.

Alternative treatments

For a cough it is quite appropriate to take the relevant remedy internally, while also applying a topical preparation to the skin.

Topical preparations

These are essential oils or creams that can be applied to the chest in order to soothe a cough and ease congestion. Choose from any of the following, bearing in mind that none of the substances mentioned for application to the skin should be taken by mouth.

Aromatherapy oils

• Gargle four times a day with four drops of tea tree (Melaleuca alternifolia) oil in spring water.

• Blend four drops of any of the following oils: tea tree, sweet green myrtle (Inula graveoleus) or Eucalyptus globulus (not to be used for small children) with two teaspoonfuls of carrier oil or one teaspoonful of gel base and rub onto the throat and chest four times daily.

Home remedies

• Tickling in the throat may be eased by gargling with lemon juice, cider vinegar or salt dissolved in warm water.

• A soothing rub for the chest may be made by

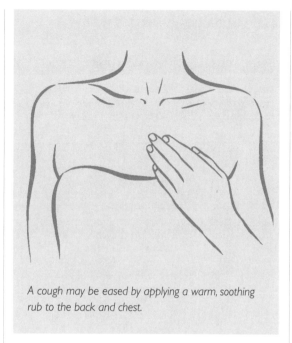

A cough may be eased by applying a warm, soothing rub to the back and chest.

chopping six cloves of garlic, placing them in a bowl and steaming them over a pan of simmering water. Add the contents of a small jar of white petroleum jelly to the same bowl as the garlic slices, cover and simmer for several hours. Use warm to rub the back and chest.

Medicines intended for internal use

These ease irritation and encourage a speedy resolution of the problem.

Home remedies

• Slice a large onion into rings and place in a bowl. Cover with clear honey and leave the mixture to stand overnight. Strain off the liquid in the morning, and use as a cough syrup. A dessertspoonful of this mixture may be taken four or five times a day as an expectorant.

• An irritating night-time cough may be soothed by dissolving a tablespoon of blackcurrant jam in a cup of warm water. The mixture can be sipped as often as needed during the night.

Anthroposophical medicine

Coughs that arise as a complication of head colds may be soothed and loosened by a cough elixir.

Biochemic tissue salts

Irritable or irritating coughs may be eased by taking Combination J, while more spasmodic, convulsive coughs may be eased by Combination H. For mild, or infrequent symptoms, take four tablets three times

HOMOEOPATHIC MEDICINES

Type	General features	Worse	Better	Remedy
Dry, irritating, tickly cough with aching chest muscles	Persistent, unproductive cough from tickling in the throat. Constant impulse to take a deep breath, which makes the cough more irritating. Presses hands firmly to painful area of chest in order to keep it still. Headache and irritability with cough	Slightest movement Deep breathing Exposure to dry cold or heat Overheated rooms Light touch	Keeping still Fresh, cool air Firm pressure Sitting upright	Bryonia
Harsh cough with established cold and congestion in sinuses	Brassy-sounding cough which begins with irritation in the throat. Unproductive coughing fits with terrible difficulty in bringing up ropy, sticky, stringy mucus. Pains radiate to back and shoulders during a coughing spasm. Raw feeling under breastbone with cough that is aggravated by eating	Undressing Cold, damp air Waking from sleep Alcohol Stooping	Movement Pressure Heat	Kali bich
Coughing spasms that are set off by touching the throat	Breathlessness and choking spasms from persistent coughing. Constant episodes of coughing prevent sleep. Burning, raw sensations in chest are made more intense by drawing a deep breath. Frothy, thin, copious phlegm	Pressure on the throat Deep breathing Moving from one temperature to another Eating Contact with cool air	Covering the mouth Wrapping up warmly	Rumex
Tight chest with loss of voice and yellow-coloured phlegm	Burning in the chest with alternating dry and loose cough. The effort of coughing leads to exhaustion and strained, aching abdominal muscles. Episodes of coughing are brought on, or made more intense by exposure to temperature changes	In the morning and evening Lying on the left side Talking Strong odours Anxiety	After a sound sleep Rest Being massaged Reassuring company	Phosphorus
Lingering cough that remains after a head cold with thick, greenish-yellow phlegm	Dry cough in the evening and night alternates with loose, phlegmy cough in the morning. Sweet, bitter or salty tasting thick phlegm. Resting, lying and keeping still make the chest feel more uncomfortable. Symptoms are generally worse for warm, stuffy, badly ventilated surroundings	Warmth Stuffy, overheated rooms After eating Rest Morning, evening	Exposure to fresh, cool air Gentle exercise in the open air Undressing Attention Sympathy	Pulsatilla

a day, and repeat the dosage at hourly intervals for more severe coughing spasms.

Herbal preparations

• Make an infusion of white horehound and marsh mallow by mixing together an equal proportion of each herb and adding a teaspoonful to a cup of boiling water. Sweeten with honey to taste and take one teaspoonful of the mixture three times daily as an expectorant.

• Coltsfoot may also be used as a valuable herb for chesty coughs, possibly because of its high vitamin C content. Steep 25g (1oz) of the dried herb in 600ml (1 pint) of cold water. Bring the liquid to boiling point, remove from the heat, cover and leave to infuse for ten minutes. Strain and drink a cupful of the infusion four times a day until coughing has eased.

• Painful coughs may be soothed by taking a mixture of honey infused with elecampane root. Place one cup of clear honey, a cup of water and one cup of elecampane root in a saucepan and bring gently to the boil. Once the root has become soft, strain the liquid and pour into a clean glass bottle.

Hay fever (allergic rhinitis)

Allergic rhinitis may occur as a seasonal problem (in the form of hay fever in the spring and summer), or it may occur all year round. Symptoms are a result of an airborne substance (such as pollen or house dust mite droppings) triggering an allergic or hypersensitive reaction in the eyes, nose and throat. Contact with the irritant (often referred to as an allergen) sets off the release of histamine, which results in inflammation and fluid production in the delicate linings of the nose and eyes.

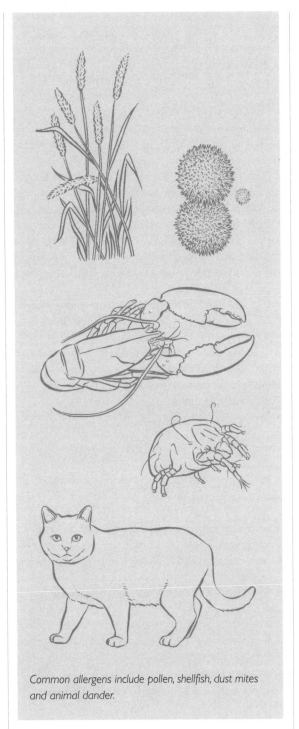

Common allergens include pollen, shellfish, dust mites and animal dander.

Symptoms can result in mild irritation or great distress, depending on the severity of the attack in the individual, and may include any of the following:

• Irritated, bloodshot, watery eyes that may feel very gritty.

• Itching of the eyes and eyelids making it very difficult to avoid rubbing the irritated area. Rubbing results in temporary relief, but usually ends up making the eyelids and the delicate area around the eyes extremely puffy and swollen.

- Nasal discharge.
- Dry, itchy throat, wheezing or itchy skin.

Practical self-help

- Bathing eyes and nasal passages as often as possible with cold water may be very soothing. Inhale steam if airways feel sensitive or inflamed.
- If pollen counts are known to be high, it is helpful to stay indoors when possible. Pollen counts are useful on a population basis, but not necessarily. A very high pollen count may not include the particular pollen that affects you, but a low pollen count at another time of year may make symptoms appear. Most pollens are seasonal, so you will know from experience which time of year is worst for you.
- Increase water intake substantially, avoiding diuretic (fluid-eliminating) drinks such as tea or coffee.
- Try to avoid rubbing your eyes.
- Where possible, avoid exposure to additional irritants such as animal fur, dust, fungal spores (from mould) or perfumes, that may aggravate eye, nose and throat symptoms.
- Wearing good-quality sunglasses may help ease eye symptoms, but contact lenses should be avoided since they can irritate the eyes, making them even more sensitive.
- A vitamin C supplement with citrus bioflavinoids works as a natural antihistamine in large doses (2–3g a day). However, the dose should be reduced if digestive upsets occur, such as acidity of the stomach or diarrhoea. Those who have a tendency to develop kidney stones should also use vitamin C supplements with caution.
- Since lack of vitamin B may intensify allergic reactions, consider taking a vitamin B complex supplement before and during the hay fever season.
- If you are sensitive to house dust mites and their droppings, dust and vacuum your house daily, keep your mattress covered with a plastic sheet, and air beds each day by exposing the bottom sheet to the fresh air.
- Increase humidity in your home by using a custom-made humidifier, or by putting a bowl of water near each radiator or heater.

Alternative treatments

In cases of hay fever, although it is perfectly appro-priate to take the relevant remedy internally while applying a topical preparation to the skin, hay fever and allergic rhinitis are chronic conditions. As a result, treatment should be sought from a trained practitioner in order to achieve the most successful, long-term outcome. However, any of the following may give temporary relief.

Topical preparations

These are lotions or tinctures that can be applied to the skin to soothe and heal. Choose from any of the following, bearing in mind that none of the substances mentioned for external use should be taken by mouth.

Herbal preparations

- Bathing the eyes with diluted Euphrasia tincture reduces inflammation and discomfort. It is especially soothing to itchy, sore eyes with or without a discharge. It can be used as a cool compress for the eyes by soaking cotton wool pads in diluted tincture, which may be applied to closed eyelids. Four drops of tincture should be added to 150ml (5fl oz) of boiled, cooled water.
- Cotton wool can be saturated with yarrow tea to bathe itchy, irritated eyelids.

Home remedies

- Cool ordinary tea bags may be very soothing to the eyes when placed on closed eyelids. Soak them in warm water and place in the fridge ready for use on irritated eyes and eyelids.
- Alternatively, soak cotton wool pads in icy-cool witch hazel and apply to the eyes.
- Red rose petals may be used as a soothing and cooling compress if eyelids feel inflamed or irritated.

Medicines intended for internal use

These ease discomfort, reduce inflammation and encourage a speedy resolution of the problem.

Biochemic tissue salts

Take biochemic tissue salt Combination H as early as possible in the season to build up resistance over the summer. Take four tablets three times a day if symptoms are mild, tailing off the dosage as symptoms improve. However, tablets may be taken at hourly intervals if symptoms are in a very severe phase.

The remedies listed above are not mentioned in order to encourage self-help prescribing for hay fever, but are suggestions of appropriate remedies that may be helpful in giving short-term relief for

HOMOEOPATHIC MEDICINES

Type	General features	Worse	Better	Remedy
Fast-developing puffy swelling of eyes and throat	Stinging, itchy feelings in the eyes and throat with heat sensitivity. Puffy, rosy-red looking eyes with waterlogged, swollen eyelids. Stinging, watery tears from eyes with sensitivity to light	Warmth or heat Resting After sleep Touch	Cool bathing Contact with open, fresh air Cool compresses Movement	Apis
Hay fever with burning nasal discharge and bland tears	Sensitivity to smells of flowers and fruit leads to repeated sneezing. Acrid, burning discharge from the nose that burns the upper lip. Extremely profuse, watery discharge from the eyes	In the evening Humid, damp weather Warmth	Cool, fresh air Bathing Motion	Allium cepa
Hay fever with burning tears from the eyes and bland nasal discharge	Hot, burning tears, with a sensation as though the eyes are swimming in water. Profuse, bland discharge from the nose. Eyelids look red, inflamed and sore	Indoors Windy conditions Warmth In the evening	Blinking or wiping the eyes Fresh, open air	Euphrasia
Hay fever with thick, bland, yellowish-green discharge	Symptoms are generally made more intense by contact with warmth in any form. Nasal obstruction at night with runny nose during the day. Craving for cool, fresh air. Depressed and weepy	In the evening At night Warmth Badly ventilated, stuffy rooms Lying down	Cool bathing Cool compresses Contact with fresh, cool air Having a good cry Attention and sympathy	Pulsatilla
Hay fever with violent symptoms from the smell or thought of flowers	Extremely sensitive sense of smell with profuse nasal discharge. Incomplete episodes of sneezing leave one nostril blocked at a time. Dry, tickling sensation begins in the nose, spreading over the whole body	Strong smells Cool air Cold drinks Mental effort	Swallowing Warmth Fresh, open air	Sabadilla

mild, acute symptoms. For long-term improvement seek professional alternative help from practitioners trained in any of the following:
- Anthroposophical medicine
- Ayurvedic medicine
- Homoeopathy
- Naturopathy
- Nutritional therapy
- Traditional Chinese medicine
- Western medical herbalism

Influenza

Those of us who have suffered from a bout of influenza will know only too well that there is a great deal of difference between the symptoms of a heavy cold and flu. The latter is a severe illness that leads to intense exhaustion and debility. As a result, we generally cannot keep on our feet when we suffer from flu, since the general sense of aching and unwellness associated with the illness gives us no choice other than to take to our beds.

flu symptoms may include any of the following:
- General feelings of lethargy and unwellness
- Feverishness
- Shivering
- Muscle aches
- Sore throat
- Swollen glands
- Nausea
- Loss of appetite
- Nasal discharge

Complications associated with flu may include any of the following:
- Depression
- Exhaustion and poor physical stamina
- Sinusitis
- Bronchitis.

However sobering this list might sound, it is important to be aware of the positive measures we can employ to boost and protect our immunity in order to fight off flu viruses effectively. On the other hand, once flu has set in, there are numerous practical steps that can speed up our rate of recovery and minimize the risks of complication or a relapse.

Practical self-help
- Friendly foods that appear to increase resistance to infection and improve vitality include the following: fresh, raw fruit and vegetables, whole grains, garlic, pulses, beans, small helpings of fish, nuts and seeds.

Filtered or mineral water should be drunk on a regular basis to encourage the detoxifying processes of the body, and fresh fruit juices should be included in the diet rather than fruit squashes or carbonated drinks. Eating sea plants or algae can remineralize the body after overexposure to processed foods. Spirulina, alfalfa, chlorella or seaweeds can be added to soups or juices in powder or capsule form.

- Increase the proportion of vitamin C-rich foods in the diet, such as tomatoes, raw green peppers, strawberries and citrus fruit. This vitamin is easily destroyed by the process of oxidation, so do not leave peeled, chopped fruit or vegetables to stand for a long time before eating. Overcooking also leads to loss of vitamin C, especially if fruit or vegetables are boiled. Vegetables and fruit are best eaten raw, and if vegetables must be cooked, steam them, which preserves essential nutrients.
- As the liver is responsible for efficient detoxification of the body, avoid food and drinks that put extra strain on it. These include convenience foods containing substantial amounts of chemicals such as colourings and preservatives, and alcohol, which also depletes the body of vitamin C.
- Taking a vitamin C supplement as soon as the first symptoms of flu develop can do a great deal to support the body in its fight against infection. Take 1000mg each day while illness lasts, ideally divided into four 250mg doses. Reduce the dosage if digestive problems occur, or if there is a history of kidney stone formation.
- Once symptoms such as aching, shivering and a general feeling of weakness or lethargy have appeared, rest as much as possible to help the body fight infection.
- Avoid exposure to extreme changes of temperature when feverish, as this puts extra strain on the body.
- In the early, feverish stages of flu it is much more important to drink rather than eat, especially since appetite is likely to be absent or diminished in this stage of the illness. Water, fruit juices and herbal teas are ideal.
- If you have a history of sinus or chest problems following a previous bout of flu, make a point of taking a garlic supplement at the first opportunity. Take two tablets three times a day until mucus production has slowed down dramatically, or until the colour of mucus becomes clear rather than yellow or green.

HOMOEOPATHIC MEDICINES

Type	General features	Worse	Better	Remedy
Slow-developing symptoms with general sense of lethargy	Extreme tiredness, heaviness and listlessness with aching and shivering. Eyes look glassy and eyelids appear heavy and drooping. Face is dusky red and lips look cracked and dry. Wants to lie down all the time and be left in peace	Physical or mental effort Chill or contact with cold draughts Becoming overheated Direct sunlight Dwelling on symptoms	Fresh air Stimulants Sweating Headache is relieved by passing water	Gelsemium
Severe flu symptoms with extreme aching deep in the bones	Bruised feeling in the muscles, with awful generalized aching pains in the bones. Chilly, restless and weak with pains in the limbs, back and chest. Soreness in chest muscles from constant coughing. General feelings of sluggishness and nausea	Lying on painful parts Mornings Becoming chilled Movement Coughing Sight or smell of food	Vomiting Sweating Being spoken to	Eupatorium perfoliatum
Secondary stage of flu with severe sore throat and swollen glands	Sweaty, achy and shivery from head to foot with severe discomfort in glands. Thick, offensive, greenish nasal discharge and phlegm. Aches and pains, anxiety and general uneasiness are all much worse at night	At night Sweating Damp, cold conditions Overheating Extreme changes of temperature	Moderate warmth Rest	Mercurius
Extreme debility with restlessness from aching muscles	Sore, aching and heavy body. Moves about the bed in an effort to get comfortable: mattress feels too hard. Dark red, swollen throat with great difficulty in swallowing solid food: can only swallow liquids	Humidity Pressure On waking Cool air		Baptisia
Lingering, well-established flu symptoms with depression and weepiness	Sinus and chest problems with thick, greenish-yellow mucus from nose and chest. Alternating dry and loose cough that is productive at night and dry in the morning. Unusual symptoms of dry mouth without thirst. Chilliness with aggravation of symptoms from warmth	Overheated, airless surroundings Rest Warm food and drinks At night or in the evening Lack of attention	Gentle movement Cool, fresh air Cool food and drinks Having a good cry Sympathy and attention	Pulsatilla

• Dairy foods and sugar should be avoided since they are thought to aggravate mucus production. Bearing this in mind, it is best to avoid a milky drink at night if you have chest problems, since this can contribute to congestion of the chest by morning.
• If a chesty cough or tight chest is a problem at night, avoid sleeping completely flat. Sleeping propped up on two or three pillows may do a great deal to help make breathing easier.

SEEK PROFESSIONAL HELP

• If you have chronic heart, lung, kidney or liver conditions or if your immune system is low.
• If sore, aching muscles and general weakness are accompanied by severe headache, stiff neck and/or sensitivity to light.
• If a high temperature (40°C/102°F) occurs in babies, small children or the elderly.
• If a sore throat develops in someone who has previously suffered from rheumatic fever.
• If persistent high temperature and exhaustion develop in an otherwise healthy adult.

Alternative treatments

For influenza it is quite appropriate to take the relevant remedy internally, while also using a topical preparation.

Topical preparations

These are lotions, tinctures or oils that can be used externally. Choose from any of the following, bearing in mind that none of the substances mentioned for external use should be taken by mouth.

Aromatherapy oils

Use ravensar (Ravensara aromatica) in a body rub under the direction of a professional aromatherapist. Influenza is a serious illness and requires specialized treatment. Use Eucalyptus globulus hydrolat (but not on small children) on a cotton wool pad to wash the chest, throat and neck.

Home remedies

See advice given in the colds section (pages 147-8).

Medicines intended for internal use

These ease feverishness, reduce congestion and encourage speedy resolution of the problem.

Anthroposophical medicines

Infludo, following directions given.

Biochemic tissue salts

Combination J or tissue salt No. 4 may be effective in reducing feverishness and inflammation of the throat, nasal passage or nerve endings (causing general aches and pains) in the early stages of influenza. If symptoms are severe, tablets should be taken every hour until relief is obtained. For milder symptoms, take four tablets three times daily until symptoms improve, tailing off the dosage accordingly.

Herbal preparations

A comforting herbal tea may be made from an infusion of equal measures of elderflowers, peppermint and hyssop. However, only small doses of hyssop should be taken (no more than 1–2g three times daily).

See additional advice under 'Herbal preparations' in the section on colds (page 148).

Consult table of homoeopathic remedies included in the colds section on page 147 for additional remedies that may be useful in the early stages of flu.

Sinusitis

Sinusitis is a painful condition that arises when the mucous membranes of the sinuses become inflamed as a result of a bacterial or viral infection. Areas most likely to be affected include the maxillary sinuses (in the cheeks) or the frontal sinuses (above the eyes). The micro-organisms responsible for sinus infection travel to the sinuses from the nose, often as a result of a cold.

Possible symptoms include:
• Breathing difficulties as a result of blockage or obstruction of the nasal passages.
• Recurrent headaches affecting the eye sockets, cheekbones or the bridge of the nose.
• A feeling of pressure or fullness in the head and face when bending forwards.
• Persistent, thick, yellow or green mucus.
• Recurring, offensive taste in the mouth and unpleasant smell in the nose.
• Pains in the upper jaw that may resemble toothache; this may be worse when walking.

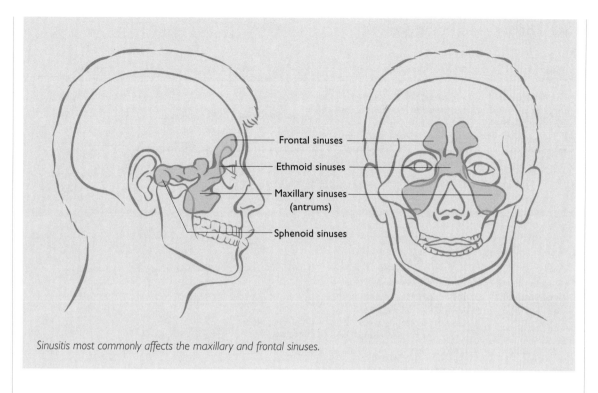

Frontal sinuses
Ethmoid sinuses
Maxillary sinuses
(antrums)
Sphenoid sinuses

Sinusitis most commonly affects the maxillary and frontal sinuses.

Practical self-help

• If you catch a cold, take a garlic supplement at the first sign of symptoms. Take two garlic tablets three times a day while symptoms persist in order to discourage infection. Also take 1000mg vitamin C supplements once or twice a day to shorten the duration of the cold and to minimize risk of complications. Reduce the dose if digestive upset occurs. Drink six to eight large glasses of water a day, and foods should be kept as light and fresh as possible, including portions of raw or steamed fruit and vegetables, salads and fresh fruit juices.

• Avoid foods that encourage mucus production: sugary foods or cows' milk products.

• Fresh air soothes blocked and congested nasal passages, and counteracts the dehydrating effect of heating systems by using a humidifier or putting bowls of water near each fire or radiator. Steamy atmospheres (such as hot showers or steam-filled bathrooms) may also be helpful in easing blocked air passages.

• Resist the temptation to blow the nose too violently if the sinuses are painful, as it may make the pain worse. Blow the nose gently into a disposable paper tissue, which should be thrown away, rather than reusing handkerchiefs, which can lead to reinfection.

• If nasal discharge is persistently bloodstained. A few drops with the original cold doesn't matter, but if persistent this may indicate a polyp or tumour.

• If general sensations of feeling ill and high temperature accompany sinus pain.

• If nasal discharge is unpleasant-smelling, yellow or green in colour.

• If severe sinus pain fails to respond to self-help measures within twenty-four hours.

• If sinus problems are well established, or occur on a recurrent basis.

Alternative treatments

For sinusitis it is quite appropriate to take the relevant remedy internally, as well as using external applications.

Topical preparations

These are essential oils that can be used in steam inhalations and aromatic baths. Choose from any of the following, bearing in mind that none of the substances mentioned for external use should be taken by mouth.

Aromatherapy oils

Make a blend of two drops of each of the following:

HOMOEOPATHIC MEDICINES

Type	General features	Worse	Better	Remedy
Discomfort, sneezing and nasal obstruction that are much worse for cold air	Offensive, thick, yellowish nasal discharge with soreness at the bridge of the nose. Pains and discomfort radiate to, or settle in the bones of the face. Bad-tempered and easily irritated when ill and in pain	Chill Contact with cold draughts of air Undressing Physical or mental effort During the night Touch Noise	Humidity Wrapping up warmly Warmth in general	Hepar sulph
One-sided sinus pain with yellow or blood-streaked nasal discharge	Eyes feel heavy, painful and tired: eye sockets feel tender. Nasal discharge alternates between dry and fluent. Congested, swollen and inflamed nasal passages with oversensitivity to smells	Lying on the back Lying on the tender side Cool, fresh air in the evening Mornings	Bathing the face in cool water Sound, uninterrupted sleep Having a massage	Phosphorus
Sinusitis with persistent or severe pain that affects the bridge of the nose	Unpleasant, offensive smell in the nostrils from impacted mucus. Pressure and pain in sinuses above the eyes and the nose. Nasal mucus is ropy, stringy, greenish in colour and is extremely difficult to dislodge	Stooping or bending forwards Contact with cold, open air Cold and damp Sleep Alcohol	Firm pressure Warmth Movement	Kali bich
Sinusitis with severely blocked nasal passages that are made worse by stuffy rooms	Sinus pain and headaches that feel considerably relieved by contact with fresh, open air. Stuffed up, congested nasal passages that feel worse at night and in the evening. Nasal discharge flows freely in the morning. Generally depressed, weepy, and in need of care and attention when ill and in pain	Warm compresses Overheated, badly ventilated rooms Lying down Evenings At night Being alone	Cool compresses Gentle exercise in the fresh, open air Attention and sympathy After a good cry	Pulsatilla

Scots pine (Pinus sylvestris), Eucalyptus globuleus (not to be used for small children) and sweet marjoram (Origanum majorana) in two teaspoons of carrier oil or one teaspoon of gel base. Gently massage a little around the nostrils and on the throat in the morning and at night.

Medicines intended for internal use
These ease pain, reduce inflammation and encourage a speedy resolution of the problem.
Home remedies
• Adding garlic, onions, mustard and aromatic herbs like oregano to food may help with overproduction of catarrh and nasal congestion.

• Hot drinks made from freshly squeezed lemon juice and hot water may also reduce excess production of mucus and catarrh.

• A soothing tea that calms the queasiness often accompanying excessive mucus production may be made by adding a quarter of a teaspoon of ground ginger and two teaspoons of honey to a cup of hot water.

Anthroposophical medicines

Silicea comp may be used to ease the discomfort of sinusitis. Take five pills four times daily until symptoms improve.

Biochemic tissue salts

Tissue salt No. 5 may be helpful in easing inflammation of the sinuses and diminishing production of catarrh. If symptoms are severe, tablets should be taken every hour until relief is obtained. For milder symptoms, take four tablets three times daily until symptoms improve, tailing off the dosage accordingly.

Herbal preparations

• A preparation of lobelia compound may ease the symptoms of sinusitis. Take one tablet at four-hourly intervals as necessary (do not exceed the recommended dose since too large a dose of lobelia may lead to nausea and vomiting). This preparation is not recommended for children under twelve years old, and should be avoided in pregnancy if the supervision of a practitioner is unavailable.

• Add a cup of boiling water to a teaspoon of powdered golden seal and infuse for fifteen minutes. This may be taken every couple of hours during an acute attack of sinusitis. Do not drink this infusion during pregnancy because golden seal stimulates the uterus. It should be avoided by those who suffer from high blood pressure.

A tendency to attacks of severe or recurrent sinusitis may be eased by professional help from any of the following therapies:

• Acupressure
• Anthroposophical medicine
• Ayurvedic medicine
• Aromatherapy
• Homoeopathy
• Nutritional therapy
• Reflexology
• Shiatsu
• Traditional Chinese medicine
• Western herbal medicine

Sore throats and tonsillitis

A sore throat may be a mild condition that causes no more than some discomfort, or a severe illness such as tonsillitis. With tonsillitis we are likely to feel extremely ill with general symptoms of feverishness, weariness, swollen glands, headache and possible vomiting.

A broad diagnosis of pharyngitis means that the area of the throat between the tonsils and the vocal chords has become painful and inflamed. This may be due to a bacterial or viral infection or because cigarette smoke, excessive talking, exposure to chemical fumes or alcohol has irritated the pharynx. Despite the fact that the symptoms are rather similar to those of tonsillitis, they are likely to be less intense or severe.

Laryngitis is an inflammation of the larynx (the voice box that is located at the top of the windpipe), and possible symptoms of laryngitis include feverishness, hoarseness, pain on speaking and loss of voice. The infection should clear up within a few days, but those who suffer from sinusitis (see page 156) or bronchitis (see page 140) may experience chronic laryngitis.

Practical self-help

• If you have a sore throat, avoid situations or activities that may aggravate it such as overusing the voice, smoking or spending a long time in a smoky atmosphere. Make a conscious effort to rest and relax the voice as much as possible, and keep in a comfortable, stable temperature that is neither too hot nor too cold.

• Support the body in fighting infection by increasing the amount of vitamin C in the diet by eating citrus fruit, strawberries, green, leafy vegetables, tomatoes and raw, green peppers. For a severe sore throat take a 1000mg vitamin C supplement up to three times a day while the acute phase of infection lasts. Reduce the dose if digestive upsets occur, such as acidity of the stomach or diarrhoea.

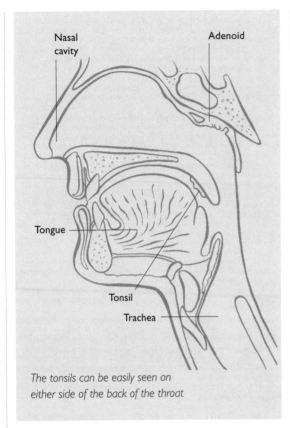

Nasal cavity

Adenoid

Tongue

Tonsil

Trachea

The tonsils can be easily seen on either side of the back of the throat

• Rest as much as possible in the early stages of illness in order to speed up recovery.
• Make sure your throat is kept well lubricated by taking regular warm or cool drinks and sucking glycerine pastilles whenever your throat feels dry. However, throat lozenges containing eucalyptus, menthol or camphor may interfere with the action of homoeopathic medicines. If you are taking a homoeopathic remedy for a sore throat, choose pastilles that have a fruit flavour such as blackcurrant.
• Take plenty of fluids to reduce feverishness and encourage the body to flush toxic by-products out as quickly as possible. Avoid diuretic (fluid-eliminating) drinks such as tea and coffee, and drink plenty of water, herb teas, lemon and honey drinks or fresh fruit juices. Remember that herb teas may be drunk warm, or as a long, cool drink after being chilled in the fridge.

SEEK PROFESSIONAL HELP

• If hoarseness persists for a month.
• If a severe sore throat develops in anyone who has previously suffered from rheumatic fever.

• If a rash or high temperature develops.
• If there are signs of pus formation or ulceration of the tonsils.
• If a sore throat is accompanied by a degree of swelling that makes swallowing difficult.
• If a severe sore throat develops in a child with a persistent high temperature.
• If there are any indications of breathing difficulties or drooling from the mouth.

Alternative treatments

For acute sore throats and tonsillitis it is quite appropriate to take the relevant remedy internally, while also using a gargle to give more localized relief.

Topical preparations

These are gargles and inhalants that can soothe pain and discomfort. Choose from any of the following, bearing in mind that none of the substances mentioned for application to the skin should be taken by mouth.

Aromatherapy oils

Add three drops each of Eucalyptus globulus (not to be used for small children), ravensar (Ravensara aromatica) and tea tree (Melaleuca alternifolia) to one teaspoonful of gel base or two teaspoonfuls of carrier oil and gently massage the throat four times a day. For tonsillitis, seek advice from a qualified aromatherapist.

Herbal preparations

• A soothing gargle may be made from sage, cider vinegar and honey. Make an infusion by adding one teaspoon of sage to a cup of warm water and leave to steep for a minute. Strain and add a teaspoonful each of cider vinegar and honey.
• Diluted tincture of Calendula and Hypericum also make a very comforting, pain-relieving gargle. One part of tincture should be added to ten parts of boiled, cooled water.

Home remedies

• If none of the above are available, make a basic gargle with lemon juice or cider vinegar and warm water.
• Alternatively, common salt may be dissolved in hot water for a simple gargle. However, make sure that the solution is not swallowed by accident, since it can induce vomiting.
• A more palatable and appetizing gargle may be made by dissolving blackcurrant or blackberry jam in hot water. The liquid should be strained and used as a gargle.

Medicines intended for internal use

These reduce inflammation, ease pain and encourage a speedy resolution of the problem.

Home remedies

Swallowing a teaspoonful of sunflower oil can ease the pain of sore throats and improve hoarseness and loss of voice.

Anthroposophical medicines

Mild sore throats or irritation and dryness of the throat may be soothed by sage pastilles. Dissolve one pastille in the mouth every one to two hours while symptoms are troublesome. For more severe symptoms of inflammation of the throat, cinnabar/pyrites may be helpful. Dissolve one tablet in the mouth up to four times a day.

Biochemic tissue salts

For the initial stage of an acute sore throat Combination J or tissue salt No. 4 may ease discomfort, pain and inflammation and encourage speedy resolution of infection. If symptoms are severe, tablets may be taken every hour initially and repeated until symptoms improve. In the case of less severe problems, take four tablets three times a day.

HOMOEOPATHIC MEDICINES

Type	General features	Worse	Better	Remedy
Rapidly developing severe, bright red sore throat	Violent onset with rapidly developing high temperature and extreme physical and mental sensitivity. Wants citrus drinks, but finds swallowing difficult: has to sit forward to do so. Bright red throat with small red spots on tongue.	Right side Chill Talking Swallowing saliva Jarring movements Drinking	Warmth Resting semi-erect in bed	Belladonna Belladonna is often needed in the initial stages of a sore throat
Established stage of sore throat with sharp, splintering pains	Swollen glands with severely painful, ulcerated throat. Sharp sensation in the throat like a fish bone or splinter. Least draught of cold air leads to a disproportionate sense of distress and discomfort. Extremely irritable and touchy with illness	Cold draughts Undressing Touch Night Physical effort	Humidity Wrapping the head up warmly	Hepar sulph
Extreme pain and swelling of the right tonsil	Bluish-red colour of the throat and greyish-white spots on the tonsils. Throbbing pains in the right tonsil. Swallowing and warm drinks aggravate burning pains	Warm drinks Movement Humid, damp conditions Warmth	Rest	Phytolacca
Left-sided sore throats	Sore throats and swollen glands that feel awful on waking from sleep. Tight, constricted sensations in the throat that are made more intense by touch or pressure. Swallowing saliva is much more painful than swallowing food	After sleep In the morning Warmth Empty swallowing Warm drinks Pressure around the neck	Contact with cool air Cold drinks Swallowing food	Lachesis

A tendency to recurrent severe sore throats or tonsillitis may respond to treatment by professionals from any of the following therapies:
- Anthroposophical medicine
- Aromatherapy
- Ayurvedic medicine
- Homoeopathy
- Nutritional therapy
- Reflexology
- Traditional Chinese medicine
- Western medical herbalism

DIGESTIVE PROBLEMS

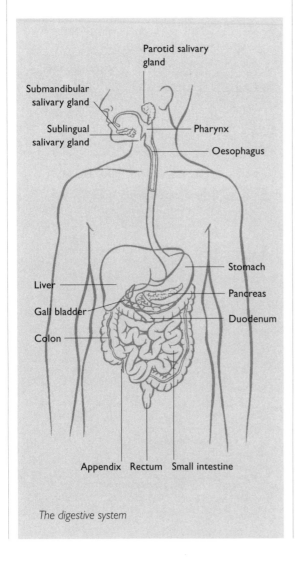

The digestive system

Parotid salivary gland
Submandibular salivary gland
Sublingual salivary gland
Pharynx
Oesophagus
Liver
Stomach
Pancreas
Gall bladder
Duodenum
Colon
Appendix   Rectum   Small intestine

Constipation

Although not serious in itself, constipation is one of those tiresome conditions that can leave us feeling sluggish, lethargic, uncomfortable and generally under par. Some of us may battle with a tendency towards constipation throughout our lives, while others begin to experience this problem as a result of taking on a sedentary job, neglecting the quality of their diet or becoming overstressed and tense. Constipation can also be caused by persistently ignoring the call to go to the toilet.

Symptoms may include any of the following:
- Infrequent or irregular stools that are painful or difficult to pass.
- A sense of discomfort or incompleteness after passing a stool.
- Frequent urging to achieve a bowel movement or complete absence of any urge to empty the bowels.
- Stools that are hard, small, dry or large.
- Associated problems that may be sparked off by habitual constipation include headaches, indigestion and nausea. Period pains may also become more uncomfortable as a result of this problem.

Sensible changes in lifestyle combined with appropriate alternative medical help can help our bodies deal with the problem at its source, rather than providing the temporary alleviation of symptoms that laxatives provide.

Practical self-help
- Avoid prolonged regular use of painkillers.
- Make sure that dietary fibre plays an important role in your daily eating plan by including regular helpings of raw vegetables, fresh fruit, whole grains, beans and pulses. Easy ways of keeping fibre intake at a healthy level include having a large salad once a day, including a substantial portion of vegetables

with lunch and dinner and frequently eating fresh fruit as a pudding or snack.

• Drink enough water each day to provide the necessary lubrication for your digestive system. Drinking six to eight large glasses of water a day discourages the formation of hard, dry stools that can result in fruitless straining and distress. Avoid tea and coffee because of their diuretic effect: in other words, they encourage the body to eliminate rather than conserve fluid.

• Foods to avoid if constipation is a problem include instant 'ready' meals high in refined ingredients such as white flour, processed rice and fat. Eggs, cheese and red meat should also be kept to a minimum because of the burden they place on the digestive tract (red meat can begin to putrefy in the gut because it takes so long to pass through). Consequently, if we eat frequent helpings of red meat and very little fibre, we are at risk of developing diseases that research suggests are linked to sluggish bowel movements, such as diverticulosis or bowel cancer.

• Consistently ignoring signals to open your bowels because you are too busy or can't be bothered, means easy, regular bowel movements will diminish. If you act on these signals as soon as possible, it is normally very easy to establish a regular time of day when the bowels can be opened without strain or difficulty.

• Avoid using laxatives where possible, and never take them on a long-term basis. Dependency on laxatives occurs because their protracted use reduces muscle tone in the bowel. As a result, once medication is discontinued, the chances of achieving a regular bowel movement are reduced rather than increased. Also, taking laxatives over an extended period can result in a distressing alternation between diarrhoea and constipation, with possible problems of a nutritional deficiency occurring as a result of malabsorption.

• Stress can also be a major factor in contributing towards problems with constipation, especially when combined with a reliance on low-fibre 'fast' foods, stimulants such as tea and coffee, painkillers and alcohol. If this pattern of living is combined with a high-pressured job that leaves little time in which to relax, constipation or irritable bowel syndrome is almost certainly going to be a problem. The latter is an increasingly commonly diagnosed condition that involves a variety of digestive symptoms, including a frustrating alternation between diarrhoea and constipation. Since it is usually seen as a stress-related condition, learning how to relax can do a great deal to ease the overall problem. Introduce relaxation as an integral part of your daily routine by using relaxation tapes, learning meditation techniques, attending yoga classes or taking up running, brisk walking or cycling. Exercise not only releases endorphins, natural chemicals that increase well-being, it actively encourages healthy working of the bowel.

• Traces of aluminium in the system may aggravate a tendency towards constipation, so avoid using tea bags (which use aluminium in the production process), aluminium cookware and aluminium-based antacids.

SEEK PROFESSIONAL HELP

• If any change in pattern of bowel movement occurs that cannot be accounted for (e.g. unexplained diarrhoea or constipation, or alternation between the two).

• If stools appear uncharacteristically light or dark in colour.

• If there is any sign of blood in the stools.

• If severe constipation occurs in pregnancy.

Alternative treatments
Medicines intended for internal use

These encourage a speedy resolution of the problem through re-balancing the system as a whole. However, if constipation is a chronic, or well-established problem, it is best to seek professional alternative medical advice.

Home remedies

• Ensure that rhubarb, figs and prunes are included in the diet to combat a tendency to constipation. Apart from eating dried fruit, it is also a help to drink the liquid in which they have been soaked in order to obtain maximum benefit from their cleansing properties.

• Blackstrap molasses taken daily in warm water, fruit juice or milk can also guard against problems with constipation.

• Agar-agar has gentle laxative properties and may be included in the diet in soups, jellies or other foods as a substitute for animal-based gelatine.

• A glass of warm or cold water taken first thing in the morning and last thing at night has a reputation for being an extremely gentle and simple way of combating a tendency to sluggish or inefficient bowel movements.

Biochemic tissue salts

Combination Remedy S may be helpful in easing constipation that is accompanied by biliousness and sick headaches. Alternatively, tissue salt No. 9 may ease persistent constipation that arises from dry, dehydrated stools. Take four tablets three times a day until symptoms improve. If there is no improvement within three or four days, consider another approach.

Herbal preparations

• Psyllium seeds may be useful in easing occasional bouts of constipation. Two teaspoons of seeds should be mixed in a cup of warm water and stirred well. Leave the mixture for five minutes before stirring once more. A cupful may be taken once or three times a day after meals, flavoured with lemon and honey.

• Constipation that is the result of muscular and emotional tension may be eased by an infusion containing the following: one part of valerian, peppermint,* chamomile and ginger, to two parts of licorice, dandelion root and wild yam. (**NB** Licorice should not be used by those who suffer from high blood pressure, and large or regular doses of valer-

HOMOEOPATHIC MEDICINES

Type	General features	Worse	Better	Remedy
Persistent constipation with large, hard, dry stools that are passed with great difficulty	Constipation with no urge to empty the bowels. Discomfort in the abdomen with irritability and throbbing headache that is intensified by the slightest movement. Generally dehydrated with thirst for long, cool drinks	Making an effort Slight movement Becoming overheated Being disturbed Stuffy, badly ventilated rooms	Cool air Long, cool drinks Lying as still as possible Peace and quiet	Bryonia
Constipation when travelling away from home	Constipation alternates with diarrhoea associated with over-reliance on laxatives. Bloated, unsettled abdomen with lots of flatulence, rumbling and gurgling: has to loosen clothing around the waist in order to feel more comfortable	Emotional stress or anticipation Tight clothing Cool drinks and food In the afternoons	Being distracted or occupied Gentle movement in the fresh air Warm drinks and food Loosening clothes	Lycopodium
Constipation from stress, over-indulgence or over-use of painkillers	'Burning the candle at both ends' leads to reliance on junk foods, alcohol and cigarettes in order to keep the pace. As a result, constipation, headaches and nausea are frequent experiences. Fruitless urging with constipation and a sense of incomplete passage of stool	Stress Coffee Alcohol Painkillers Poor sleep pattern In the morning Noise and disturbance	Sound, uninterrupted sleep Peace and quiet Warmth By the evening and night	Nux vomica
Constipation with soft stools that are passed with great difficulty	Persistent, insidiously developing constipation with marked straining and bleeding when achieving a bowel movement. Knotted, soft, dry or hard stools.	Potatoes and starchy foods Cold Alternate days Sitting	Warm drinks Eating Warmth in general	Alumina Alumina is particularly recommended for constipation that develops in the elderly

ian should never be taken as it may cause muscular spasms, headaches and/or palpitations. Herbs marked with a * may interfere with the action of homoeopathic remedies.)

• The following infusion may benefit those whose constipation is due to poor muscle tone. One part of damiana, raspberry leaves, licorice, rhubarb root, golden seal and ginger, may be added to two parts of dandelion root. (**NB** Damiana should not be used on a regular basis by those who suffer from headaches or insomnia, while golden seal should be avoided in pregnancy.)

Recurrent problems with constipation may benefit from consulting a practitioner of one of the following therapies:
• Acupressure
• Anthroposophical medicine
• Aromatherapy
• Ayurvedic medicine
• Chiropractic
• Homoeopathic medicine
• Massage therapy
• Naturopathy
• Nutritional therapy
• Osteopathy
• Reflexology
• Shiatsu
• Traditional Chinese medicine
• Western medical herbalism

Diarrhoea

Diarrhoea, as many of us may have experienced, is a debilitating, often exhausting condition. It frequently occurs as a temporary problem in response to having eaten contaminated food or water, and may often be accompanied by episodes of vomiting as the body expels the toxic stimulus.

Alternatively, short-lived episodes of diarrhoea, nausea or vomiting may occur in response to emotional triggers such as anticipatory anxiety (as in the case of exam nerves), or if we are in severe pain. The latter can provoke a short-lived need to empty the bowels and stomach, although nothing toxic has been eaten.

Chronic conditions that can lead to periodic bouts of diarrhoea or loose stools over an extended period include irritable bowel syndrome (see page 177), Crohn's disease, ulcerative colitis and coeliac disease.

Practical self-help

• It is important to avoid eating if the body is attempting to rid the digestive tract of toxic matter. Eating will slow this process down making the discomfort of diarrhoea more protracted than it needs to be. However, make sure you drink enough liquid to prevent dehydration. This is particularly important if diarrhoea and vomiting occur together, since this combination can cause rapid loss of body fluids.

• Avoid drinks that irritate the stomach lining, such as coffee, tea, alcohol, acidic drinks such as orange or grapefruit juice, and sugar-laden fizzy colas. Choose still mineral or filtered water and herbal teas that soothe the digestive tract such as fennel or peppermint.

• Where possible, find effective alternatives to conventional antidiarrhoea formulations available from pharmacies. Although these may provide initial temporary relief, they hamper the body's attempts to rid itself of toxic or irritant material. By interfering with this process, we are likely to feel unwell and nauseated even though diarrhoea is not present.

• Make a point of resting as much as possible when feeling generally out of sorts with a bout of diarrhoea. Making extra demands on your body at a time like this will prolong the process of getting well.

• If appetite remains unaffected during an episode of diarrhoea, ensure that the food that is eaten is as light and easily digestible as possible. Rice and clear broths made from vegetable stock, puréed vegetables, home-made soups and poached or steamed fish are suitable. Avoid fatty foods such as cheese, red meat, sausages or salami, fried or battered foods, or creamy puddings. If vegetables or fruit appeal, they should be lightly steamed in order to make them more digestible.

SEEK PROFESSIONAL HELP

• If severe or persistent diarrhoea occurs in the very young or the elderly.

- If episodes of diarrhoea are accompanied by abdominal pain and/or vomiting.
- If there are any traces of blood, pus or mucus in loose stools.
- If the pattern of bowel movements changes for no obvious reason, and remains unsettled for an extended period.
- If signs of dehydration are apparent. These may include any of the following:
  - Drowsiness (this does not mean feeling sleepy or sleeping a lot, which is normal, but feeling not quite with it when you are awake) i.e. not reacting to things going on around you, answering simple questions slowly with an abnormally slow voice pattern.
  - Sunken eyes.
  - Concentrated or reduced urine output.
  - Reduced saliva or tears.
  - Depressed fontanelle (the soft area at the crown of the head in young babies).
  - Loose or slack skin that does not spring quickly back into place after being pinched.

Alternative treatments

In the case of diarrhoea and digestive upsets, it is quite appropriate to take the relevant internal remedy while also applying a soothing topical application to the skin.

Topical preparations

These are compresses that can be applied to the skin to soothe, comfort and ease distress.

Home remedies

A warm compress made from chamomile tea may be very soothing when applied to tense or uncomfortable areas of the abdomen.

Medicines intended for internal use

These ease inflammation, soothe discomfort and encourage a speedy resolution to the problem.

Home remedies

- Rice water has a reputation for soothing the distress and discomfort of an irritated bowel. Boil 28g (1oz) rice in 1l (1¾ pints) water for one-and-a-half hours. Strain off the liquid and drink as frequently as needed.
- A similar, soothing gruel may be made by boiling oatmeal or barley and straining off the liquid.
- Grape juice diluted in water may be a comforting drink for sufferers of diarrhoea as a result of food poisoning.

- A teaspoon of honey dissolved in a small amount of warm water makes a soothing drink for small children who have an upset stomach. Note that this should not be given to babies under one year old.
- Diarrhoea sufferers should take warm rather than cold drinks, because warm drinks aid the digestive process, while cold drinks may aggravate spasms and irritation of the gut.

Anthroposophical medicine

Episodes of diarrhoea in babies may be eased by using a homoeopathic potency of chamomile root (Matricaria chamomilla). Use in 3x potency every hour or two until symptoms improve. If there is no improvement after three or four hours, consider a different medical strategy.

Biochemic tissue salts

Biochemic tissue salt No. 5 may be helpful in easing diarrhoea that is triggered by eating too many fatty foods. Alternatively, Combination Remedy S may be more helpful for bouts of summer diarrhoea that develop in hot, sultry conditions. For rapidly developing symptoms tablets may be taken hourly until symptoms improve. For more low-grade symptoms, take four tablets three times a day until the situation eases.

Herbal preparations

- Soothe abdominal discomfort by taking a drink made from powdered slippery elm mixed with warm milk or water. Mix a teaspoonful of the powder with a little cold water or milk before adding the rest of the warm liquid, making sure that the mixture is stirred constantly to avoid the drink becoming lumpy.
- If diarrhoea is accompanied by nausea, take frequent sips of any of the following herbal teas to help settle the stomach: chamomile, peppermint* or fennel. Adding a pinch of any of the following spices will also serve to ease nausea: ginger, cardamom, cinnamon or coriander. (Items marked with a * may interfere with the action of homoeopathic remedies.)

A tendency to severe or recurrent (chronic) diarrhoea may benefit from treatment from any of the following therapies:
- Anthroposophical medicine
- Ayurvedic medicine
- Homoeopathic medicine
- Naturopathy
- Nutritional therapy
- Shiatsu
- Traditional Chinese medicine
- Western medical herbalism

HOMOEOPATHIC MEDICINES

Type	General features	Worse	Better	Remedy
Diarrhoea with extreme thirst for drinks of cold water	Simultaneous bouts of severe diarrhoea and vomiting. Straining, exhaustion, cramping pains and clammy sweat with diarrhoea. Extreme pallor and chilliness after episodes of diarrhoea. Unusual symptom of hunger pangs with diarrhoea	After drinking Cramping pains Motion Pressure	Rest Warmth Being wrapped up well	Veratrum album
Diarrhoea with extreme flatulence and wind production	Severe, cramping diarrhoea that leads to state of near collapse due to exhaustion and weakness. Faintness and clamminess with pale, bluish-tinged skin. Noisy passage of wind with bouts of diarrhoea. Sensitivity and intolerance of tight, restrictive clothing around waist	Chilly surroundings Stuffy, badly ventilated rooms Extreme variations of temperature Tight clothes	Fresh, cool air Being fanned Passing wind upwards or downwards Resting with feet slightly higher than the body	Carbo veg
Severe, watery diarrhoea with little, or no pain	Alternating episodes of diarrhoea and headache. Weakness and nausea after emptying bowels. Sense of urgency is preceded by noisy gurgling in abdomen. Diarrhoea may be aggravated or brought on by an excess of milk or fruit	Movement After eating Early morning Before, during or after a bout of diarrhoea	Massage Stroking Lying on abdomen	Podophyllum
Painless diarrhoea from anticipatory anxiety	Headache and dizzy, giddy feeling with diarrhoea. Exhaustion and lethargy with heavy feeling in the limbs. Quiet, morose, and withdrawn when feeling anxious	Anxiety Anticipation Physical or mental effort	Bending forward Rest Passing urine	Gelsemium
Watery, gushing diarrhoea that is especially urgent on waking	Rushes on waking to pass violent, frothy diarrhoea. Frequent passage of diarrhoea leaves the anus burning, sore, inflamed and itchy. Because of sensitivity of this area, achieving a bowel movement is put off until the very last moment	Standing Warm bathing Heat of bed Becoming chilled Exertion Sweets Milk	Moderate temperature Drawing knees up Fresh, cool air Perspiration	Sulphur
Diarrhoea and vomiting from food poisoning with extreme chilliness and restlessness	Food poisoning symptoms develop after eating contaminated meat or fruit. Burning sensations in stomach and gut are soothed by taking frequent sips of warm drinks, or by warm compresses applied to sensitive areas. Anxious, fussy and fearful when unwell	At night When alone Becoming chilled Cold drinks	Warmth Sitting propped up in bed Company or distraction Frequent sips of warm, soothing drinks	Arsenicum album

Flatulence

See advice given for indigestion on pages 172-6.

Gallstones

Many of us may have gallstones without being aware of them, only discovering the fact they are there when we have a routine scan or X-ray. On the other hand, those who have experienced pain as a result of gallstones will know how excruciatingly uncomfortable it can be.

This pain occurs when gallstones move from the gall bladder (where they cause relatively little pain) to the duodenum. If they block the exit from the gall bladder, or become stuck in the duct leading to the duodenum, the gall bladder may become inflamed and swollen. As a result, right-sided pain may occur beneath the ribcage, or between the shoulders, possibly accompanied by pain when eating too fatty a diet, nausea and vomiting. Symptoms of jaundice may develop, including a yellowish tinge to the whites of the eyes, skin and urine.

Women have a reputation for being at a higher risk of developing this problem than men, especially if they are middle-aged and overweight. Using the contraceptive pill may also increase the risk of developing gallstones.

If severe attacks of pain and inflammation occur, it is often suggested that the gall bladder should be removed in order to prevent a repetition of the problem in the future. An alternative option is to shatter gallstones by using shock waves, or to dissolve them by the use of chemicals.

Practical self-help

• Make a drastic reduction in the amount of fatty foods in your diet by cutting out fried foods, full-fat cheeses, cream, chocolate and red meat. It is also helpful to reduce or eliminate foods from the diet that are made from refined ingredients such as white sugar, white flour and fat. Biscuits, cakes and

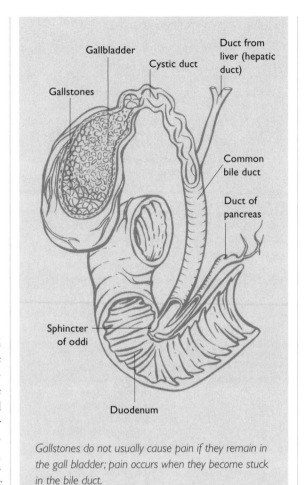

Gallstones do not usually cause pain if they remain in the gall bladder; pain occurs when they become stuck in the bile duct.

puddings tend to be the worst offenders in this category.

• Replace the items mentioned above with plentiful helpings of fresh fruit, vegetables, pulses, whole grains and small portions of fish or poultry.

• If gallstones have been a problem that have required surgical removal in the past, it is worth consulting an alternative practitioner in order to establish a strategy for preventing a recurrence of the problem in the future.

• It may be helpful to include asparagus, artichokes, barley water and kelp in the diet. A small amount of alcohol drunk on a daily basis may also reduce the concentration of bile salts. The recommended amount is not more than two units a day (a single unit being half a pint of beer, a small glass of wine or a measure of spirits).

• Make sure that enough water is drunk on a daily basis: ideally six to eight glasses a day.

- If pains are severe, especially if they are accompanied by vomiting and/or nausea.
- If any signs of jaundice occur such as yellowness of the whites of the eyes or skin.
- While the self-help measures above may ease problems with gallstones, it must be stressed that gallstones are only one potential cause of pain in the abdomen. As a result, if pain persists for more than four hours, medical help must be sought rather than relying on home prescribing. If a diagnosis of gallstone colic is confirmed, help should be sought from an alternative medical practitioner in order to deal with the underlying predisposition to the problem, rather than relying on self-help measures.

Recurrent problems with gallstones may benefit from consulting a practitioner of one of the following therapies:

- Anthroposophical medicine
- Homoeopathy
- Naturopathy
- Nutritional therapy
- Traditional Chinese medicine
- Western medical herbalism

Haemorrhoids (piles)

Haemorrhoids occur when the veins of the anus become swollen, usually as a result of stubborn constipation, with resulting fruitless urging and straining when attempting to pass a stool. This puts extreme pressure on the veins in this area, encouraging them to become distended and inflamed. Being overweight can also contribute to this distressing and uncomfortable condition, as can pregnancy and childbirth.

Bleeding often accompanies or follows a difficult bowel movement when haemorrhoids are present.

The blood is typically bright red in appearance, and may appear as streaks on the stool that has been passed and/or may stain the toilet paper.

If haemorrhoids become protruding (prolapsed), they may only emerge as a temporary effect of a stressful bowel movement. However, if the problem goes on long enough, and if constipation is not remedied, protruding haemorrhoids may become chronic, resulting in pain, irritation or itching affecting the area around the anus, as well as frequent passage of blood and/or mucus during or after a bowel movement.

If haemorrhoids are a mild or infrequently occurring problem, the self-help measures suggested below in combination with an appropriate alternative medical approach may do a great deal to improve the situation. However, well-established, severe or prolapsed haemorrhoids should be treated by a trained alternative medical therapist.

Practical self-help

Constipation is the most common cause of haemorrhoids and can be caused by a low-fibre, high-fat diet, insufficient fluid intake, laxative misuse, a sedentary lifestyle and stress. See 'Practical self-help' in the section on constipation (pages 162-3) for advice on eliminating constipation.

- If stools are unnaturally dark in colour or otherwise changed in appearance.
- If heavy or persistent bleeding occurs from the rectum.
- If any change in pattern of bowel movements occurs that cannot be explained by any modifications in daily routine.

Alternative treatments

In the case of haemorrhoids it is quite appropriate to take the relevant remedy internally, while also applying a topical preparation to the skin. In this way, the healing process is simultaneously being encouraged on the surface and internally.

Topical preparations

These are creams, ointments, lotions and tinctures that can be applied to the skin to soothe and heal. Choose from any of the following, bearing in mind that none of the substances mentioned for application to the skin should be taken by mouth.

HOMOEOPATHIC MEDICINES

Type	General features	Worse	Better	Remedy
Inflamed, full sensations in haemorrhoids and rectum	Haemorrhoids aggravated by constant, fruitless urging and straining when constipated. Incomplete feeling after passing a difficult stool. Stitch-like pains radiate up spine, with tight, constricted feeling in the rectum. Sensitivity to touch with easy-bleeding haemorrhoids	Poor diet Stress Over-use of painkillers In the morning Coffee Alcohol Chill	Rest By the evening Sound, uninterrupted sleep Warmth	Nux vomica
Haemorrhoids with irritation and itching after bowel movement	Constipation and haemorrhoids may be aggravated by a stodgy diet that includes too much starch. Burning, stinging pains that shoot upwards. Great distress, straining and painful urging when attempting to pass even a soft stool	Lifting Exertion Sitting Starchy foods Alternate days Smoking	Bathing with cool water Rest Fresh air	Alumina
Prickling, stinging pains with easy-bleeding haemorrhoids	Tense feeling in piles as though they are about to burst. Rectum feels terribly sore and uncomfortable with haemorrhoids that bleed profusely for the slightest reason. General tendency to varicose veins of the abdomen	Jarring Pressure Touch Cool air Motion		Hamamelis
Prolapsed, protruding piles that look like a bunch of grapes	Bluish-tinged haemorrhoids with feeling of fullness and congestion. Pulsating in rectum following a meal. Bearing-down, burning sensations aggravated when sitting down, and eased by movement	Eating Drinking Warmth Sitting Jarring	Cool air Cool compresses Cool bathing Passing wind	Aloe
Haemorrhoids with sharp, sticking pains in the rectum that remain long after passing a stool	The rectum feels it is full of sharp sticks or splinters. Swollen, congested feeling with discomfort and burning in anus. Haemorrhoids may develop or become worse as a result of the menopause	Movement Standing Stooping Lying down In the morning	Cool bathing Contact with fresh, cool air Physical effort	Aesculus hippocastanum

Anthroposophical medicine
Antimony praep. ointment.

Aromatherapy oils
Add ten drops of niaouli (Melaleuca quinqueneriva) and ten drops of cypress to 30ml (1fl oz) gel base and apply four times a day to the affected area.

Herbal preparations
• Herbal haemorrhoid ointments contain a combination of soothing ingredients, such as horse chestnut, aloe and witch hazel in bland base. Applying the

ointment as often as necessary to the sensitive area can do a great deal to ease distress and discomfort.

• Pilewort ointment may be made by adding 350g (12½oz) of chopped pilewort to three times its weight of melted lard. (Vegetarians can use an unscented cream base.) Decant into a jar, cover and leave in a warm place for twenty-four hours. Then remove, strain and replace in its container ready for use.

Home remedies

• Cool compresses or warm bathing may do a great deal to temporarily ease the pain and irritation of haemorrhoids. Salt baths may be especially soothing and can easily be prepared by adding common salt to the water.

• Witch hazel may be applied diluted on cotton wool to the affected area in order to ease inflammation.

• Applying alternating hot and cool compresses may feel soothing, while also encouraging circulation to flow more freely in the affected area.

Medicines intended for internal use

These ease pain, reduce inflammation and encourage a speedy resolution of the problem.

Biochemic tissue salts

A combination preparation called Elasto may be helpful in easing the pain and distress of haemorrhoids. It may be taken three times daily until symptoms improve. If symptoms are resistant to improvement after a few days, switch to tissue salt No. 1, using the same instructions for dosage.

Herbal preparations

Calendula or blackberry leaf tea may be taken to soothe inflammation and improve circulation.

Home remedies

Plentiful amounts of garlic should be included in the diet in order to improve circulation.

If haemorrhoids are severe or do not respond swiftly to self-help measures, professional help may be obtained from any of the following:

• Anthroposophical medicine
• Aromatherapy
• Ayurvedic medcine
• Homoeopathy
• Naturopathy
• Nutritional therapy
• Traditional Chinese medicine
• Western medical herbalism

Hiatus hernia

This is a condition that often arises in pregnancy or in older people, especially if they are overweight. A hiatus hernia is a protrusion of the stomach lining (gastric mucosa) above the level of the diaphragm. The term is commonly misused to describe symptoms of other problems, but a hiatus hernia itself is symptom-free unless massive, when it may cause respiratory problems. However, its presence means that the normal 'valve' mechanism preventing the stomach acid and contents regurgitating into the oesophagus is disrupted.

Symptoms of a hiatus hernia may include any of the following:

• Digestive uneasiness and discomfort that is much worse when bending or stooping.

• Burping, with acidity that rises into the gullet.

• Discomfort and burning in the chest that may also affect the neck and arms.

A hiatus hernia, although not a serious condition in itself, predisposes the sufferer to oesophagitis, inflammation of the oesophagus (although it is possible to get oesophagitis – often referred to as gastro-oesophageal reflux disease, or reflux – without having a hiatus hernia). Oesophagitis incorporates the symptoms caused by the presence of a hiatus hernia and can lead to an intolerance of hot or cold drinks and very cold foods like ice cream, the stomach contents being aspirated into the lungs, or ulceration of the oesophagus.

If possible, avoid the use of anti-inflammatory drugs, which will aggravate, not relieve the pain.

Practical self-help

• It is best to eat small amounts at regular intervals, rather than large meals with long gaps in between. Eating rich or heavy meals late at night can also

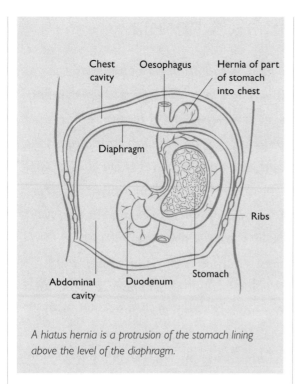

A hiatus hernia is a protrusion of the stomach lining above the level of the diaphragm.

Labels in figure: Chest cavity · Oesophagus · Hernia of part of stomach into chest · Diaphragm · Ribs · Abdominal cavity · Duodenum · Stomach

result in digestive discomfort that may cause great distress and prevent sleep.

• Provided swollen ankles are not a problem, it may be helpful to prop up the head of the bed by approximately 10cm (4in). Alternatively, sleeping semi-upright on a couple of square continental pillows may ease acid reflux and digestive pain.

• Take time to eat food in a relaxed way and try to avoid gulping down air with each mouthful. Chew each mouthful thoroughly in order to make the job of digestion less stressful for the stomach.

• Where possible avoid coffee, cigarettes and alcohol, which can make digestive problems more intense by irritating the stomach lining and causing nausea, acidity and general discomfort in the stomach.

• Avoid bending and stooping when the stomach is full, since this can aggravate acidity and cause acid to wash from the stomach into the gullet.

• If you are overweight, symptoms of a hiatus hernia may be greatly improved by shedding excess pounds. For ideas on how to lose weight sensibly, see the section on weight loss, pages 324-6.

SEEK PROFESSIONAL HELP

• If food sticks when swallowed.

• If severe pains occur, radiating from the chest to the shoulder blades. This is especially important if the discomfort has not eased within an hour or two.

• If pains occur in the chest that radiate to the neck and arms.

• If there is a combination of indigestion and weight loss.

Alternative treatments

Because of the chronic nature of this problem, it is important to seek help from an alternative therapist if self-help measures have not yielded positive results within a short time.

Biochemic tissue salts

Tissue salt No. 1 may be of help in discouraging the flabbiness and sagging of tissues that may lead to hernias. A low dose (two tablets twice daily) may be taken for a number of weeks, tailing off as symptoms improve, or increasing the dosage if there are any signs of symptoms becoming more troublesome.

Herbal preparations

• The following infusion may ease the discomfort of a hiatus hernia: add one part of meadowsweet to half a part each of gentian and golden seal (do not use during pregnancy), plus two parts each of comfrey and marsh mallow. To make the infusion, place the measured amounts of herbs in a warmed teapot, add boiling water and cover. Leave to stand for fifteen minutes before straining.

• Stomach acidity and pain may be eased by drinking warm milk in which a teaspoonful or two of powdered slippery elm has been dispersed (see instructions in the section on diarrhoea, page 166).

Suitable professional help may be obtained from any of the following:

• Anthroposophical medicine
• Naturopathy
• Nutritional therapy
• Traditional Chinese medicine
• Western medical herbalism

Indigestion

Most of us will have experienced the discomfort of indigestion from time to time, usually as a result of poor eating habits, such as skipping meals or eating in

HOMOEOPATHIC MEDICINES

Type	General features	Worse	Better	Remedy
Discomfort in the stomach that develops soon after eating	Weight and nausea in the stomach with possible heartburn and acidity. Saliva tastes bitter. Very thirsty for long, cool drinks. Irritable, bad-tempered and antisocial with digestive problems	Even slight movement After eating Overheating Sitting up Touch Pressure	Lying down Keeping as still as possible Cool surroundings Warm drinks	Bryonia
Digestive uneasiness and acidity that develops at night, or in the early hours of the morning	Burning pains and discomfort in the stomach that are eased by frequent sips of warm drinks. All symptoms are aggravated with the approach of night. Extremely restless, chilly and anxious with digestive problems	Being alone At night Chill or cold Cold food or drinks Alcohol	Sips of warm drinks Warmth Gentle movement Company and distraction	Arsenicum album
Digestive uneasiness from eating an excess of fatty, rich foods	Acidity, heaviness and flatulence occur after eating too much cheese, red meat or creamy sauces. Burping with taste of foods eaten long before. Nausea and uneasiness develop an hour or two after eating, or in the evening. Weepy, restless, and in need of attention and sympathy when feeling sick	Overheated, poorly ventilated rooms Warm food or drinks Being too heavily clothed Resting	Gentle movement Fresh, open air Undressing or loosening clothes Sympathy Having a good cry	Pulsatilla
Digestive discomfort with heartburn and acid reflux	General uneasiness of the digestive tract with very noisy gurgling and rumbling. Stomach fills very quickly: sits down to eat feeling hungry, but feels full very quickly. Constant belching is unable to relieve discomfort in the stomach	Pressure of clothes around the waist Cold drinks Chill Overheated rooms Stress Physical or mental effort	Loosening clothes Warmth Warm drinks Gentle exercise in the fresh air Distraction	Lycopodium
Digestive disturbance that is aggravated by eating too much sugar	Stomach pain and flatulence come on soon after eating. Severe discomfort is not relieved by violent belching. Nausea is eased by eating light, easily digested food. Symptoms caused by anticipatory anxiety, stress or emotional strain	Sugar At night On waking Warmth Poorly ventilated surroundings	Walking in the fresh air Cool surroundings Light clothing	Arg nit

too great a hurry. A stressful lifestyle can also contribute to problems with digestive discomfort. This often occurs because high stress levels compromise our ability to relax when eating, and frequently lead us to rely too much on convenience foods, cigarettes, alcohol and caffeine in order to keep the pace. As a result, increased acidity and tension in the stomach make the job of digestion very much harder than it should be.

Symptoms of indigestion may include any of the following:
• Discomfort or sharp pain in the stomach after eating.
• Wind and flatulence.
• Nausea, fullness or a sensation of weight in the stomach.
• Acidity and burning that may rise into the throat or mouth.

Factors that increase the likelihood of indigestion include:
• Eating beans, pulses, raw onions, peppers, cabbage, red meat or rich, overly fatty dishes.
• Chewing food too quickly.
• Pregnancy.
• Anxiety, nervousness or depression.
• Smoking and being overweight.

Although indigestion is a commonly occurring problem and is not a serious condition in itself, recurrent episodes of digestive discomfort of this kind should not be overlooked. If any obvious change in the pattern of indigestion occurs, such as daily episodes of pain instead of intermittent discomfort, it is essential to seek medical advice.

Practical self-help

• Avoid foods that have a reputation for aggravating indigestion, and concentrate instead on those that assist the process of easy digestion. The former include the foods listed above, plus full-fat hard cheeses, spicy foods such as chillies and curries, Brussels sprouts, strong coffee, tea and alcohol (espe-cially spirits). Digestive-friendly foods include home-made soups, purées and broths, lightly steamed or stir-fried dishes, salads made from raw, grated vegetables, non-citrus fruit, pasta and small portions of fish or chicken. Still mineral or spring water should also be drunk at frequent intervals during the day to flush out the system.

• Chew food thoroughly and slowly to allow saliva to penetrate the ground-down food in the mouth. Salivation lubricates the ground-up food, making it easier to swallow, while digestive enzymes in the saliva begin the process of digestion in the mouth. This makes digestion easier for the stomach, so bolting down inadequately chewed food is likely to cause excess wind, acidity and fullness in the digestive tract.

• Eat small meals at regular intervals rather than large, heavy meals separated by long gaps. Be especially vigilant about this pattern during times of pressure and stress when it may seem more convenient to gulp down snacks while working, speaking on the telephone or running for the next appointment. Missing regular meals and habitually snatching snacks is usually disastrous for the digestive processes, due to a combination of problems that stem from inadequately chewed food, and the accumulation of wind, flatulence and bloating that arise from long gaps between meals.

• Avoid reliance on antacids, which may ease symptoms in the short term, but can cause worrying problems if used too frequently. Products with a bicarbonate of soda base may intensify water retention or high blood pressure. Aluminium-based gels and liquids may produce constipation as a side effect. Some antacids should also be avoided in pregnancy since they may interfere with vitamin absorption. Long-term use of antacids may result in acid rebound, which is caused when the body registers that stomach acid levels have been reduced (by the antacid) and responds by pumping in extra acid to rectify the balance. This puts the sufferer back where he started, beginning a vicious cycle in which long-term medication is necessary to keep indigestion at bay.

• Try to avoid eating when feeling uptight or tense, since this can directly contribute towards or intensify indigestion. If something irritating, anxiety-making or stressful has happened, avoid eating straight away. Instead, consciously take a few minutes to breathe slowly and steadily in order to relax and reduce tension before starting to eat.

• Consider avoiding combinations of food that may make digestion more difficult. These include red meat combined with starchy foods like potatoes, followed by a sweet pastry, or fatty foods such as cheese, combined with bread. These items eaten together are thought to make the digestive process much more of an uphill struggle.

SEEK PROFESSIONAL HELP

• If persistent indigestion occurs that is not improved by self-help measures.
• If unexplained weight loss and/or loss of appetite occur for no apparent reason.
• If nausea and pain are accompanied by episodes of vomiting, especially if there are traces of blood in the vomit.
• If occasional bouts of indigestion change their pattern, or begin to happen on a daily rather than a sporadic basis.

Alternative treatments

Infrequent or mild episodes of indigestion may improve considerably as a result of making straight-forward adjustments in lifestyle that deal with the problem at its root cause. Short-term use of self-prescribed alternative treatments should also be effective. They are not intended for long-term use, so if indigestion becomes a persistent feature of life, it is important to seek advice from an alternative practitioner.

Aromatherapy oils
Add two drops each of mandarin, ginger, peppermint, black pepper and Roman chamomile (Chamaemelum nobile) to two teaspoons of carrier oil or gel base and rub over the solar plexus (just beneath the ribcage) to ease discomfort. If indigestion continues, seek advice from a qualified aromatherapist. **NB** Do not use this remedy for heartburn during pregnancy.

Medicines intended for internal use
Anthroposophical medicines
One or two carvon tablets (including a mixture of birch charcoal and caraway seed oil) may be taken immediately after eating.
Biochemic tissue salts
Tissue salt No. 8 or Combination E may ease the discomfort of indigestion. The former is suitable for digestive discomfort that is made worse from contact with cold and touch, but eased by firm pressure, warmth and bending, while the latter may be

useful in situations of intermittent, colicky pains and flatulence. Take four tablets three times a day until relief is obtained, when dosage should be tailed off.
Home remedies
• It has been suggested that fresh pineapple or celery eaten at the end of a meal can aid the process of digestion, as can regular portions of raw, grated carrot.
• Add spices to food that have a reputation for aiding digestion. These include cumin, coriander, cinnamon, fenugreek and cayenne.
• Cardamom seeds may be chewed to ease symptoms of flatulence and discomfort, or simmered with ground ginger or grated nutmeg in two cups of water and then drunk.
Herbal preparations
• An infusion of any of the following herbs may ease digestive discomfort and flatulence: fennel, mint, * dill, chamomile, aniseed or lemon balm. To make an infusion, use one teaspoon of dried herb for each cup of water. Measure the required amount of herb into a warmed teapot, adding the required amount of boiling water, cover and leave for ten to fifteen minutes before straining.
• Marjoram, fennel, skullcap, rosemary or peppermint* herb teas soothe indigestion. (Herbs marked with a * may interfere with the action of homoeopathic remedies.)
• Powdered slippery elm has a very soothing effect on the stomach lining. It should be taken daily in milk as a hot drink as long as symptoms persist. (See the section on diarrhoea, page 166, for instructions.)
• Colicky pains and flatulence may be eased by sipping an infusion of warm water and dill seeds.

Alternative help, treatment and advice suitable for indigestion may be obtained from practitioners of any of the following therapies:
• Acupressure
• Anthroposophical medicine
• Aromatherapy
• Ayurvedic medicine
• Homoeopathy
• Naturopathy
• Nutritional therapy
• Reflexology
• Shiatsu
• Traditional Chinese medicine
• Western medical herbalism

HOMOEOPATHIC MEDICINES

Type	General features	Worse	Better	Remedy
Indigestion resulting from 'nerves' or anxiety	Extremely loud gurgling and rumbling that is intensified by pressure of a waistband. Pain, burning and acidity rise into the gullet from the stomach. Severe flatulence that moves upwards and downwards	Indigestible foods: beans, cabbage and Brussels sprouts Cold food and drinks Tight clothing Anxiety about a coming event In the afternoon	Diversion or occupation Gentle exercise out of doors Warm food and drinks Passing water After midnight	Lycopodium
Burning and acidity in the stomach that are soothed by sips of warm drinks	Acid indigestion, nausea, vomiting and diarrhoea develop as a result of a period of tension and anxiety. Finds difficulty in relaxing and sleeping because of perfectionist tendencies. Restless and chilly with digestive problems	Anxiety about health Being chilled Cold food and drinks During the night Physical effort	Warmth Regular sips of warm drinks Distraction or company Sitting propped up in bed	Arsenicum album
Indigestion that follows over-indulgence in food and drink	Digestive discomfort and nausea that develops after an excessive amount of food, alcohol, coffee, cigarettes, prescription drugs or stress. Symptoms generally aggravated by a lifestyle of 'burning the candle at both ends'	Being disturbed Excessive levels of mental and emotional stress In the morning Noise Eating Poor-quality sleep Chilly, draughty surroundings	Peace and quiet Sound, uninterrupted sleep Warmth Passing a stool By the evening	Nux vomica
Heavy, full sensation in the stomach with severe flatulence	Violent burping with nausea and extreme swelling and bloating of the waist and abdomen after eating anything, however small. Symptoms are generally aggravated by being in airless, stuffy surroundings	Tight clothes around the neck, waist and abdomen Rich food Movement Alcohol	Burping Fresh, cool air Being fanned Sleep Resting with feet elevated	Carbo veg
Indigestion that follows eating an excessive amount of fatty foods	Stomach pains and uneasiness develop from an eating pattern that includes too many rich foods such as creamy sauces, red meat, cheese or rich cakes. Dry mouth without thirst and 'repeating' of food eaten hours before. Stomach pains are very sensitive to jolting or jarring	Rest In the evening or night Dairy products Lying down Warm food or drinks	Gentle movement in the fresh, open air Cool drinks and food Undressing Rubbing	Pulsatilla

Irritable bowel syndrome

Irritable bowel syndrome (IBS) is a diagnostic term frequently used to cover a range of symptoms that may include any of the following:

- Alternation between diarrhoea and constipation.
- Straining, pain or discomfort when attempting to pass a stool.
- Excess wind or flatulence.
- Bloating, swelling or distension of the abdomen.
- Cramping, colicky pains in the abdomen.

The diagnosis of IBS is usually made only when the possibility of other conditions has been ruled out through a range of tests, such as X-rays or endoscopy as well as checking for the presence of infection or parasites such as threadworms, tapeworms or amoebae. A tendency to candida overgrowth that can upset the smooth functioning of the digestive tract, leading to symptoms of flatulence, constipation and abdominal bloating will also form part of the normal investigations prior to a diagnosis being reached. If IBS has been diagnosed, it can be very helpful to identify the triggers that may aggravate the condition in order to help deal with the problem at a fundamental level. Possible contributory factors may include:

- Long-term anxiety or stress.
- A diet that is low in fibre and/or nutritionally deficient.
- Some people may find that certain foods aggravate the problem such as wheat, dairy products, citrus fruit, tea or coffee. However, if wheat appears to be the predominant culprit, you may need to be checked for coeliac disease, rather than IBS.

If symptoms of IBS are well established, severe or persistent, it is important to consult an alternative medical practitioner who will attempt to rectify the underlying source of the problem, rather than simply providing temporary relief of symptoms.

On the other hand, if infrequent or mild symptoms emerge in response to specific, limited situations (such as anticipatory anxiety about a coming stressful event), the self-help measures outlined below, combined with an appropriate alternative remedy, may be all that is needed in order to enable you to deal with the situation easily and effectively.

Practical self-help

- Certain foods have a reputation for aggravating IBS symptoms. Offending items may include any of the following: wheat products such as pasta or bread, sugar (including 'hidden' sugars in carbonated drinks, sauces or processed foods), cows' milk products, pulses, beans and Brussels sprouts. If you have a suspicion that one or more of these items may be upsetting your digestive system, try eliminating the suspect food from your diet for a month. If during this time there is a noticeable improvement in your symptoms, reintroduce the suspect food. If your problems return, eliminate the offending food a second time. Should your digestive symptoms improve once again, you are probably sensitive to this food, and should avoid it while your digestive system is in an overreactive state.
- Drink plenty of filtered or still mineral water (carbonated varieties can contribute to abdominal distension and flatulence), avoiding other drinks that may irritate the digestive tract such as alcohol, coffee or strong tea. It is also worth eliminating or drastically cutting down on cigarettes, which can irritate the lining of the stomach.
- Although an excess of fibre may aggravate a tendency towards diarrhoea, a certain amount is vital to keep the digestive system in good order. If you experience a problem with frequent, overenthusiastic, loose bowel movements, always grate or chop and steam fresh vegetables to make them more readily digestible. Home-made soups and purées are also an excellent way of adding a healthy proportion of vegetables to the diet (excluding the use of pulses such as beans and peas, which may aggravate flatulence and loose stools).
- High-fat foods can be difficult to digest, so avoid red meat, cream, butter and full-fat cheeses. If you are not a vegetarian choose fish or poultry, making sure that you discard the skin which has a very high fat content.
- If you experience occasional problems with constipation, always avoid the temptation of using laxatives. Instead, try to stimulate bowel function more gently and naturally by making appropriate dietary and lifestyle changes, which are outlined on pages 162-3 in the section on constipation.

HOMOEOPATHIC MEDICINES

Type	General features	Worse	Better	Remedy
Irritable bowel symptoms with colicky pains that are eased by bending double	Intermittent abdominal pains that come in waves after drinking or eating. Excessive wind and diarrhoea with discomfort in the abdomen. Watery diarrhoea may be triggered by anger or emotional stress. Faint and chilly with pain	In bed Becoming chilled At night Stress Anger	Warmth Firm pressure Bending over Passage of wind or stools Rest Gentle movement	Colocynthis
Irritable bowel syndrome with constipation and unproductive urging	Bowel pains are aggravated by coughing and jarring movements. Indicated in tense, overstressed people who choose to 'live in the fast lane'. Long-term reliance on alcohol, cigarettes, coffee and painkillers leads to indigestion, headaches, constipation and bowel spasms	Cold draughts Alcohol Coffee Smoking Lack of sleep Laxative use Stress Tight clothes In the morning	Peace and quiet Sound sleep As the day goes on	Nux vomica
Irritable bowel syndrome symptoms that are aggravated or triggered by eating too many sweet things	Severe diarrhoea soon after eating sugary foods and/or drinks. Alternating diarrhoea and constipation with swelling and discomfort of the abdomen that feels as though it is about to burst. Severe, noisy passage of wind in an upward and downward direction. Digestive symptoms are combined with nervous tension and anxiety	Sugar Drinking Ice cream Warmth Emotional stress and strain Anxiety	Cool, fresh air Firm pressure Passing wind Bending double Motion	Arg nit
Irritable bowel syndrome with gurgling, rumbling and bloating of the abdomen	Sensitivity and uneasiness of the digestive tract with heartburn, acidity and burning in the stomach. Alternating diarrhoea and constipation with excessive production of wind. Digestion reacts badly to anticipating a future stressful event	Tight, restrictive clothing Chill Cold food or drinks Extreme temperature changes Afternoons Anticipatory anxiety	Loosening clothes at the neck and waist Moderate warmth Gentle exercise in the fresh air Warm food and drinks Distraction from worry and anxiety	Lycopodium

• Stress can often be a cause of irritable bowel syndrome. Many of us may find that digestive problems do not arise when we are under extreme strain, but experience symptoms when the immediate source of stress has eased off. However, low-grade stress on an extended basis can lead to ongoing problems with acidity, indigestion and a troublesome tendency to diarrhoea and/or constipation. For advice on how to cope, see the section on psychological and stress-related conditions on page 236.

SEEK PROFESSIONAL HELP

• If foods containing wheat aggravate the symptoms.
• If persistent, unexplained weight loss occurs, especially if it is combined with long-term pain or discomfort in the stomach or abdomen.
• If there are traces of blood in stools, or if stools have an unusually pale, black or tarry appearance.
• If severe abdominal pain occurs combined with high fever and/or vomiting.
• If a change in bowel habit occurs that cannot be linked to any modifications in lifestyle or diet.
• If severe or persistent swelling of the abdomen occurs, accompanied by any of the other symptoms listed above.

Alternative treatments

Medicines intended for internal use
Herbal preparations
• Infusions of peppermint* or chamomile may soothe a sensitive digestive tract, especially if combined with a little ginger. (Items marked with a * may interfere with the action of homoeopathic remedies.)
• Mix two teaspoons of powdered slippery elm with a cup of warm milk and take morning and evening until the digestion feels more settled. If an allergy to cows' milk is suspected, mix the slippery elm with a little warm water instead.
• Aloe vera juice also has a reputation for soothing the digestive tract and encouraging a more regular bowel movement. It may be taken in liquid or capsule form.

Alternative help, treatment and advice may be obtained from practitioners of any of the following therapies:
• Anthroposophical medicine

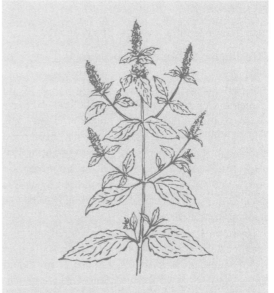

When taken in an infusion, peppermint is very soothing to the digestive tract.

• Aromatherapy
• Ayurvedic medicine
• Biochemic tissue salts
• Homoeopathy
• Naturopathy
• Nutritional therapy
• Reflexology
• Shiatsu
• Traditional Chinese medicine
• Western medical herbalism

Vomiting

Vomiting can be caused by food poisoning, a fever, over-indulgence in food and/or alcohol, appendicitis, emotional shock or trauma, morning sickness in pregnancy and eating disorders such as bulimia nervosa, in which sufferers induce vomiting. Extended bouts of vomiting leave the sufferer feeling sore, exhausted and weak, but a great deal can be done to help by following the 'Practical self-help' measures below, plus any appropriate alternative therapeutic measures.

You will discover that alternative medicines are of immense support in encouraging the body to carry out its natural functions as efficiently as possible. This may result in a speedy end to dry, protracted retching, or briefly increased bouts of vomiting that resolve the situation decisively. If the latter reaction occurs, it is likely to be rapidly followed by a deep sleep from which the patient wakes feeling refreshed and considerably better.

However, because vomiting can sometimes be a symptom of a serious disorder, it is always best to seek prompt medical advice if there is any doubt about the severity of the situation. This is particularly the case if vomiting and diarrhoea occur together in babies and small children, or in the elderly.

Dehydration is the only danger from straight forward vomiting, with or without diarrhoea, but as dehydration can be serious, check the symptoms below, under 'Seek professional help'.

SEEK PROFESSIONAL HELP

• If abdominal pains occur with vomiting, especially if they affect the area around the navel and gradually settle in the right-hand side of the abdomen.
• If vomiting is accompanied by a severe headache, light sensitivity, stiff neck or high temperature.
• If traces of bright, or dark 'coffee-ground' blood are visible in vomit.
• If nausea and vomiting occur after an accident or head injury.
• If there is any indication of blurred vision or severe pain in or around one eye.
• If easy vomiting occurs with no nausea, especially if it is accompanied by recurrent headaches on waking.
• If any signs of dehydration are visible in the very young or very old. These may include any of the following:
  • Drowsiness (this does not mean feeling sleepy or sleeping a lot, which is normal, but feeling not quite with it when you are awake), not reacting to things going on around you, answering simple questions slowly and speaking with an abnormally slow voice pattern.

• Sunken eyes.
• Dry skin.
• Reduced or concentrated urine output.
• Dry mouth.
• Depressed fontanelle (the soft spot at the crown of the head in newborn babies).

Practical self-help

• It is better to drink small amounts of fluid frequently, even only a sip at a time, as large amounts can cause a rise in stomach pressure and contribute to vomiting.
• Make sure that dehydration is kept at bay by keeping body fluid levels up (this is especially important if vomiting and diarrhoea occur together, since this results in a substantial volume of liquid being expelled from the body within a short space of time). Drink water frequently to avoid dehydration.
• It is important to bear in mind that when vomiting and/or diarrhoea occurs, the body is attempting to rid itself of something toxic, so it is essential to avoid putting further strain on the system by eating. In reality, most of us are unlikely to feel very hungry in between bouts of being sick because of the nausea that frequently accompanies vomiting.
• When the sickness has subsided and appetite gradually returns, it is important to introduce light, easily digestible foods slowly, avoiding those that are oily, fatty, spicy, stimulating (such as tea and coffee) or acidic. Appropriate foods include yoghurt, steamed fruit and vegetables, non-acidic fruit juices and vegetable broths.

Alternative treatments

Anthroposophical medicines

Nausea may be eased by taking fifteen Amara drops dissolved in water every few hours. This mixture of herbal bitters contains gentian, chicory, wormwood and yarrow.

Biochemic tissue salts

Queasiness and vomiting may be eased by using Combination Remedy E or tissue salt No. 2. The latter is suitable for general uneasiness of the digestive tract, which is made worse from becoming chilled, and better from bed rest; the former is suitable for vomiting and queasiness with colicky pains and flatulence. Take four tablets at hourly intervals if symptoms are very acute, tailing off the dosage as the situation improves. In less severe situations, take four tablets three times a day.

HOMOEOPATHIC MEDICINES

Type	General features	Worse	Better	Remedy
Chilliness, extreme anxiety and restlessness with vomiting	Severe nausea with extreme distress from the smell, sight or thought of food. Craving for cold water with burning thirst: vomits it back as soon as it is drunk.	Being alone Chill Cold drinks At night Physical effort	Small regular sips of warm drinks Warmth Lying propped up in bed Wrapping up well Company and distraction	Arsenicum album. Indicated for vomiting and diarrhoea that occur together
Exhaustion, pallor and prostration with vomiting and diarrhoea that occur together	Extremely forcible episodes of vomiting with constant craving for cold water that is vomited back soon after drinking. Nausea and vomiting are made much worse for the least movement. Pale, sweaty and clammy during and after vomiting	Pressure Effort Drinking Touch	Covering up Warmth Resting Milk	Veratrum album
Nausea and vomiting after over-indulgence in food and alcohol	Awful difficulty in bringing up vomit which seems to want to return to the stomach. Severe retching with cold sensitivity and 'morning after' feeling. Irritable, headachy and constipated	Cold, draughty surroundings Physical effort Noise Touch Pressure of clothing In the morning	As the day goes on At night Sound sleep Being left undisturbed After vomiting or passing a stool	Nux vomica
Nausea with vomiting of water as soon as it becomes warmed by the stomach	Marked thirst for ice-cold drinks which are returned after a while. Anxious and fearful with vomiting with a great need for reassurance.	Contact with cold air Warm drinks Talking Effort Lying on the back	Sound sleep Cool drinks (until they become warmed) Sponging or bathing the face with cool water	Phosphorus is suitable for vomiting that occurs as a result of anaesthetic
Extremely severe nausea and vomiting that are much worse for the slightest movement	Continuous, awful nausea that is no better after vomiting. Sensitive, bloated abdomen with colicky, intermittent pains. Thirstless with frothy or mucus-streaked vomit. Sickness is aggravated by stooping. Miserable, depressed or sinking sensations with illness	Motion Warmth Overeating or too great a mixture of foods Vomiting	Resting Fresh air Cold drinks Closing eyes	Ipecac

Home remedies

• Spices such as clove or nutmeg can be very soothing for the stomach when dissolved in warm water and sipped as needed.
• Sucking a piece of ginger root or crystallized ginger can also ease nausea and settle the stomach.

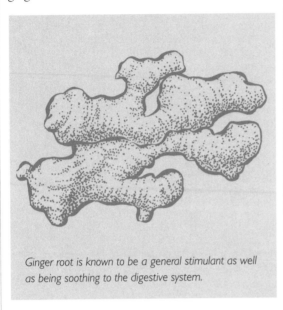

Ginger root is known to be a general stimulant as well as being soothing to the digestive system.

• Provided it is not unappetizing to a sensitive stomach, apple cider vinegar or lemon juice dissolved in warm water may settle an upset stomach.

Herbal preparations

The following teas may ease the nausea that occurs between bouts of sickness: chamomile, mint* or catnip. (Teas marked with a * may interfere with the action of homoeopathic remedies.)

Alternative help, treatment and advice may be obtained from practitioners of any of the following therapies:

• Anthroposophical medicine
• Homoeopathy
• Naturopathy
• Nutritional therapy
• Reflexology
• Traditional Chinese medicine
• Western medical herbalism

PROBLEMS OF THE REPRODUCTIVE SYSTEM AND URINARY TRACT

Cystitis

Cystitis is a distressing and painful condition that can affect both sexes. It is rare in children, so children with cystitis should be checked to ensure that they have no structural abnormalities and to prevent kidney damage later in life. It is also uncommon in men, so the cause should be checked (for example, enlarged prostate). In the elderly it is usually caused by incomplete emptying of the bladder. Women tend to be more subject to this problem, especially during pregnancy. Unfortunately, cystitis has a tendency to appear on a recurrent basis, with the result that many women find they are subject to flare-ups of this unpleasant condition on a long-term basis.

Cystitis is the inflammation of the bladder, usually in response to the presence of a bacterial infection. Symptoms can cause varying degrees of discomfort and distress and may include any of the following:
• Stinging, smarting or burning before, during or after passing urine.
• Strong, dark, concentrated urine.
• Unpleasant-smelling urine.
• Frequent urge to pass water even though there is very little in the bladder.
• Heavy or dragging feeling in the abdomen.
• A general sense of malaise or feverishness.
• Incontinence, particularly if due to urgency.
   Alternative measures can do a great deal to ease

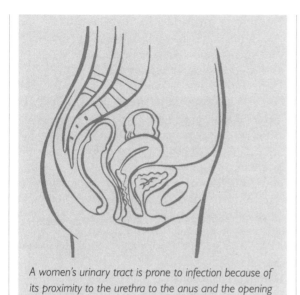

A women's urinary tract is prone to infection because of its proximity to the urethra to the anus and the opening of the vagina.

the misery of an acute bout of cystitis, especially when combined with the practical self-help measures (below). However, if cystitis has become a well-established or recurrent condition, seek help from a trained practitioner in order to deal with the underlying predisposition to the problem.

Practical self-help

• Rest as much as possible during the initial phase of cystitis; this is especially important if there are any signs of feverishness or malaise. By resting and staying in a stable temperature during the onset of symptoms it is often possible to help the body fight illness more effectively and decisively. On the other hand, making extra demands on vital energy reserves at this time can prolong the time taken to overcome infection and illness.

• If you suffer from cystitis on a recurrent basis, never delay the urge to pass water. Allowing urine to build up can encourage infection to spread to the kidneys, so regular and complete emptying of the bladder is an important and simple way of discouraging any problems from developing.

• Emptying the bladder completely before and after intercourse can also discourage recurrent infection. Combining this with washing the genital area gently with warm water after intercourse can do a great deal to keep recurrent attacks of cystitis at bay.

• Avoid cross infection by always wiping from front to back and not vice versa after emptying the bowels. This avoids transferring bacteria from the anus to the genito-urinary area.

• In severe cases 'bottle washing' can help. Each time after urinating or a bowel movement, pour a bottle full of water between the legs from front to back.

• If cystitis becomes a persistent or well-established problem, it may be helpful to reconsider another method of contraception if using a diaphragm. If the diaphragm fits overly snugly it can interfere with the free flow of urine from the bladder, encouraging a residue to remain, which can encourage infection. In addition, the delicate balance of micro-organisms in the vagina can be adversely affected by the use of barrier methods, especially when used in conjunction with spermicidal creams, gels or pessaries. The resulting imbalance can promote the growth of E. coli bacteria, one of the most common triggers for bladder infections.

• It is best to avoid wearing tight jeans, tights, leggings and figure-hugging underwear made from artificial fibres such as nylon if cystitis (or thrush) are a problem. They all create a warm, poorly ventilated environment that encourages the growth of fungal or bacterial infections. However, loose-fitting clothes made from natural fibres such as cotton, linen or silk allow the genital area to remain as cool and airy as possible.

• Vitamin C supplements may discourage infection if recurrent bouts of cystitis are a feature of life, but they should not be used routinely if there is any history of kidney stone formation.

• Increase the amount of garlic in the diet, since it is claimed to have antibacterial properties, and may be useful in aiding the body in fighting the micro-organisms that are responsible for bladder and urinary-tract infections. If the taste of garlic is unpalatable or unacceptable, use garlic supplements, available in capsule or tablet form.

• Constipation can increase general discomfort and pressure. Make sure it does not become a problem by including a high proportion of fibre-rich foods in the diet and drinking six to eight large glasses of water a day. Although fresh fruit and vegetables are a natural source of fibre (especially when eaten raw), some of them can aggravate problems with cystitis, especially strawberries, spinach, grapes, citrus fruits, asparagus, raw carrots and tomatoes.

• Any of the following drinks may also aggravate problems with cystitis and are best avoided, or taken infrequently in small quantities if cystitis is a well-established or recurrent problem: sugary carbonated drinks, caffeinated drinks, alcohol, tea and coffee.

• If there are any signs that an acute bout of cystitis is developing, drink a large glass of water at the first twinge, repeating the process at hourly intervals until the situation has eased. Cranberry juice can also be invaluable in easing the misery and discomfort of cystitis by making urine more alkaline and easier to pass as a result. Drink cranberry juice at hourly intervals while symptoms are acute, cutting down to two glasses a day until the situation has cleared completely.

• An effective alternative drink to cranberry juice may be obtained by drinking home-made barley water. Add two tablespoons of pearl barley to a litre of cold water, bring to the boil and strain off the liquid, which should be kept in the fridge until needed. Although home-made barley water is an excellent alkaline drink, it should not be confused with the commercially prepared, flavoured barley waters that resemble fruit squashes. Because these contain a high proportion of sugar, they can irritate the bladder, making the problem worse rather than better.

SEEK PROFESSIONAL HELP

• If there are any traces of blood in the urine.
• If pain occurs in the back or sides, especially if combined with feverishness, nausea and vomiting.
• If symptoms are persistent, do not respond to self-help measures or increase in severity.
• If the problem occurs in men or in children.

Alternative treatments

Topical preparations

For cystitis these are essential oils used in the form of aromatic baths and warm compresses to soothe and ease discomfort. Choose from any of the following, bearing in mind that none of the substances mentioned for external use should be taken by mouth.

Aromatherapy oils

A daily bath to which four tablespoons of crystal sea salt has been added is very helpful. A blend of two drops each of tea tree (Melaleuca alternifolia), lavender (Lavendula angustifolia), niaouli (Melaleuca quinqueneriva), thymus linalol and thymus thujanol in four teaspoons of carrier oil can be made up by a qualified aromatherapist and massaged over the stomach and lower back.

Medicines intended for internal use

These ease pain, reduce inflammation and encourage a speedy resolution of the problem.

Anthroposophical medicines

Chamomile tea may soothe the discomfort and cramping pains of cystitis. Steep half a teaspoonful of the dried flowers in 300ml (10fl oz) boiling water and strain after three minutes. Drink a mugful of this tea every few hours until symptoms improve.

Biochemic tissue salts

Tissue salt No. 6 may be helpful in easing cramping pains of cystitis that are brought on by anxiety or stress and made worse from moving about and being left alone too long. Tablets may be taken hourly while symptoms are acute, tailing off the dose as the situation improves.

Herbal preparations

The following infusion may be taken three or four times a day while symptoms of cystitis are present: add one part of marsh mallow root, cornsilk, couch grass, horsetail and bearberry with two of buchu to 600ml (1 pint) boiling water. Leave to steep for ten to fifteen minutes before straining and drinking hot. Avoid using bearberry for an extended period of time since it can give rise to toxic side effects if used for too long.

Home remedies

• Drink the cooled water in which potatoes have been boiled (avoiding using an aluminium saucepan).
• A soothing tea may be made from the silky tassels of corn of the cob. Alternatively, ample portions of the vegetable may be included in the diet.
• Cherries also have a reputation for easing symptoms of bladder or kidney problems.

Professional alternative medical help may be obtained from any of the following:
• Anthroposophical medicine
• Aromatherapy
• Ayurvedic medicine
• Homoeopathy
• Naturopathy
• Nutritional therapy
• Reflexology
• Shiatsu
• Traditional Chinese medicine
• Western medical herbalism

HOMOEOPATHIC MEDICINES

Type	General features	Worse	Better	Remedy
Cystitis that follows surgery involving catheterization	Inability to completely empty the bladder. Constant sensation of a few persistent drops remaining in the bladder that cannot be voided. Concentrated, dark urine with stinging, burning pains that occur after passing water. Bad-tempered and irritable with cystitis	Intercourse After surgery or childbirth Touch Pressure In the early morning	Warmth Rest After breakfast	Staphysagria
General state of fluid retention and lack of thirst with cystitis	Stinging, burning pains with scalding sensation on passing urine. Extreme urging with a violent need to pass water immediately. Awful sensitivity to heat with increased distress and discomfort. Fidgety, irritable and fussy when unwell	Warmth Contact with warm air Warm bathing Hot-water bottles Restricting clothes Touch Rest Night	Gentle movement Exposure to cool air Removing clothes or covers Cool bathing Cool compresses	Apis
Cystitis with violent burning pains that develop abruptly	Discomfort and distressing scalding sensations occur before, during and after passing water. Constant urge to urinate but only a few drops of concentrated urine are passed. Pain and discomfort extends from bladder to kidneys. Shivery, feverish and chilly when ill	Urination Drinking Coffee Movement	Warmth Soothing massage Night	Cantharis
Anxiety, extreme restlessness, nausea and shivering with cystitis	Severe burning when urinating that is relieved by warm bathing and warm compresses (e.g. hot-water bottles). Extreme distress and anxiety about health when unwell. All symptoms become more intense during the night	Chill Cool rooms Long, cool drinks As night comes on Alcohol Physical effort that exhausts	Warmth Sips of warm drinks Gentle movement Company and distraction Fresh air	Arsenicum album
Cystitis that develops after exposure to cold, damp conditions	Pain and urgency are intense when resting or lying still. Dribbling of urine if the urge to urinate is delayed or ignored. Chilly, but worse for being warm. Cystitis with thrush. Weepy and in need of sympathy and attention when feeling ill	Stuffy, rooms Warmth Rest Feeling neglected	Fresh, cool air Cool drinks Sympathy After having a good cry Company Gentle exercise	Pulsatilla

Heavy periods

Heavy or flooding periods may often be combined with an erratic or unpredictable monthly cycle, with periods often being early or late. The characteristic time for a previously regular monthly cycle to become irregular is usually approaching the menopause, when intervals between bleeding may become shorter or longer, while the nature of the flow may change from moderate to extremely heavy. Heavy periods can leave the sufferer feeling fragile and exhausted, while the frequent need to change sanitary protection can make the practicalities of life seem much more difficult to cope with.

Symptoms of heavy periods may include any of the following:
- Nausea or vomiting.
- Fainting or dizziness.
- Severe period pains.
- Gushing, heavy menstrual flow that seeps through most forms of sanitary protection.

If extremely heavy and frequent periods go on for an extended period of time, symptoms of anaemia may also emerge, such as:
- Weariness, light-headedness and persistent exhaustion.
- Pallor.
- Breathlessness.
- Palpitations.

If previously average periods have suddenly become very heavy or irregular for no apparent reason, it is important to discuss this change with your family doctor, who is likely to want to check that there is no underlying cause leading to this problem, such as fibroids, pelvic inflammatory disease (PID) or endometriosis. Once these possible triggers are ruled out, it is worth considering alternative medical help to ease the problem in addition to adopting the suggestions included in 'Practical self-help' section.

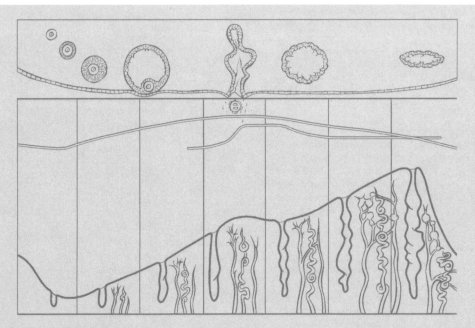

On average, ovulation occurs at day 14 and menstruation at day 28. Oestrogen from the ovary maintains the womb lining and when the level drops the lining breaks down (menstruation). If pregnancy occurs the corpus luteum enlarges and produces oestrogen to maintain the lining.

Practical self-help

• If anaemia has been identified as a problem, it is important to include the following foods in the diet to boost iron levels: pulses, eggs, green, leafy vegetables, oatmeal, blackstrap molasses, wholemeal bread, nuts, seeds and fish.

• Cut down on dairy foods, alcohol and strong tea and coffee, while increasing quantities of whole, fresh foods such as whole grains, raw fruit and vegetables.

HOMOEOPATHIC MEDICINES

Type	General features	Worse	Better	Remedy
Extremely heavy bleeding with awful nausea	Steady heavy flow, or alternation between gushing and oozing menstrual flow. Faint and nauseated from loss of blood, with marked intensification of symptoms from the slightest movement. Craving for fresh air when feeling dizzy and faint	Being exposed to extreme heat or cold Movement Eating	Resting Keeping as motionless as possible Closing the eyes	Ipecac
Heavy, dark, clotted menstrual flow with feelings of faintness	Extreme pain in pelvis before the flow starts, with obvious improvement as soon as the bleeding begins. Flooding periods with palpitations and hot flushes. Strong aversion to warmth and tight clothing around the neck and waist. Mood swings, depression and left-sided pre-menstrual headache or migraine	Before a period After sleep Stuffy rooms Hot baths Cold draughts Contact with extreme heat or cold	Exposure to fresh, open air As soon as the flow begins Gentle exercise Eating Cool drinks	Lachesis
Persistent backache and pain at base of spine with heavy bleeding	Strong tendency to puffiness, fluid retention and bloated abdomen. Extremely heavy bleeding persists even after corrective surgery (e.g. D and C), leading to anaemia and extreme tiredness. Painful areas feel cold. Chilly and exhausted to the point of not wanting to talk	Cold draughts Chill Lying on painful area Pressure Touch	Leaning forwards Warmth	Kali carb
Gushing, hot flow of bright red, clotted blood	General sense of congestion with cramping, dragging pains that set in before and during a period. Hot, dry, flushed skin with throbbing pains, restlessness and irritability	Lying flat Physical effort Jarring movements	Resting sitting propped up in bed Warmth	Belladonna
Early, heavy periods with anaemia and vertigo	Chilly with alternating episodes of shivering and flushes of heat. Very heavy, dark, clotted flow. Faintness and buzzing in the ears from profuse loss of blood. Antisocial, irritable and touchy with exhaustion	Physical effort Cold and chill At night Exposure to fresh air	Sleep Resting Warmth Firm pressure	China

• Take regular, stress-reducing exercise in the open air (if possible), in order to improve circulation and muscle tone. However, it is important during the initial phase of a period when blood loss is likely to be heavy to avoid overly vigorous exercise, since this can stimulate bleeding.

SEEK PROFESSIONAL HELP

• If any persistent change in bleeding pattern occurs for no apparent reason.
• If symptoms are severe and adversely affecting quality of life.
• If breakthrough bleeding or 'spotting' occurs in between periods.
• If bleeding occurs after the menopause.
• If bleeding becomes irregular or more frequent.
• If bleeding occurs with intercourse.

Alternative treatments

Medicines intended for internal use
These help to regulate blood loss.
Biochemic tissue salts
Tissue salt No. 4 may be useful for excessively heavy periods that resemble a haemorrhage in severity. Take four tablets three times a day while symptoms are present. Seek professional help if the symptoms do not improve within a short period of time.
Herbal preparations
• If heavy bleeding is due to a hormone imbalance, a decoction of chaste tree and false unicorn root may be useful. Chop, grind or pound the items in a pestle and mortar, then place 28g (1oz) of each herb in a little over 600ml (1 pint) water in a saucepan. Bring the mixture to the boil, simmer for ten minutes and strain.
• Golden seal may help to regulate the shedding of the lining of the uterus, due to its astringent, tonic properties. It works quickly. To be avoided in pregnancy.

Professional alternative medical help may be obtained from any of the following:
• Anthroposophical medicine
• Ayurvedic medicine
• Homoeopathy
• Naturopathy
• Nutritional therapy
• Shiatsu
• Traditional Chinese medicine
• Western medical herbalism

Impotence

Although a basic definition of impotence may sound fairly straightforward (an inability to achieve or maintain an erection), the potential causes of the problem can be extremely varied. These triggers may include anything from emotional stress, exhaustion, guilt, anxiety, taking drugs or an excess of alcohol. In addition, experiencing difficulty in achieving an erection can occur as men go through the ageing process.

Almost every man occasionally suffers from impotence at some time or another. Since most men tend to equate a great deal of their self-confidence and self-esteem with satisfactory sexual performance, persistent problems with lack of ability to achieve an erection can cause great psychological distress. As a result, it is extremely important to seek professional help if a problem of this kind is adversely affecting quality of life. In addition, some of the following suggestions may be of help.

Practical self-help

• If stress has become a major problem, consider ways of unwinding and relaxing. These may include relaxation techniques, meditation or attending a yoga class. Any of these may be extremely helpful where there is a risk of physical or psychological 'burn-out' developing.
• In addition, see general advice given in the 'Practical self-help' section for burn-out on page 240.
• Avoid items that have a reputation for restricting blood vessels such as alcohol, recreational drugs and caffeine.
• If the problem is occurring on a regular basis and causing distress, counselling may explore and resolve the problem.

SEEK PROFESSIONAL HELP

If impotence is persistent professional help is needed to exclude diabetes, vascular disease, etc.

This is especially true if there is an absence of morning erections; if these are present, a physical cause is far less likely.

Alternative treatments

Since this is a problem that can arise from a wide range of potential causes, it is best to seek help and advice from a trained alternative therapist. Appropriate therapies include any of the following:
- Acupressure
- Anthroposophical medicine
- Aromatherapy
- Ayurvedic medicine
- Flower remedies
- Homoeopathy
- Massage therapy
- Nutritional therapy
- Reflexology
- Traditional Chinese medicine
- Western medical herbalism

Infertility

Difficulty in conceiving a baby is a relatively common problem, which affects one couple in ten in Western countries. The causes are equally distributed between male and female, or may affect both, so it is essential that both are checked, even if one has previously had children. It has been suggested that it might be more accurate to describe some of these couples as experiencing sub-fertility rather than infertility, since many of them do eventually manage to conceive.

However, if a couple have been enjoying regular sexual intercourse for at least a year without protection from contraception, and conception has not taken place, your family doctor may suggest tests to investigate potential problems.

Factors that can adversely affect fertility may include any of the following:
- Cigarette smoking.
- Regular or excessive alcohol consumption.
- Emotional and physical stress.
- Strenuous or excessive exercise.
- Anxiety.
- Long-term illness.

Factors that may influence fertility in women may include any of the following:
- Age; low body weight; early menopause.
- Problems with ovulation: this may be the result of a hormonal imbalance, ovarian disease, severe weight loss or extreme stress and anxiety.
- Blockage of the fallopian tubes: problems of this nature usually occur because of a current or past infection. As a result of the obstruction, sperm are unable to make contact with the egg, and the latter is prevented from making its way to the womb.
- A problem with progesterone levels: if too little of this hormone is produced, the embryo is prevented from implanting itself securely in the womb.
- Irregularities with cervical mucus: a sticky mucus is secreted around the opening of the entrance to the womb in order to prevent infection from developing. During ovulation (a woman's most fertile time), this mucus becomes thinner in consistency so that sperm are able to penetrate. However, in some women this mucus may contain antibodies that kill off the sperm.
- Structural problems of the womb: the most common problems of this kind include fibroids (non-malignant tumours of the womb), an abnormally-shaped womb or scar tissue in the lining of the womb (adhesions).
- Endometriosis: this is a condition in which small pieces of the womb lining become attached to areas outside the womb. The main symptom is usually severe period pains, but fertility problems can also be a symptom.

Male infertility, on the other hand, may be caused by one of the following:
- Low sperm count or abnormality of sperm: some men may produce sperm that are unable to fertilize an egg. Co-factors that may aggravate these problems may include developing mumps (see page 292) in adulthood, being overweight (see page 324), having problems with varicose veins (see page 321) near the groin and testicles, or wearing very close-fitting underwear or tight jeans that cause the genital area to become overheated. Being under severe

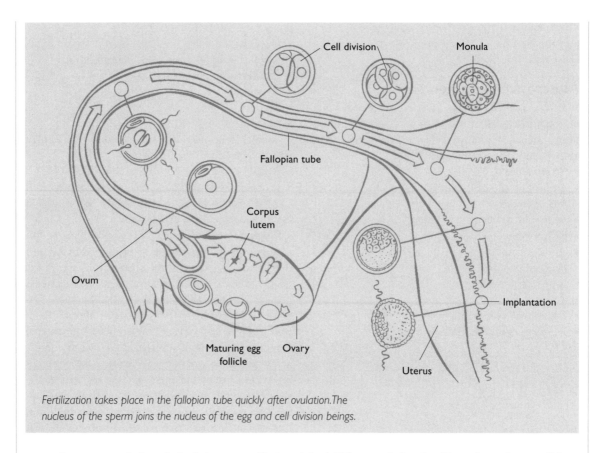

Fertilization takes place in the fallopian tube quickly after ovulation. The nucleus of the sperm joins the nucleus of the egg and cell division beings.

stress for an extended period of time or suffering from a hormone imbalance can also have an adverse effect on sperm production. Problems can also occur after reversal of a vasectomy, when sperm may begin to clump together so that they are unable to move as freely as they need to.

• Ejaculation problems: these may include premature ejaculation (where ejaculation precedes penetration), blockage of the sperm ducts, or a disorder called retrograde ejaculation, in which sperm pass into the bladder instead of out of the penis.

Practical self-help

• If stress is a problem, see the section on burn-out (page 240) for general advice on optimum nutrition and positive lifestyle changes.

• If you are feeling generally uptight about conceiving, the general advice given in the anxiety section (page 238) may also be helpful.

• It is extremely useful for a woman to know when she is ovulating to maximize the possibility of conception. Using a digital thermometer, take your temperature on waking each morning, before getting out of bed. When ovulation is taking place, there will be a rise in temperature of approximately 0.4–0.5°C (0.5–1°F), accompanied by a change in vaginal secretions, which should become thin and transparent, a little like raw egg white. Provided other problems are not present, the optimum time for conception lasts for two to three days around the time of ovulation. If this method proves unreliable, it is now possible to buy commercially produced kits that can identify when ovulation is taking place.

• If a low sperm count is suspected, men should make sure that they wear loose-fitting underwear and avoid clothing that is too tight.

If problems with conception have been continuing for more than a year, a professional medical opinion should be sought.

Alternative treatments

Problems with fertility require professional alternative help because of the complex nature of the problem. Any of the following therapies may be helpful in addition to exploring conventional medical help:

- Acupressure
- Anthroposophical medicine
- Aromatherapy
- Ayurvedic medicine
- Homoeopathy
- Nutritional therapy
- Traditional Chinese medicine
- Western medical herbalism

Irregular or absent periods

Temporary, long-term or permanent disruption of a woman's menstrual cycle may occur as a result of any of the following:

- Pregnancy (see page 259).
- Anaemia (see page 328).
- Eating disorders (see page 245).
- Hormone imbalances.
- The menopause (see hot flushes, page 307, vaginal dryness, page 319, and osteoporosis page 208).
- Emotional stress (see 'Psychological and stress-related conditions', pages 236–59).
- Surgical intervention such as a hysterectomy.
- Excessive exercise.

If periods remain absent or irregular with no apparent cause, professional medical help should be sought.

In addition, alternative medical help may be obtained from any of the following:
- Anthroposophical medicine
- Aromatherapy
- Ayurvedic medicine
- Homoeopathy
- Naturopathy
- Nutritional therapy
- Shiatsu
- Traditional Chinese medicine
- Western medical herbalism

Painful periods

Anyone who has suffered the misery of painful periods will understand why the monthly bleed is sometimes referred to as 'the curse'. However, although period pains can cause a great deal of distress and discomfort, this is by no means inevitable. If you are one of the unlucky ones, there are a number of practical steps you can take to improve your situation, which are listed in the practical self-help section below.

There are identifiable phases when women may be especially prone to painful or difficult periods, especially the onset of menstruation, when periods may be both painful and irregular, or during the approach of the menopause, when bleeding may become much more sporadic and heavy. Women prone to painful periods in their early teens may discover that the problem decreases in their twenties or following pregnancy.

The degree of pain that menstruation causes can vary a great deal: some people experience the odd twinge of discomfort, while others may be in such distress that they cannot function in a normal way at all, and find that life is severely disrupted every month.

Those women who experience painful periods may also have to cope with:
- Dizziness
- Fainting
- Clammy sweats
- Vomiting
- Diarrhoea
- Exhaustion
- Severe headaches or migraines
- Anxiety
- Tearfulness or irritability.

If you are unhappy about taking painkillers, or using other conventional medical strategies, you would do well to explore alternative remedies. If painful periods are a long-standing or severe problem, it is advisable to consult a trained alternative practitioner, but for occasional discomfort, some of the alternative measures outlined below may do a great deal to improve the situation.

Practical self-help

• A tendency to constipation or fluid retention can aggravate painful periods. Fluid retention can be combated by avoiding foods that are high in sodium such as convenience foods, crisps, nuts and other salted snacks. It is also helpful to avoid adding extra salt to food, and instead using alternative seasonings such as toasted sesame or sunflower seeds. Fluid retention can also be discouraged by taking regular exercise to stimulate the circulation such as brisk walking, cycling or running. Fresh parsley should also be added to the diet because of its diuretic (fluid-eliminating) qualities. To avoid constipation see advice on pages 162–5.

• Warmth is often soothing and pain relieving when applied to the lower abdomen and the back. The easiest way of achieving this is to soak in a warm bath, or to wrap a hot-water bottle in a towel and apply it to the painful area. Alternatively, a custom-made heating pad may be applied to the area in which the pain is centred. Since each of these methods of pain relief work by stimulating circulation in the painful area, a similar effect may be obtained by having a lower back or abdominal massage.

• The following supplements may be helpful in easing painful periods that occur within the general context of pre-menstrual syndrome (PMS): vitamin C, vitamin B complex, vitamin E and oil of evening primrose.

• Improving the circulation can also do a great deal to ease the misery of painful periods. Brisk, rhythmical exercise encourages the large muscles of the legs to work hard and ensures that the heart and lungs are given a thorough conditioning. Brisk walking, swimming, cycling, rowing or weight training will improve all-round fitness, as well as stimulating the circulatory system.

• Many of us instinctively respond to pain by tensing up and contracting our muscles, which can make the pain more severe and protracted. However, breathing techniques or becoming aware of simple ways of tensing and relaxing the main muscle groups can do a great deal to ease the distress of a painful period. Learning effective relaxation techniques can also relieve the anxiety that may surface when we are in severe pain.

• TENS (transcutaneous electrical nerve stimulation) machines ease pain without the side effects of conventional painkillers. Although very simple to use, TENS machines are used to positive effect in clinics dedicated to relieving the misery of chronic pain. The machine is made up of a battery-operated unit roughly the size of a personal stereo, to which two or four adhesive pads may be attached. The pads are placed over the site of the pain, and once the machine is switched on, a small electrical current passes between them. The resulting sensation should not be unpleasant, but feels rather like a gentle tingling, which should last for only a short time. As the tingling passes away, the pain should also subside. TENS machines work by producing low-level electrical stimulation that prevents or slows down the transport of messages reaching the nervous system and brain. The versatility of the TENS machine is considerable, since it can provide effective pain relief in labour, after surgery, for back pain or discomfort in the joints.

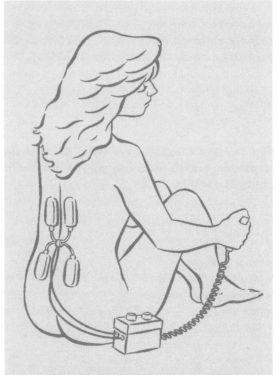

TENS machines ease pain without the side effects of conventional painkillers.

HOMOEOPATHIC MEDICINES

Type	General features	Worse	Better	Remedy
Rapidly developing period pains that come in waves	Weak, faint and doubled-over with pains that build quickly in severity. Unable to get comfortable when moving or at rest. Pains come on and leave very rapidly. Agitation and anger make the pains more intense and distressing	Resting Cool drinks when overheated Cold and damp Becoming angry or agitated	Warmth Firm pressure Bending over	Colocynthis
Painful periods that become more intense as the flow increases	Periods that occur too early or too frequently with shooting, flitting pains that affect the abdomen and extend down the thighs. Dark, heavy, severely clotted flow with extreme restlessness and desire to change position. Very low and depressed with pre-menstrual tension	As the flow goes on First movement after rest Chill or damp Night	Contact with warmth in any form Fresh air While eating After a bout of diarrhoea Walking about	Cimicifuga
Period pains that are eased as soon as the flow begins	Severe symptoms that are at their most intense from ovulation to the days leading up to the period. Distressing cramping pains extend to back and radiate down the thighs. Dark-coloured, clotted flow. Severe insomnia and emotional instability before period begins	Stuffy, overheated conditions Heat On waking from sleep Restrictive clothing If the flow is irregular or delayed, e.g. at menopause or during puberty	Fresh, cool air Loosening tight clothing As soon as the period starts Gentle exercise	Lachesis
Severe period pains with vomiting and diarrhoea	Extremely chilly, anxious and restless with periods. Although prostrated and exhausted, the severity of pain leads to an inability to keep still. Exposure to chill makes the pain more intense while warmth is very soothing. Fussy, fearful, and fidgety when in severe pain	At night Cold in any form Physical effort Being alone Alcohol	Local application of heat Warmth in general Sips of warm drinks Company Gentle movement	Arsenicum album
Violent labour-like contractions with period pains	Periods occur too frequently with bearing down sensations accompanying severe cramping pains. Gushing, clotted, bright-red flow that feels hot. Irritable and bad-tempered with pain	Lying on the painful part Jarring Being disturbed Noise Bright light	Warmth Keeping as still as possible When well wrapped up Being left in peace and quiet	Belladonna

• If previously easy periods have become painful, irregular or heavy for no obvious reason.
• If period pains are regularly incapacitating because of their severity.
• If painful periods are a well-established or persistent problem.

Alternative treatments

Topical preparations

For painful periods these are essential oils that can be applied to the skin to soothe and ease pain. Choose from any of the following, bearing in mind that none of the substances mentioned for application to the skin should be taken by mouth.

Aromatherapy oils

A blend of three drops each of lavender (Lavendula angustifolia), clary sage (Salvia sclarea), Roman chamomile (Chamaemelum nobile) and honey myrtle can be added to a bath of warm water, or a gentle, aromatic rub of three drops of each of the above added to four teaspoons of carrier oil may be applied to the abdomen and lower back. **NB** Only use clary sage on the day before a period plus the first two days of the period, but for no longer.

Home remedies

• A warm (but not too hot) bath can do a great deal to soothe muscle cramps. Alternatively, a warm compress or hot-water bottle can be applied to the painful area.

Medicines intended for internal use

These ease discomfort and encourage a speedy resolution of the problem.

Biochemic tissue salts

Crampy period pains that are worse from contact with cold and eased by warmth, pressure and bending forward may respond to tissue salt No. 8. Alternatively, the general distress and discomfort of difficult periods may require Combination N. Take tablets at hourly intervals if pains are severe, tailing off to four tablets three times a day for less severe symptoms.

Herbal preparations

• If painful periods are due to muscular stress and tension, the following herb teas will be a soothing aid to relaxation: chamomile, lemon verbena or lemon balm.

• An infusion of wild yam may ease muscular spasms associated with painful periods. Since wild yam also has a slight diuretic (fluid-eliminating) effect, it may be helpful when fluid retention exaggerates painful periods. Use 28g (1oz) dried herb to 600ml (1 pint) hot water, and leave to steep for ten to fifteen minutes before straining.
• Cramping period pains may also benefit from an infusion made from the stem bark of cramp bark. It soothes pains by acting as a muscle relaxant. The fresh berries should not be used because of their potentially toxic effect.

Home remedies

• Taking to bed with a soothing drink such as hot milk and nutmeg or chamomile tea can feel very comforting as well as encouraging muscular relaxation.
• Safflower or linseed seeds may reduce pain when they are made into a tea and drunk every five hours or so. Steep 7g (¼oz) of seeds in 600ml (1 pint) of boiling water, strain and drink by the teacupful.

Professional alternative medical help may be obtained from practitioners of any of the following:

• Acupressure
• Anthroposophical medicine
• Aromatherapy
• Ayurvedic medicine
• Chiropractic
• Homoeopathy
• Naturopathy
• Nutritional therapy
• Reflexology
• Shiatsu
• Traditional Chinese medicine
• Western medical herbalism

Pre-menstrual syndrome

Pre-menstrual syndrome (PMS) affects about 40 per cent of women. Symptoms can cover the full spectrum of physical, emotional and mental problems, and, although these may not be considered serious in a life-threatening way, they can have a profound adverse effect on the day-to-day quality of life.

Many women feel emotionally stable and secure for the first half of the menstrual cycle, but extremely vulnerable, volatile and insecure for the remainder of the time leading up to a period. Rapid or violent changes of mood can occur, with marked swings between euphoria and depression, irritability, violent anger, weepiness, lack of confidence and self-destructive impulses.

The following may also occur as common symptoms of PMS:
- Low energy levels.
- Lack of libido.
- Clumsiness and poor co-ordination.
- Mental and physical fatigue.
- Apathy and lack of direction.
- Breast tenderness and swelling.
- Fluid retention with puffiness of feet, ankles, fingers, waist and abdomen.
- Food cravings and disrupted appetite.
- Pain and discomfort when ovulating at mid-cycle.
- Painful periods.
- Recurrent headaches and/or migraines.
- Poor skin quality or acne.
- Cystitis.
- Thrush.
- Disrupted sleep patterns and insomnia.

Generally speaking, when women are enjoying optimum health they should experience little difficulty with their menstrual cycles, and certainly should be free of a large proportion of the miseries outlined in the list above. However, if PMS is a severe or well-established problem, treatment should be sought from an alternative practitioner in order to re-establish order and harmony in the system as a whole.

Alternative therapists who approach treatment of PMS from a holistic perspective are likely to give general advice to boost overall levels of vitality, health and well-being. This will usually include suggestions of dietary adjustments, relaxation techniques, appropriate forms of exercise for stimulating energy levels and sensible advice on reducing stress. On the other hand, if symptoms are infrequent or very mild, paying attention to the general self-help measures advocated below, as well as judicious use of an appropriate alternative medical remedy may do a great deal to ease the situation.

Practical self-help

- Concentrate on foods that are as nutritious as possible, avoiding those that have a reputation for aggravating symptoms of PMS. The latter include foods and drinks that contain a large proportion of sugar (e.g. cakes, biscuits, ice cream, colas and other carbonated drinks), convenience foods that include chemical additives, preservatives, flavourings and sodium, strong tea and coffee, and alcohol. Many of these items have a destabilizing effect on blood-sugar levels, leaving us open to exhaustion, poor concentration, dizziness, irritability and rapid changes of mood. Ways of stabilizing blood-sugar levels include the following simple steps: eat small amounts every couple of hours, avoiding going for long periods of time without eating; when snacking, avoid sugary items that may initially give a sense of increased energy, but rapidly leave the body feeling tired and sluggish as insulin is secreted into the bloodstream to combat the sugar; snack instead on fresh fruit (fruit sugar is less destabilizing than refined sugar), raw vegetables, rice cakes with savoury toppings such as vegetarian pâté, brown rice salad or wholemeal bread.
- Foods that should form the mainstay of the diet include those that are as close to their whole, natural state as possible; those that have been refined, preserved, tinned, freeze-dried or dehydrated should be avoided. Concentrate on whole grains and cereals, fresh fruit, raw or steamed vegetables, sprouted and unsprouted seeds, unsalted nuts, freshly squeezed fruit juices, fish, poultry, pulses and regular helpings of live natural yoghurt. By opting instead for a high proportion of fresh, raw foods in the diet, we are likely to increase our intake of essential vitamins and minerals while also avoiding some of the symptoms that may be aggravated by a diet that is mainly made up of junk foods. These symptoms may include recurrent headaches, indigestion, constipation, bloating of the abdomen, fluid retention, unstable energy levels, irritability and lack of concentration.
- Symptoms of PMS such as headaches, constipation and fluid retention may be aggravated by dehydration that results from drinking too little water during the day. It is important to drink six to eight large glasses of filtered tap water or still mineral water each day, especially when exposed to environ-

ments that are centrally heated, air-conditioned and double-glazed, since these can contribute to a very dry atmosphere. Herbal teas and grain-based coffee substitutes are also good additions to the diet.

• If fluid retention is a problem, avoid high-sodium foods such as salted nuts, crisps and convenience foods. Use alternative seasonings to make the flavour of food more interesting, such as toasted herbs, tahini and ground sesame or sunflower seeds.

• Symptoms of PMS may be eased by supplementing with oil of evening primrose, vitamin B complex and vitamin C. If your diet has recently been less nutritious than it should be, taking a good-quality multi-vitamin and mineral supplement may help PMS symptoms. Avoid high doses of vitamin B6 on its own, since it may have toxic effects if taken to excess over an extended period of time. Use a vitamin B complex in preference.

• Transient depression, anxiety and mood swings that are linked to PMS may be eased by taking up regular exercise. To derive maximum benefit the form of exercise chosen should involve rhythmic

HOMOEOPATHIC MEDICINES

Type	General features	Worse	Better	Remedy
Extreme mood swings that are relieved as soon as bleeding starts	Severe headaches and left-sided migraines that occur in days leading up to a period. Severe problems with insomnia with PMS, with all symptoms being much worse on waking from sleep. Heavy, dark, clotted flow. Violent alternation of mood from euphoria to depression	If onset of a period is delayed Waking from sleep Left side of the body Stuffy, poorly ventilated conditions Restrictive clothing around the waist or neck	Onset of a period Cool surroundings Movement in the fresh air Firm pressure Sitting bending forwards	Lachesis
Extreme weepiness and emotional vulnerability with PMS	Irregular periods with indigestion, headaches, backaches or diarrhoea occurring before or during the flow. Severe PMS at puberty, following pregnancy or the menopause. Persistent vaginal discharge and irritation. Constantly shifting, changeable symptoms	Stuffy, airless rooms Night Resting Heavy clothing Fatty foods Feeling neglected Solitude	After a good cry Sympathy and attention Gentle exercise Cool bathing Undressing	Pulsatilla
PMS with recurrent headaches, fluid retention and extreme introversion	Irregularities of fluid levels in the body lead to generally dry skin and persistent vaginal dryness. Lips are also cracked and dry and prone to recurrent cold sores. Severe headaches or migraines develop before or after periods. Extremely depressed, withdrawn and weepy with a strong dislike of sympathetic, supportive company	Displays of sympathy and affection Crying in public Touch Exposure to warmth and sunlight	Solitude Peace and quiet Sitting in the cool and shade Resting Going without regular meals	Natrum mur

working of the muscles, such as brisk walking, running, cycling, weight training or low-impact aerobics. Choose an activity that you can enjoy often, as regularity is more important than the time spent involved in the activity: in other words, a half-hour session of exercise enjoyed three or four times a week is likely to be more beneficial than a couple of hours spent once a fortnight. Aerobic exercise, which conditions the heart and lungs, has an important bearing on energy levels and sense of emotional stability and well-being because it causes chemicals called endorphins to be produced in the brain, which have a natural antidepressant effect. So, regular aerobic exercise is likely to relieve the depressive, self-destructive feelings that are often a part of PMS.

• If difficulty in coping with stress is contributing to PMS, it may be very helpful to take up a relaxation technique or meditation. Yoga is an excellent option for people who want to combine stress reduction through relaxation with an effective exercise programme that encourages suppleness, strength, improved muscle tone and stamina.

Type	General features	Worse	Better	Remedy
PMS with deep depression and lowered libido	Symptoms may develop if there is insufficient time to recover between pregnancies. Heavy, drooping pains with feeling as though contents of pelvic cavity are about to fall out. Extreme changes of mood with screaming, shouting, weepiness, feeling on edge and unable to cope	Sitting still Touch Going without regular meals Morning Emotional responsibilities and demands	Rhythmic, aerobic exercise Brisk walking in the fresh air Elevating the legs Eating small amounts at regular intervals	Sepia
PMS with digestive disturbance and marked sugar cravings	Extreme bloating of the abdomen with a strong need to pass wind. Curious sensation of wind passing through the vagina. Alternating constipation and diarrhoea with rumbling and gurgling. Painful, heavy periods with dark-coloured, clotted flow. Extreme insecurity, anxiety, bad-temper and depression before a period begins	Tight clothes around the waist or abdomen Too much fibre in the diet Too many physical demands Becoming too hot or too cold Stress and anticipation In the late afternoon	Loosening clothes Gentle exercise in the fresh air Being distracted Moderate, stable temperatures	Lycopodium

• If there is any sign of breakthrough bleeding, or 'spotting' between periods.
• If symptoms of PMS are severe, persistent or well established.
• If intercourse is painful and accompanied by a persistent vaginal discharge.
• If emotional symptoms are very severe or distressing.
• If symptoms have not responded positively to self-help measures within a reasonable period of time.

Alternative treatments

Topical preparations

Essential oils can be used externally to induce well-being and relaxation. Choose from any of the following, bearing in mind that none of the substances mentioned for external use should be taken by mouth.

Aromatherapy oils

A massage blend of four drops each of Roman chamomile (Chamaemelum nobile), lavender (Lavendula angustifolia) and honey myrtle added to four teaspoons of carrier oil or gel base can be used four times a day. If symptoms continue, seek advice from a qualified aromatherapist.

Medicines intended for internal use

These ease discomfort and encourage a speedy resolution of the problem.

Anthroposophical medicines

Cramp-like pains preceding a period may be eased by chamomile root. Two tablets of 3x potency may be used hourly for up to three doses, or until symptoms improve.

Herbal preparations

• Agnus castus (chaste tree) taken in tincture form appears to ease problems with PMS by acting on the pituitary gland to balance sex-hormone production. A half teaspoon of the tincture is recommended before breakfast each day, probably for three months.
• Alternatively, a decoction of false unicorn root has a balancing effect on the production of the female hormones oestrogen and progesterone, and also has a tonic effect on the ovaries. To make the decoction, 28g (1oz) of dried herb should be used to 600ml (1 pint) of boiling water.

Home remedies

• If fluid retention is a problem, try boiling lemon rind in water, leaving to stand overnight and drinking the strained liquid on waking.
• Alternatively, dandelion tea is a powerful diuretic that encourages the body to rid itself of excess fluid very effectively. This may ease symptoms of bloating and breast tenderness.
• Headaches and tension may be eased by sipping vervain tea (lemon verbena), while peppermint* or fennel tea may ease digestive problems associated with PMS. (Teas marked with a * may interfere with the action of homoeopathic remedies.)

Professional alternative medical help may be obtained from any of the following:

• Acupressure
• Anthroposophical medicine
• Aromatherapy
• Ayurvedic medicine
• Homoeopathy
• Massage therapy
• Naturopathy
• Nutritional therapy
• Reflexology
• Shiatsu
• Traditional Chinese medicine
• Western medical herbalism

Thrush

Thrush is caused by an overgrowth of Candida albicans, a yeast-like micro-organism normally kept in healthy check by the bacteria living in the gut. However, if this balance is adversely affected, candida can begin to proliferate beyond the confines of the gut, causing problems in the genital area, and/or in the mouth.

Although not considered a major medical disorder, genital thrush in women can wreak havoc on general quality and enjoyment of life. Possible symptoms include any of the following:

- Soreness, sensitivity and burning when passing water.
- Increased urgency of urination.
- Itching and irritation of the vagina and vulva.
- Pain and discomfort during intercourse.
- A thick, cottage-cheese-type discharge that may have a yeasty smell.

Additional general problems that accompany a predisposition to repeated bouts of thrush may include any of the following:
- Persistent urinary tract infections.
- Fatigue.
- Skin rashes.
- Joint pains.
- Digestive problems such as alternating constipation and diarrhoea, indigestion, abdominal bloating and heartburn.
- Unstable or low blood-sugar levels.
- Fluid retention.
- Mood swings.

Taking antibiotics can be a trigger for developing the symptoms of genital thrush as they adversely affect the acid-producing bacteria that keep candida at bay. The vagina's delicate balance can also be affected by using any of the following:
- Perfumed vaginal deodorants.
- Douches.
- Perfumed soaps and foam baths.
- Condoms, which can cause vaginal inflammation and, therefore, an increased tendency to develop thrush.

Being pregnant or suffering from diabetes can also lead to a predisposition to developing thrush.

Infrequent or mild outbreaks of thrush may be eased greatly by using the self-help techniques suggested below. However, if symptoms are recurrent, persistent or severe in nature, treatment should be obtained from an alternative medical practitioner who will have the necessary experience and expertise to assess and treat the problem at a fundamental level.

Practical self-help

- Natural live yoghurt, inserted vaginally on a tampon, can increase natural lactobacilli levels, thereby reducing the vaginal pH. Vaginal pH levels are one reason why sexually active women are vulnerable, as semen is fairly alkaline to allow the sperm to survive long enough to escape a hostile region (in the male) to survive the higher pH-level area of the female's vagina. In the process the semen increases the pH level in the vagina. Since men also carry candida asymptomatically on the glans from intercourse, and give it back to the woman during subsequent intercourse, any treatment should involve sexual partners as well.
- There appears to be a link between certain foods and candida overgrowth. The following items increase the possibility of developing a problem with thrush: alcohol, sugary foods and drinks, mushrooms, cheeses, vinegar, pickles, malted foods, white bread, tea, red meat that has been treated with antibiotics and growth hormones, and any foods that go through a fermenting process.
- Foods that play a positive, rather than negative role in supporting the body in coping with candida include the following: whole, unrefined foods that are as close to their natural state as possible, raw fruit and vegetables, brown rice, fish, pulses, natural live yoghurt, herb teas and filtered or mineral water.
- Avoid using strongly perfumed foam baths and soaps, which can aggravate irritation and discomfort of the vagina. Contraceptive gels, creams and pessaries can also have a similar effect.
- Garlic is considered to have anti-fungal properties, and therefore may be useful in easing an acute bout of thrush. Add garlic to meals as seasoning during the cooking process, or, since supplementation is often the best practical way of obtaining a large enough amount of garlic to be therapeutically useful, two tablets of powdered garlic should be taken three times a day as long as symptoms persist.
- If thrush has a tendency to recur, it may also be helpful to consider supplementing with acidophilus, oil of evening primrose, or caprylic acid. Vitamin C and B complex may also be of value if the immune system has been undermined by emotional or physical stress and strain. During an acute episode of thrush, between 1000 and 3000mg of vitamin C may be taken daily, reducing the dose if acidity of the stomach or diarrhoea occur. It is also important to ensure that the vitamin B complex taken should be yeast-free.
- Do not be tempted to make use of creams that provide a localized anaesthetic effect. While they may be effective in the short term, they unfortunately cannot do more than mask the symptoms without solving the problem. You may also develop a sensitivity to the cream that can cause increased irritation.

HOMOEOPATHIC MEDICINES

Type	General features	Worse	Better	Remedy
Thrush with persistent, uncomfortable vaginal dryness	Vaginal discharge may be thin, clear and watery or thickened like uncooked egg white. Burning pain, lack of lubrication and general discomfort in vagina lead to disinclination for love-making. Depressed, despondent and withdrawn with thrush symptoms	Touch Heat During or following a period Waking from sleep Sympathy and attention	Cool bathing Cool compresses Exposure to fresh, cool air Gentle movement Being left alone	Natrum mur
Thrush with urgent desire to pass water	Chilliness and low back pain with thrush symptoms which are more intense before a period and when feeling cold. Vaginal discharge is burning and leads to irritation and itching. General cramping pains in muscles when unwell	Becoming overheated Movement Physical effort After intercourse Pregnancy Touch	Contact with warmth Fresh air Daytime	Kali carb
Awful smarting, burning and yellow discharge with thrush	Terrible discomfort that extends deep into the vagina. Offensive, irritating discharge that stains underwear. Great uneasiness in genital area and back with pulling, dragging sensations. Restless and bad tempered when unwell	Becoming chilled Lying down Touch Bathing with cool water Standing	Warmth Sitting	Kreosotum
Recurrent thrush that dates from onset of periods or pregnancy	Thrush may be accompanied by general symptoms of pre-menstrual syndrome including headaches, bloating and severe bouts of tearfulness. Vaginal discharge may be thick, bland and yellow, or may cause intense discomfort when warm. Craving for attention and sympathetic company when ill	Overheating Hot, stuffy conditions Rest in bed Night Dairy foods	Undressing Cool compresses Contact with fresh, cool air Gentle exercise Sympathy After a good cry	Pulsatilla
Episodes of thrush that develop at ovulation	Sensitivity, irritation and burning with swollen feeling in vagina. Vaginal discharge is thin, irritating, bland or like uncooked egg white. Feels as though warm water is flowing down thighs	Touch Ovulation Following a period Uncovering genital area	Cool In the evening	Borax

SEEK PROFESSIONAL HELP

• If there is any tendency to well-established, severe or recurrent problems with thrush.

• If a vaginal discharge or unexplained irritation and itching emerge for the first time, a medical opinion is needed to diagnose thrush. By establishing the nature of the problem at an early stage it is possible to rule out other possible reasons for infection.

• If symptoms have not yielded to self-help measures within a couple of days.

Alternative treatments

For thrush it is quite appropriate to take the relevant remedy internally, while also applying a topical preparation to the skin.

Topical preparations

These are tinctures, creams or lotions that can be applied to the skin to soothe and heal. Choose from any of the following, bearing in mind that none of the substances mentioned for external application should be taken by mouth.

Aromatherapy oils

A daily bath to which four tablespoons of crystal sea salt has been added is very helpful, or make a massage blend from four drops each of tea tree (Melaleuca alternifolia), lavender (Lavendula angustifolia), niaouli (Melaleuca quinqueneriva), thymus linalol and thymus thujanol added to four teaspoons of carrier oil or gel base. Use four times a day. If symptoms persist, seek the advice of a qualified aromatherapist.

Herbal preparations

• An infusion of chamomile may be very soothing when used to wash the genital area.

• Alternatively, an infusion of any of the following anti-fungal herbs may be used for bathing: marigold (Calendula), golden seal (**NB** Not to be used during pregnancy), rosemary, hyssop, thyme or fennel. To make the infusion, add one teaspoonful of the dried herb to a cup of boiling water and leave to infuse for fifteen minutes. Once the liquid has been strained add it to the bathwater to relieve itching and irritation.

Home remedies

• If irritation and itching are severe, taking a salt bath can be very soothing. Dissolve a tablespoonful of common salt in the bathwater as the hot tap is running and soak in the bath as long as it is comfortable.

• Douching with a mixture of vinegar and water can also relieve troublesome itching.

Medicines intended for internal use

These ease irritation, reduce inflammation, and encourage a speedy resolution of the problem.

Herbal preparations

Blackberry leaf tea has a reputation for easing the irritation of thrush, as well as soothing the discomfort of haemorrhoids and cystitis.

Professional alternative medical help may be obtained from any of the following:

• Anthroposophical medicine
• Aromatherapy
• Ayurvedic medicine
• Homoeopathy
• Naturopathy
• Nutritional therapy
• Reflexology
• Traditional Chinese medicine
• Western medical herbalism

Vaginal discharges

See thrush (page 199) and vaginal dryness (page 319).

MUSCULAR AND SKELETAL PROBLEMS

Cramp

Cramp is caused by muscular spasms that usually affect the calf muscles, feet and hands. Painful periods can cause a similar sensation in the abdomen. During an acute episode, the affected muscles contract suddenly, with resulting severe pain that can last for several minutes.

Those who are especially vulnerable to developing cramp include athletes, swimmers, joggers and those who do taxing physical work that involves repetitive movement (such as gardeners). Poor circulation or calcium, magnesium or potassium deficiency can also cause cramp.

Practical self-help

• Avoid eating the following foods on a regular basis, since they appear to increase our risk of developing narrowed, or 'furred up' arteries: animal fats such as red meat, any full-fat dairy products and eggs.

• If cramp occurs in the thigh, sit down and straighten the knee. Ask a helper to lift the heel of the foot of the affected leg with one hand, while pressing down firmly on the knee on the same side with their other hand. If a cramp occurs in the hand, slowly straighten the fingers and spread them apart while pressing down on a solid, hard surface.

• If cramps are occurring on a regular basis, pay attention to the quality of your diet, making sure that you are deriving maximum benefit from a regular intake of essential vitamins and minerals. The following foods should be included on a regular basis: green, leafy vegetables, whole grain cereals, seeds, unsalted and unroasted nuts, and soya products. Bananas, which are high in potassium can also be helpful. If your diet has been suffering as a result of an unduly stressful lifestyle, it may be helpful to consider taking a high-quality multivitamin and

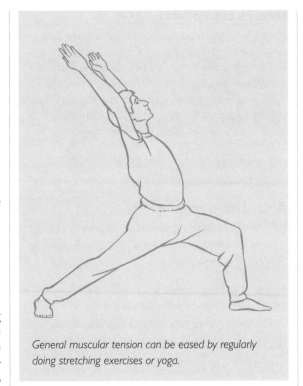

General muscular tension can be eased by regularly doing stretching exercises or yoga.

mineral supplement on a temporary basis as you are setting about improving the quality of your daily intake of food. As low salt levels can cause cramp, ensure that your diet contains enough salt.

• Specific mineral supplements that may help with a general tendency to develop cramp include the following: calcium, magnesium, potassium and iron. Helpful vitamins include vitamin B complex, vitamin C, vitamin D and vitamin E. However, caution should be used by those who have high blood pressure with regard to dosage of vitamin E, since the latter can aggravate the problem when used in large amounts.

• If you suffer from physical, mental or emotional stress, consider taking up yoga or exploring relaxation techniques. Both activities should increase your sensitivity to areas where muscular tension is being held, and as a result, it should lead to increased ability to 'let go' of physical pockets of stress and tension.

SEEK PROFESSIONAL HELP

If episodes of cramp are occurring on a regular basis, especially if they are combined with symptoms that suggest circulatory problems may be developing.

Alternative treatments

Topical preparations
These include compresses, essential oils or tinctures, that can be applied to the skin to soothe localized pain.

Aromatherapy oils
Add three drops each of French basil and honey myrtle to two teaspoons of carrier oil and gently massage the affected area as necessary.

Herbal preparations
• A hot compress of ginger may ease the pain and discomfort of muscle cramps when applied to the appropriate area, due to the circulation-stimulating properties of the spice. To make the compress, soak a clean cloth in a hot infusion and apply as warm as possible to the painful area.
• Poor circulation may be eased by using regular ginger or mustard footbaths. To make a mustard footbath add a tablespoon of powdered mustard to 2l (3½ pints) hot water.

Medicines intended for internal use
These ease pain and encourage a speedy resolution of the problem.

Anthroposophical medicine
Abdominal cramps that are associated with digestive upsets or diarrhoea may be eased by using a homoeopathic preparation of chamomile root (in 3x potency). Five pills may be taken every two to three hours until pain eases.

Biochemic tissue salts
Tissue salt No. 8 may be helpful in easing cramping, spasmodic pains that are aggravated by cold and touch, and eased by warmth, pressure and bending double. Alternatively, Elasto may be useful to those who experience cramps in combination with varicose veins and a general tendency to aching legs.

Herbal preparations
Nettle (Urtica) tea may ease a general tendency to cramp. Boil 50g (2oz) dried nettle leaves in 1l (1¾ pints) water for three minutes. Remove from the heat and leave to stand for ten minutes, strain and drink a cup of the warm tea three times a day.

HOMOEOPATHIC MEDICINES

Type	General features	Worse	Better	Remedy
Violent cramps that begin in, or only affect the left side	Trembling and weakness with severe cramp. Pains affect the chest, fingers, toes and calf muscles. Cramps make muscles feel knotted and are severe enough to make patient cry out	Mental and physical burn-out; Touch; Movement; Lack of sleep; Emotional stress	Cool drinks	Cuprum met
Cramping pains that come on after muscular overexertion	Muscle pains that set in when someone unfit takes up taxing physical exercise. Strained muscles feel bruised and very sensitive.	Jarring movements; Too much exercise; Touch; After sleep; Movement	Lying with head lower than the body	Arnica Specifically helpful for writer's cramp in the fingers
Muscular cramps that set in at night	Spasmodic, cramping pains with severe state of general muscular tension. Constant desire to stretch the feet due to tightness in muscles of calf and soles of the feet. Numb, stiff sensations in arm muscles that go to sleep easily	Contact with cold draughts; Mental and physical exhaustion; Lack of sleep; Too much coffee, tea or alcohol	Warmth; Sound sleep	Nux vomica

Home remedies

• Include celery in your diet regularly to make the most of its potassium and natural salt content. This can be especially important in hot summer weather when an excessive amount of salt may be lost from the body as sweat levels increase.

• Flagging calcium levels may be boosted by eating sesame seeds and including tahini paste in your diet.

• A warm drink made from hot water, one teaspoon of cider vinegar and one teaspoon of organic honey may reduce a tendency to cramp in the muscles at night.

Alternative help, treatment and advice may be obtained from practitioners of any of the following therapies:

• Acupressure
• Anthroposophical medicine
• Aromatherapy
• Ayurvedic medicine
• Chiropractic
• Homoeopathy
• Massage therapy
• Naturopathy
• Nutritional therapy
• Osteopathy
• Reflexology
• Shiatsu
• Traditional Chinese medicine
• Western medical herbalism

Osteoarthritis

Osteoarthritis has long been regarded as part and parcel of the ageing process, with vulnerable joints becoming immobile, stiff and sore as a result of general wear and tear. The areas most predictably affected include the large weight-bearing joints of the hips, knees and/or spine. The misshapen appearance of the joint develops as a result of the smooth cartilage that covers the ends of bones becoming distorted

and thickened. Once this process gets well under way, the damaged area becomes painful and stiff.

From a conventional medical standpoint, a rather fatalistic viewpoint has been adopted with regard to the incidence of osteoarthritis: it has been estimated that some degree of osteoarthritic change has occurred in

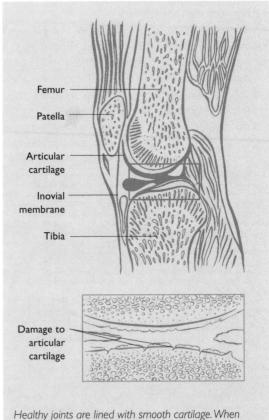

Healthy joints are lined with smooth cartilage. When osteoarthritis develops, the cartilage becomes roughened and eroded.

90 per cent of people aged forty years and over. However, it has also become increasingly clear that there are positive steps that can be taken to safeguard the mobility and smooth running of our skeletal systems. This information is listed in the 'Practical self-help' section opposite.

Occasional twinges of pain and discomfort in joints may be relieved by using some of the self-help measures included in the 'Alternative treatments' section (pages 205–7). However, if problems with osteoarthritis have become well established or severe, it is very important to seek help and advice from a trained practitioner.

Practical self-help

• Since there appears to be a strong link between eating certain foods and aggravation of arthritic problems, it makes sense to try to drastically reduce, or eliminate these items from the diet. They include red meat, products made from refined (white) sugar or flour, citrus fruit (including oranges), dairy foods, tomatoes, potatoes, aubergines, tea, coffee, alcohol, or 'instant' meals that tend to contain a hefty amount of artificial preservatives, colourings or flavourings. If you are unsure which of the above may be causing a potential problem, adopt an elimination diet for a few weeks to clarify the picture. Cut out any suspect foods or drinks and introduce each one systematically, waiting to see if there are any adverse reactions after they have been reintroduced to your diet. If a problem occurs in reaction to one specific item, eliminate it for a few weeks, reintroducing it again once your joints are more comfortable. If a problem occurs in reaction to this item for the second time, there is a good chance that you have a sensitivity to this food and should avoid it whenever possible.

• Your diet should concentrate on pulses, brown rice, whole grains, rye bread, sugar-free oatcakes, modest helpings of free-range chicken, fish, eggs (discarding the yolk), fruit (except for citrus), home-made muesli, unroasted, unsalted nuts, freshly pressed fruit juices (avoiding citrus varieties), home-made soups, vegetable purées, coffee substitutes, mineral water and herb teas. By using imagination and ingenuity it should be possible to make sure that eating remains enjoyable and varied, and you should not feel deprived and restricted as far as food options are concerned.

• Although it may seem obvious, it is important to remember that constipation can aggravate joint problems, due to the system becoming overloaded with toxic waste. See the section on constipation (page 162) for measures to alleviate this.

• A number of supplements have a reputation for alleviating stiffness, discomfort and immobility in the joints, and also discouraging further degeneration of the affected areas. These include cod liver oil, oil of evening primrose, vitamin A, vitamin B complex and vitamins C and E. However, it is important to remember that although vitamin B complex and C are water-soluble and can be efficiently flushed out of the body if too much is taken, vitamins A and E are quite different. The latter are fat-soluble, with the result that when an excessive amount is taken, the body stores the extra, which can lead to a toxic build-up and potentially serious side effects. To avoid this, always make a point of checking that you are safely within your recommended daily limit for the vitamin concerned.

• It is vital to keep as flexible and mobile as possible to guard against possible joint problems in the future and to cope with minor aches, pains and stiffness in the joints. Always make a point of choosing an activity that is fun, absorbing and enjoyable instead of dutifully taking up a form of exercise that you drop very quickly because you are bored with it. Avoid any activity that involves jarring, repetitive, pounding movements such as jogging on a hard surface. Swimming is an excellent choice, since the buoyancy of the water provides support for the large, weight-bearing joints while they are being exercised, reducing the possibility of damage. Other appropriate activities to consider include yoga, brisk walking or cycling.

• Arthritis of the large, weight-bearing joints of the hip and knees can be made more of a problem by being overweight. See the section on weight gain on pages 324–6 for advice on a healthy weight-loss plan.

• If joint and muscle pains occur on a regular or frequent basis it may be of help to seek treatment and advice from a chiropractor or osteopath. In addition, if there is any suspicion that aches and pains are being compounded by muscular tension, a regular massage of the back, neck and shoulders may be helpful in relieving pain and stiffness.

SEEK PROFESSIONAL HELP

• If persistent and/or severe joint pains occur with increasing stiffness or lack of mobility in the affected joint or joints.
• If general feelings of feverishness, malaise or fatigue occur in association with joint pains.
• If heat, redness or swelling occur in the small joints of the fingers, toes, knees or ankles.

Alternative treatments

For osteoarthritis it is perfectly appropriate to take the relevant remedy internally while also applying a topical preparation to the skin.

Topical preparations

These include tinctures, lotions or essential oils that can be applied to the stiff or painful area in order to soothe and increase mobility. Choose from any of the following, bearing in mind that none of the substances mentioned for application to the skin should be taken by mouth.

Aromatherapy oils

There are many oils that can help, but always seek advice from a qualified aromatherapist when dealing with inflammatory conditions.

Herbal preparations

• Inflamed joints may respond well to the application of a capsicum compress. Make a hot infusion by adding 28g (1oz) dried herb to 600ml (1 pint) water. Bring to the boil, simmer for fifteen minutes and strain before soaking a clean piece of linen or towel in the hot liquid. Apply the compress as warm as is comfortable to the painful area and replace it with a fresh hot compress as soon as it has cooled.

• A warm comfrey poultice may also ease the discomfort of stiff, inflamed joints. To prepare the poultice, mix the dried herb and warm water or cider vinegar before wrapping the mixture in clean, thin gauze. Apply the poultice warm to the painful joint, replacing it with a fresh one as soon as it has cooled down.

Home remedies

• Epsom salt baths have a reputation for relieving aches and pains and stiffness in the joints and muscles. Dissolve 450g (1lb) Epsom salts in a few pints of boiling water and add to comfortably warm bathwater. Soak in the bath for no more than fifteen minutes once or twice a day. Do not use soap, since it can interfere with the therapeutic action of the salts.

• Inflamed joints that feel more comfortable for cool contact may be greatly relieved by the application of cabbage leaves to the painful area. Make them into cool compresses by wrapping them in thin gauze and fastening around the affected joint with a safety pin, or place the leaves directly over the inflamed area. Once the leaves have warmed up replace them with fresh, cool ones.

Medicines intended for internal use

These reduce inflammation, ease pain and discourage further degeneration.

Biochemic tissue salts

Arthritic pain combined with muscular stiffness may respond to Combination I, while generally rheu-matic pains may be eased by Combination M. If neither of these appear to be suitable, Zeif may be more appropriate. This combination is regarded as being particularly helpful for arthritic and rheumatic pain. Acute flare-ups of joint pain require frequent repetition of tablets (e.g. every hour), while more low-grade symptoms are more likely to respond to tablets taken three times a day, discontinuing their use as symptoms improve.

Herbal preparations

Extracts of green-lipped mussel or devil's claw have a reputation for easing pain and inflammation of arthritic joints. They may be obtained in tablet form, or a decoction may be made by chopping or grinding 28g (1oz) dried tuber and adding it to just over 600ml (1 pint) water. Bring to boiling point in an enamelled pan, cover and simmer for fifteen minutes. Strain the liquid and take warm three times a day for a maximum of six weeks. **NB** The use of devil's claw should be avoided in pregnancy because of its uterine tonic properties.

Home remedies

• Cabbage juice has a reputation for acting as a detoxifying agent in reducing the production of catarrh as well as easing joint pains.

• One teaspoonful of cider vinegar and honey diluted in a small cup of warm water taken each morning is recommended as a way of warding off arthritic pain and stiffness.

Alternative help, treatment and advice may be obtained from practitioners of any of the following therapies:

• Acupressure
• Anthroposophical medicine
• Aromatherapy
• Ayurvedic medicine
• Chiropractic
• Homoeopathy
• Massage therapy
• Naturopathy
• Nutritional therapy
• Osteopathy
• Shiatsu
• Traditional Chinese medicine
• Western medical herbalism

HOMOEOPATHIC MEDICINES

Type	General features	Worse	Better	Remedy
Puffy, swollen joints that are sensitive to heat in any form	Stiff, painful, rosy-red, inflamed joints with stinging, prickling pains. Ankles in particular become enlarged and puffy. Severe pain flares up rapidly and severely, leading to fidgetiness and restlessness. Terrible sensitivity and overreaction to warmth	Bathing with warm water Contact with warm air Touch Resting After sleep	Bathing with cool water Contact with cool air Gentle exercise Undressing	Apis
Arthritic pains that date from an injury or fall	Bruised pain, aching and stiffness that are aggravated by the slightest touch or movement. Aching in hip joints leads to a sense of weakness and difficulty in walking. Morose, exhausted and touchy when in pain	Old accidents and injuries Jarring movement Touch or pressure After sleep Making too much of an effort Cold, damp conditions	Resting with head lower than the body	Arnica
Painful, stiff arthritic joints that feel cold to the touch	Discomfort and pain in joints is soothed and calmed by bathing with cool water. Pains move from the feet upwards.	Warmth Being wrapped up or covered too snugly Movement At night Too many eggs in the diet Alcohol	Resting Bathing with cool water Applying cool compresses	Ledum May be needed after a painkilling or steroid injection if the general symptoms fit
Stiff, painful joints that limber up well for gentle exercise	Painful joints that feel at their worst when resting in bed, or on initial movement: once continuous exercise is under way they feel much better. Stiffness and pain are aggravated by damp, cold weather. Depressed, restless and despairing when in pain	Rest in bed At night Damp, cold weather Chill or overheating First movement Jarring or jolting movement	Continuous, gentle movement Warm bathing Support to painful area Stretching Gentle massage	Rhus tox
Stiff, painful joints that are much more comfortable for resting as much as possible	Red, swollen, hot joints that get more and more uncomfortable during the day. They are most comfortable after a night's rest. Arthritic pains develop following injury to affected joints. General toxic state of the system leads to headaches and constipation	Getting up after sitting for a while Movement Stooping Jarring Sudden movements such as coughing Touch or light pressure	Firm support to painful joint Resting Warmth locally applied Lying on painful part	Bryonia

Osteoporosis

Although osteoporosis has attracted a great deal of publicity as a problem that primarily is a matter of concern for women in their post-menopausal years, it is also important to realize that men can also suffer from this condition as they get older, as can younger people with severely deficient diets (such as those suffering from anorexia nervosa). However, women are especially vulnerable to this problem once they experience the menopause and their fertile years draw to a close.

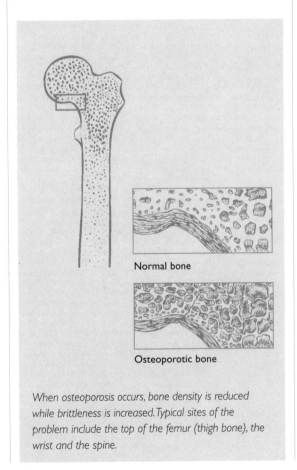

Normal bone

Osteoporotic bone

When osteoporosis occurs, bone density is reduced while brittleness is increased. Typical sites of the problem include the top of the femur (thigh bone), the wrist and the spine.

The increased risk of developing osteoporosis after the menopause appears to be linked to a dramatic drop in levels of the hormone oestrogen. Additional co-factors that indicate vulnerability to the onset of osteoporosis include:

• An inherited tendency to poor bone density with a significant number of close relations having suffered from osteoporosis.

• An early menopause, especially if it occurs before the mid-thirties. An especially early menopause may occur in exceptional circumstances as a natural development or, more commonly, as a result of surgical intervention such as a hysterectomy, or intense drug treatment, such as chemotherapy. Those who have had both ovaries removed during a hysterectomy are at greater risk of osteoporosis than those who have been left with one or both ovaries intact following surgery.

• Long-term steroid use.

• A history of alcohol excess, smoking (especially in women), thyroid disorders and immobility for any reason, for example, rheumatoid arthritis.

• A history of eating disorders such as anorexia nervosa or bulimia nervosa (see page 245) can be more vulnerable to developing osteoporosis. If oestrogen and body-fat levels plummet to a point where periods stop, especially in teenagers, the risk is higher, since this is the time when our bone density is being built up.

Although it has been estimated that fifty is the average age for the menopause to occur, bone density can begin to suffer at any point after the mid-thirties, due to calcium steadily leaching from the bones, leaving them less resilient to physical stress. Those who suffer from this problem find that their bones become thin and brittle, with the result that fractures may happen spontaneously, or as a result of very little stress or trauma. Common symptoms include:

• In advanced cases of osteoporosis, a characteristic stooped appearance. The curvature of the spine that develops is often referred to as a 'dowager's hump', and can affect men as well as women.

• Easy fractures from minor accidents that should not be expected to do much damage. Bones may be broken as a result of minor falls (this may include a simple accident such as falling off a chair), or following severe jolting or jarring movements. The bones most subject to injury are those of the hip, wrist, neck and spine. If a fracture occurs in any of these areas for a minor reason, investigating overall bone density is definitely to be advised.

• Restricted movement in the spine and chest and/or severe pain in the weight-bearing joints of the spine, hips and knees.

• Muscle spasms and/or weakness of the muscles of the pelvic floor in women.

Although this makes rather sobering and alarming reading, it is important to adopt a positive perspective and investigate alternative medical treatments. Holistic approaches such as herbalism, homoeopathy and acupuncture have a very positive role to play in helping deal with osteoporosis. For women, since problems can precede the menopause, it is wise to seek help from a qualified practitioner as a preventative measure, especially if recurrent pain, weakness or fragility of the bones become apparent well before symptoms of the menopause have begun.

The advice given below may also be helpful in giving a broad perspective on the self-help measures that can be adopted if you appear to have a high risk of osteoporosis. However, it is also important to stress that due to the serious consequences that may arise as a result of this condition, long-term management of the problem should be put in the hands of a trained practitioner, and you should not attempt to deal with the situation alone.

Practical self-help

It is essential to make an effort to include calcium-rich foods in the diet beyond the most obvious source, dairy foods. The following should be eaten on a regular basis as an alternative way of boosting calcium intake: tofu, spinach, kale, broccoli, chick peas, wild greens, whole grains, hazelnuts, almonds, sea vegetables (kelp, etc.) and molasses.

• Since it is vital to keep a healthy balance between calcium and magnesium in the diet (in order to ensure that maximum absorption of calcium occurs), make sure that magnesium-rich foods are not ignored, such as pulses, black-eyed peas, green, leafy vegetables, liver, eggs, almonds and whole grains. When using a calcium supplement the same rules apply, so it is important to take a combined formula of calcium and magnesium together.

• Try to avoid eating too many foods that contain phosphorus such as tinned meats, processed cheese and 'instant' foods such as packet soups and puddings. Although this mineral taken in small quantities will encourage calcium absorption, when too much is present in the diet it will have the reverse effect, encouraging leaching of calcium deposits from the bones.

• It is also important to remember that although protein-rich foods are essential for building, maintenance and repair of body tissues, including too much animal protein in the diet aggravates problems with osteoporosis.

• It is usually preferable to make sure that essential vitamins and minerals are obtained from a well-balanced, healthy diet, rather than becoming over-reliant on vitamin and mineral supplements to meet basic nutritional requirements. However, there are certain situations where it may become necessary to boost vitamin and mineral intake temporarily by judicious use of supplements. Bearing this in mind, the following supplements can have a positive part to play in protecting sound bone density: vitamins C, D and E, zinc, silicon and boron.

• Care should also be taken with regard to consumption of caffeine, alcohol and cigarettes, since they can cause calcium to leach from the bones. Smoking also reduces oestrogen production, as well as being linked to a host of potential health problems, including an increased risk of heart and/or lung disease.

• Never underestimate the importance of regular, weight-bearing exercise in protecting bone density. The beneficial effects of exercise include increased strength, flexibility, stamina, as well as encouraging the production of small amounts of oestrogen in women. In men, it could be linked to lowered testosterone levels in mid-life (any time between the ages of forty and seventy). Regular physical activity should ideally begin before the mid-thirties, when bone density has usually reached its peak mass. Regular exercise and a healthy diet from the early to mid-twenties provides the best chance of preserving strong, healthy bones in later years. The ideal form of physical activity includes anything that involves repetitive, rhythmical movement, especially of the weight-bearing joints. Good examples of this kind of exercise include any of the following: cycling, brisk walking, low-impact aerobics, dancing, weight training, tennis, badminton and yoga. Avoid putting excessive strain on the weight-bearing joints of the hip, ankle and knee by jogging on a hard surface or playing a violent game of squash. If you are unfit, build up to a regular exercise routine slowly and steadily, since regularity of physical activity is the most important thing.

SEEK PROFESSIONAL HELP

• If there is any obvious pain or weakness in the joints of the hip, knee, ankle, spine or neck.
• If stress fractures occur.

Alternative treatments

Medicines intended for internal use

These discourage further loss of bone density and ease pain and discomfort.

Herbal preparations

• Herbs containing calcium should be included in the diet, such as parsley, dandelion leaves, kelp and horsetail. These may be used as garnish, flavourings, or in salads.
• Certain herbs have a reputation for discouraging loss of calcium from the bones. They include marigold (Calendula), false unicorn root, wild yam, hops, licorice,* sage* and blue cohosh.* They may be taken in the form of herbal infusion. (*Never to be

HOMOEOPATHIC MEDICINES

Type	General features	Worse	Better	Remedy
Osteoporosis with severe pains in the long bones	Restless from pains that feel deep in the bones. Weak feelings in the legs that are most noticeable on rising out of a sitting position. Cracking sounds in the joints	Stretching Physical exertion Cold, damp weather Lying Getting up from a sitting position Stooping Climbing steps	Warmth Rubbing sensitive area Lying on back Changing position	Ruta
Osteoporosis with burning pains in bones	Aching pains in knees with cold sensations in limbs. Painful, contracted, shortened feeling in legs. Difficulty in achieving fine movements of the hands because of joint problems	At night Warmth Contact with cold air Movement Touch	Wrapping up well	Mezereum
Osteoporosis with chilly, numb sensations in limbs	Tendency to rheumatic pains in cold weather. Weakness and pain in hip joints. Fractures knit slowly and with difficulty from childhood. Pain and burning in affected bones	Change of weather Exposure to cold, draughty conditions Brooding on symptoms Lifting Climbing stairs	Warm, dry weather During the summer Lying down	Calc phos
Osteoporosis with lightning-like, stabbing pains	May be indicated in those who show signs of premature ageing. Painful erosion of strength and density of the long bones. Permanent sensation of being overheated: constantly wants to bathe in cool water	Becoming overheated At night Drinking alcohol (especially red wine) Sour foods	Bathing with cool water Rapid movement A short sleep	Fluor ac

taken in pregnancy or when breastfeeding.)

• Uptake of calcium from the diet may be increased by the use of herbs that stimulate digestion and mineral absorption and support effective functioning of the liver and gall bladder. They include dandelion root, yellow dock root, marigold (Calendula), rosemary, yarrow* and wormwood. (*Never to be used in pregnancy.)

Alternative help, treatment and advice may be obtained from practitioners of any of the following therapies:
• Anthroposophical medicine
• Homoeopathy
• Massage therapy
• Naturopathy
• Nutritional therapy
• Traditional Chinese medicine
• Western medical herbalism

Rheumatism

This is a term that tends to be used more by the layperson than the medical profession to describe stiffness of the joints and muscles. It is a condition that can be part and parcel of the ageing process, with pains often being located in the neck and shoulder.

For practical self-help and general advice on alternative medical approaches see the sections on osteoarthritis (pages 204-7) and rheumatoid arthritis (page 341). Visiting a practitioner of any of the following therapies may be of help:
• Acupressure
• Anthroposophical medicine
• Aromatherapy
• Chiropractic
• Homoeopathy
• Massage therapy
• Naturopathy
• Nutritional therapy
• Osteopathy

• Reflexology
• Shiatsu
• Traditional Chinese medicine
• Western medical herbalism

Sciatica and back pain

Back and sciatic pain can occur at any age, but are more common in middle age as a result of compression or pressure of the sciatic nerve. This may occur as a related problem when osteoarthritis has developed, if a disc in the spine is protruding (often referred to as a prolapsed disc) or if the vertebrae in the spine have become fused together.

Symptoms may vary in severity and may include any of the following:
• Shooting pains in the back, leg and buttock.
• Discomfort and pain that are made more intense

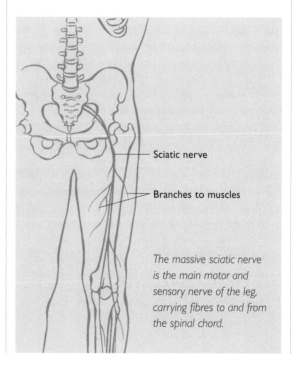

Sciatic nerve

Branches to muscles

The massive sciatic nerve is the main motor and sensory nerve of the leg, carrying fibres to and from the spinal chord.

and distressing when bending, or making jarring movements when sneezing or coughing.

• Back and sciatic pain that are sometimes eased when standing.

Since backache and sciatica are chronic problems with a tendency to repeated flare-ups of acute pain, they are best treated by a qualified alternative practitioner. However, the advice given below gives a general overview of the appropriate therapies available, and suggests practical lifestyle changes that are likely to ease the condition and discourage its recurrence.

Practical self-help

• It is best to avoid wearing high heels most of the time: always make a point of spending some time in flat shoes that provide good support. Also avoid carrying your shoulder bag always on one side, as this can cause twisting or uneven alignment of the spine.

• Choose a comfortable mattress that is neither so soft that it is unable to provide adequate support, nor so hard that it feels too uncomfortable to encourage a good night's rest. The ideal mattress should never sag in the middle, but should provide an even surface of support.

• Since poor posture can contribute to or compound problems with back pain or sciatica, consider taking Alexander Technique lessons for preventative advice. Once problems have surfaced, consulting an osteopath, chiropractor or acupuncturist may be very helpful in easing pain and discomfort.

• If warmth is soothing to the painful area, make a simple warm compress by wrapping a hot-water bottle in a soft cloth and applying it to the affected area, or invest in a commercially produced electric heating pad specially designed for this purpose.

• Consider using a TENS (transcutaneous electrical nerve stimulation) machine as an alternative method of pain relief, which appears to work by stimulating nerve pathways and blocking other sensory input (such as pain). A TENS machine can be a remarkably effective way of easing pain without resorting to frequent use of painkillers.

SEEK PROFESSIONAL HELP

If sciatic pain is recurrent, persistent or severe.

Alternative treatments

For back pain and sciatica it is quite appropriate to take the relevant internal remedy while also applying a topical preparation to the skin.

Topical preparations

These include essential oils and herbal tinctures that can be applied to the skin to soothe and ease pain and discomfort. Choose from any of the following, bearing in mind that none of the substances mentioned for application to the skin should be taken by mouth.

Aromatherapy oils

There are many oils that can help, but you should always seek advice from a qualified aromatherapist when dealing with inflammatory conditions.

Herbal preparations

If pains are sharp or shooting in character, the painful area may benefit from a massage with Hypericum oil . However, overfrequent use of the oil should be avoided, since it can cause a skin reaction in hypersensitive patients.

Home remedies

• A warm poultice made from ivy leaves may ease pain and discomfort from back pain or sciatica. Take a couple of generous handfuls of ivy, chop finely and mix with twice the amount of bran. Add 300ml (10fl oz) water, place in a small saucepan and mix to a paste over a low heat. After ten minutes, place the warm mixture on a soft, clean cloth and apply warm to the painful area.

• Alternatively, an equally warming, soothing poultice may be made by making a paste from crushed fenugreek seeds mixed with warm milk. Place on a piece of clean, soft cloth over the painful area.

Medicines intended for internal use

These ease pain and reduce stiffness and inflammation.

Biochemic tissue salts

Both back pain and sciatica may respond to Zeif. However, sharp, shooting sciatic pain may respond better to Combination A.

Herbal preparations

If back pain is aggravated by a tendency to tense muscles that have a habit of going into spasm, white clover and lime tea provide a soothing drink that encourages relaxation.

HOMOEOPATHIC MEDICINES

Type	General features	Worse	Better	Remedy
Back pain and sciatica that are most severe when sitting	Violent, shooting, sharp pains that turn into tingling, burning, numb sensations in the affected leg. Pains may be left-sided or worse on the left side than the right. Problems may set in after a fall or accident that damages the bones at the base of the spine	Effort or exertion Cold, damp conditions Jarring movements Change of weather After a fall or injury	Lying on stomach Massage to painful area	Hypericum
Tearing pains in thighs with sciatica and back pain	Weakness in the legs with pains that extend from the hip to the knee on the painful side. Muscles in the painful part feel weak and may be subject to jerking, spasmodic twitching. Cold sensation in painful area. Sharp, throbbing, stabbing pains when lying on the painful side	Overheating Effort and exertion In the winter Stooping Touch Movement Contact with cold draughts	Warmth	Kali carb
Sciatica and back pain with shooting pains that dart quickly from place to place	Unbearable, cutting, twisting, griping pains with anxiety and severe trembling. Right-sided sciatica with burning pains that shoot and radiate down the thigh on the affected side. Discomfort is relieved by lying as still as possible	In the evening At night Motion Sitting up Bending double	Firm pressure Bending backwards Standing Stretching	Dioscorea
Constricted, band-like sensations with sciatica and back pain	Awful, distressing pains that pinch, gnaw and cut, leading the patient to toss, turn, twist and cry out in pain. Pain is rapidly followed by numb sensation that is quickly eased by pressure applied to the affected area. Shooting pains extend from top of the leg to the foot	In bed During the night Chill Contact with cold draughts Lying on the painless side	Warmth Firm pressure applied to painful area Rest Bending double	Colocythis
Heavy, trembling sensations in legs with backache or sciatica	Pain from back or sciatic nerve makes legs feel weak, unsteady or heavy. Pain is especially problematic at night, preventing sleep. First movement after rest is very painful	Initial movement Damp, cold weather Overheating	Continuous movement Bending forwards Rest Being propped up in bed	Gelsemium

Alternative help, treatment and advice may be obtained from practitioners of any of the following therapies:

- Acupressure
- Anthroposophical medicine
- Aromatherapy
- Chiropractic
- Homoeopathy
- Massage therapy
- Naturopathy
- Osteopathy
- Shiatsu
- Traditional Chinese medicine
- Western medical herbalism

SKIN PROBLEMS

Acne

Acne is an embarrassing and irritating condition that most often develops in the teenage years. This is a most unfortunate situation, since this is the phase of life when most people are likely to be unsure of themselves and suffer from poor confidence and self-esteem. As a result, developing acne can make the turbulence and self-consciousness of being a teenager much more intense than it needs to be.

The outbreaks of spots that are characteristic of acne often start around puberty, and may spontaneously clear up by the time we reach our twenties. However, this troublesome skin condition may remain as a problem throughout the adult years, with women being especially affected premenstrually or during the menopause.

A classic bout of acne will involve the emergence of spots, blackheads, pimples, or inflamed, lumpy eruptions that most often affect the hairline, forehead, chin, jawline, shoulders, back or chest. Pimples and blackheads form as a result of an excess of sebum

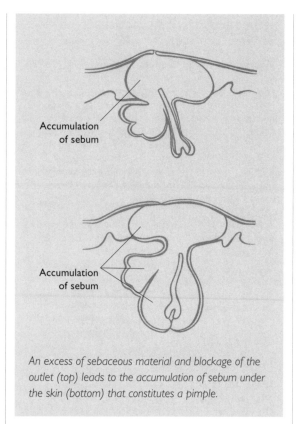

An excess of sebaceous material and blockage of the outlet (top) leads to the accumulation of sebum under the skin (bottom) that constitutes a pimple.

being produced by the sebaceous glands. If the blocked glands become infected, large pimples or cysts form, which can leave unsightly or persistent scarring.

Practical self-help

- Make sure that six to eight large glasses of filtered or still mineral water are drunk each day, which assists the eliminatory and detoxifying processes that are carried out by the body via the bowel and kidneys. When these eliminatory functions are sluggish or inefficient, skin problems often arise, or may become more severe and troublesome. Coffee, tea and carbonated drinks are not a substitute for water since the first two encourage the body to eliminate fluid (due to their diuretic properties), and the last tend to have a large amount of sugar or sweeteners added, which can also aggravate skin problems.
- Vitamin C is vitally important in preserving healthy skin texture and tone. Because vitamin C is very easily destroyed (for example, it is easily lost from fruit and vegetables during cooking) and is often in short supply in the average diet during the winter months, consider taking a supplement. An

initial dosage of 500mg a day is suitable if the stomach and bowel tolerate the dosage well, and provided there is no history of kidney stones. Although any excess vitamin C should be flushed out in the urine or faeces, too high a dosage may cause acidity of the stomach and/or loose stools. If these develop, reduce the dosage until symptoms disappear.

• Poor circulation may also contribute to skin disorders such as acne. Regular aerobic exercise that stimulates the heart and lungs (ideally taken in the fresh air) can play a positive role in preserving or improving skin tone and quality. Taking regular aerobic exercise increases the amount of oxygen available in the bloodstream and encourages the efficient elimination of toxins through the skin surface.

• If acute outbreaks of acne are more intense or severe after a period of mental, emotional and/or physical stress, consider exploring relaxation or visualization techniques, meditation, yoga or counselling.

• Poor-quality or insufficient sleep may also aggravate a general tendency to poor skin quality. See the section on insomnia (pages 252-5) for general advice on how to improve sleep patterns.

• Avoid fatty, greasy foods that have a reputation for aggravating acne, and make sure that fresh fruit and vegetables are eaten on a regular basis each day. Foods to cut down or eliminate include full-fat dairy products, battered or fried foods, chocolate, crisps, roasted nuts and convenience foods that have a high proportion of fat included. Also avoid sugary foods and drinks, which also have a reputation for irritating skin disorders. Concentrate instead on raw or stir-fried vegetables using cold-pressed, virgin olive oil, plentiful quantities of fresh, raw or steamed fruit (avoiding citrus fruits, which may aggravate sensitive skin), whole grain breads and cereals, pulses and occasional helpings of poultry and fish.

• Avoid using abrasive skin washes and creams. Although it is important to keep the skin surface thoroughly cleansed, some of the stronger acne preparations can disturb the acid mantle of the skin, which may make oiliness and congestion a greater problem in the long run. Use a gentle clay exfoliator to refine the skin surface and help unblock clogged pores, avoiding the harsher, wash-off formulations containing grains that claim to 'polish' the surface of the skin. Toners and cleansers should be thorough but gentle in their action, while moisturizers need to be water-based and light in texture.

Alternative treatments

Topical preparations

These include lotions, tinctures or creams that can be applied to the skin to soothe and heal. Choose from any of the following, but bear in mind that none of the substances mentioned for application to the skin should be taken by mouth.

Aromatherapy oils

Use hydrolats to wash the face and any other affected areas and allow to air dry. There are many helpful oils, petit grain and niaouli (Melaleuca quinqueneriva) being two of the most useful, but also lavender, chamomile, rosewood and thymus linalol. Seek advice from a qualified aromatherapist for the best choice for you.

Herbal preparations

• A herbal cleansing lotion for greasy skin can be made by mixing equal proportions of rose or elderflower water and fresh lemon juice.

• Gently steaming the face can also help unblock the clogged pores that can aggravate acne. Pour 600ml (1 pint) boiling water onto a tablespoon of any of the following herbs: chamomile, elderflowers, limeflowers, lady's mantle, lavender or yarrow (not to be used during pregnancy). Make sure that you do not continue for too long (this may make an existing tendency towards open pores more pronounced): five to eight minutes should be quite long enough. Afterwards, gently wipe the blocked pores or blackheads with clean cotton wool to which a diluted solution of Calendula tincture has been added.

• Apply aloe vera gel to any areas that have been damaged by acne or vitamin E oil to remaining scars.

Home remedies

• If skin is feeling inflamed and sensitive, boiled lettuce leaves applied warm to the skin can be extremely soothing.

• Make a simple face mask from oatmeal and yoghurt mixed to the consistency of a thick paste, spread on the affected area and leave to dry.

• A soothing, healing lotion can be made from dried marigold petals and wheatgerm oil. Add two tablespoons of pounded marigold petals to four tablespoons of warmed wheatgerm oil. Strain the liquid well into a stoppered container and apply to blemished skin.

Medicines intended for internal use

These soothe, reduce inflammation and encourage a speedy resolution of the problem.

Biochemic tissue salts

For an acute flare-up of acne, or an isolated bout of

HOMOEOPATHIC MEDICINES

Type	General features	Worse	Better	Remedy
Bright red spots that develop abruptly and violently with sensation of heat	Intensely sensitive, throbbing, red spots which feel extremely hot. Oversensitive, irritable and intolerant	Touch Jarring movement Chill Pressure to affected area	Warmth Peace and quiet Rest	Belladonna Helpful in early stages of inflammation.
Oily, greasy skin with dry patches and bouts of acne that flare up premenstrually	Blocked pores and blackheads from excess oil and sebum. Dry, sensitive skin with easy cracking and chapping (especially around the lips). Itchy, irritated spots on cheeks and back. Emotional strain and hormonal fluctuation make skin problems worse	Exposure to sunlight Warmth Touch Emotional stress or grief Before or after a period	Peace and quiet Solitude Cool air Cool bathing	Natrum mur
Unhealthy skin with a tendency to easy infection and slow healing	Large, pus-filled spots that are extremely sensitive and painful from the slightest touch or contact with cold air. Thick, yellow discharge with 'drawing' sensations in spots. Dry, chapped, cracked skin that heals very slowly	Cold air Touch Pressure During the winter Cold, dry winds	Warmth Damp heat	Hepar sulph
Slow-healing spots with a tendency to scar formation	Poor-quality skin, hair and nails with a tendency to brittleness and lack of strength. Blind spots and boils that remain inflamed and sensitive, or that may produce clear, watery pus. Poor circulation with easy sweating and flushing of the head and face	Humid conditions Cold draughts of air Touch or pressure	Dry, warm weather In summer Warmth Rest Warm compresses	Silica
Changeable spots that are much worse at times of hormonal change (e.g. puberty, premenstrually or during the menopause)	Spots change their location and character, moving from one site to another. Sensitivity to over-rich, fatty or greasy foods. Feels worse from becoming overheated. Tearful and depressed about skin condition	Resting Hot, humid conditions Premenstrually During the menopause When alone	Contact with fresh, cool air Gentle exercise in the open air Cool bathing Sympathy Having a good cry	Pulsatilla

spots, four tablets of the following may be taken three times daily for a few days, tailing off as soon as symptoms improve: tissue salt No. 3 or Combination D.

It is important to stress that the remedies listed above are not mentioned in order to encourage self-help prescribing for acne. They are intended to provide suggestions of appropriate remedies that may be helpful in giving short-term relief for mild, acute symptoms. For the best chances of long-term improvement, seek professional alternative help from practitioners trained in any of the following:
• Anthroposophical medicine
• Aromatherapy
• Ayurvedic medicine
• Homoeopathy
• Naturopathy
• Nutritional therapy
• Shiatsu
• Traditional Chinese medicine
• Western medical herbalism

Athlete's foot

This persistent and irritating condition arises as a result of a fungal infection that usually attacks the skin between the toes (it can also affect other parts of the body in the form of ringworm).

Common symptoms include the following:
• Itchy, irritated skin and/or blistery rashes between the toes.
• Cracked, flaky skin texture that exposes sore, red skin beneath.
• Distortion or crumbling of the toenails once the nail bed is affected.

Once contracted, athlete's foot can be very difficult to get rid of for those who enjoy sports activities, since reinfection is common from public places such as communal changing rooms or swimming pools.

Practical self-help
• Poorly ventilated shoes can contribute to the problem by keeping the feet in warm, moist conditions (an environment that is excellent for encouraging infection). As a result, exposing the feet to fresh air and sunshine whenever possible can do a great deal to improve the condition.

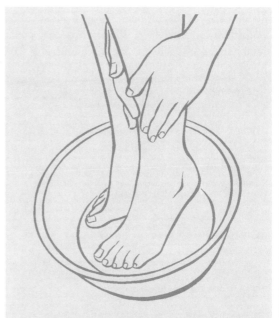

A footbath made with a decoction of sage or thyme can soothe the irritation of athlete's foot.

• Observing scrupulous hygiene is also an important way of discouraging aggravation of the condition, as well as keeping the feet as dry as possible.
• Avoid wearing socks and tights whenever possible in order to ventilate the feet. Avoid synthetic materials, opting instead for materials that allow the skin to breathe, such as cotton.

SEEK PROFESSIONAL HELP
If the condition is persistent, spreading rapidly or shows signs of infection.

Alternative treatments
For an acute flare-up of athlete's foot, it is quite appropriate to take the relevant remedy internally while also applying a topical preparation to the skin. However, bear in mind that this condition is best treated by a trained practitioner for long-term relief.

Topical preparations

These include lotions, tinctures or creams that can be applied to the skin to soothe and heal. Choose from any of the following, bearing in mind that none of the substances mentioned for application to the skin should be taken by mouth.

Aromatherapy oils

Add ten drops of tea tree (Melaleuca alternifolia) and ten drops of thymus linalol to a warm salt-water footbath and soak the feet. Check with a chiropodist the minute ulcer problems are present.

Herbal preparations

• Feet may be soaked in a decoction of sage or thyme, both of which are reputed to have antiseptic properties. Cut up the fresh herb or grind the dried ingredients, measuring the desired amount into an enamelled pan. Add water, bring to boiling point, cover, and simmer for fifteen minutes before straining off the liquid. Use 28g (1oz) of dried herb/84g (3oz) of fresh herb to 600ml (1 pint) water.

• After bathing and drying thoroughly, Calendula cream may be applied to irritated, itchy or cracked

HOMOEOPATHIC MEDICINES

Type	General features	Worse	Better	Remedy
Sweaty, cold, clammy feet with athlete's foot	Cold, unhealthy, slow-healing skin that chaps and cracks readily. Sweats from the least effort: sweaty scalp and feet	Cold, raw air Bathing Pressure of clothes	Rubbing or scratching Dry, warm weather Wiping with hands	Calc carb
Sore and raw, rapidly developing cracks in folds of skin	Terrible itching between the toes: healed-over cracks re-open easily. 'Restless legs' at night with difficulty in keeping the legs still	Extreme temperatures Dry, cold air	Washing Warmth of the bed Gentle movement	Causticum
Dry, hard, cracked skin with athlete's foot	Symptoms may be worse periodically (e.g. every spring). Terribly itchy blistery eruptions that settle in folds of skin (e.g. between the toes). Distortion of nails with athlete's foot	Cold draughts of air Before periods During pregnancy Touch Getting wet Scratching	Warmth of the bed Cool bathing	Sepia
Moist athlete's foot that is much worse from getting damp	Severe itching with blistery, crusty rash that causes extreme restlessness at night. Hot, burning, itching skin with terrific sensitivity to contact with draughts of cold air	Damp and cold Undressing Rest At night Jarring movement	Warmth Rubbing Changing position Warm, dry conditions	Rhus tox
Intolerably itchy athlete's foot which is much worse after a warm bath	Itching rapidly changes place when being scratched. Affected area feels cold. Burning, irritation and smarting of the skin with extreme sensitivity to contact with air	At night Warmth of the bed Cool draughts of air Touch Movement	Wrapping up	Mezereum

skin in order to soothe, heal and discourage infection.

Home remedies
A tablespoon of lemon juice or two tablespoons of cider vinegar added to water makes a soothing, anti-infective footbath.

Medicines intended for internal use
These reduce irritation and ease discomfort.

The remedies listed above may be helpful in giving short-term relief for mild, acute symptoms. For the best chances of long-term improvement it is important to seek professional alternative help from practitioners trained in any of the following:
- Anthroposophical medicine
- Aromatherapy
- Biochemic tissue salts
- Homoeopathy
- Naturopathy
- Nutritional therapy
- Reflexology
- Traditional Chinese medicine
- Western medical herbalism

Boils

A boil is most likely to develop if a hair follicle becomes infected, leading to inflammation and the formation of pus as the follicle and skin cells are attacked by bacteria. Resolution of the situation should usually take place within a week or two of the onset of symptoms, by the discharging of pus from the boil.

Boils and carbuncles (a crop of boils clustered together) usually appear on the hairy parts of the body, or areas where they are subject to pressure or friction. As a result, the parts most likely to be subject to boils or carbuncles include the armpits, neck, nostrils, wrists, between the legs or the buttocks. Abscesses (a form of boil) and gumboils are most commonly to be found in the mouth.

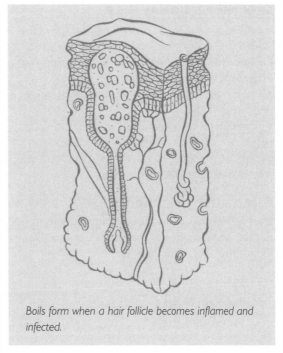
Boils form when a hair follicle becomes inflamed and infected.

Boils or carbuncles are most likely to develop if we are stressed, run down or generally out of sorts. A poor diet high in junk foods, or diabetes (see page 335-7) may also leave us vulnerable to recurrent boils or abscesses.

Practical self-help
- Make sure that good-quality wholefoods are eaten on a regular basis. Avoid making convenience or junk foods a central part of the diet, concentrating instead on fresh fruit, vegetables, whole grains, pulses and small quantities of fish or poultry. Avoid sugar, and tea and coffee should be kept to a minimum. Most important of all, drink six to eight large glasses of filtered or still mineral water each day.
- If a boil or abscess has developed, it is helpful to adopt a detoxifying regime for the first few days (up to a week). Drink plenty of water and eat mainly salads, and raw, grated or steamed vegetables, as well as a wide variety of fresh fruit (raw, or lightly steamed, with a little honey).
- Never share towels or flannels with anyone who is suffering from boils, especially if they are discharging pus. The bacteria present in boils and abscesses can also cause food poisoning if they contaminate warm food. Consequently, anyone with this problem should be scrupulously careful about personal hygiene in order to avoid spreading the condition.

SEEK PROFESSIONAL HELP

• If there are any signs of inflammation spreading or developing (redness, heat and throbbing) without the boil coming to a head, or if no pus is released even though a head has formed.
• If there are any signs of fever and/or symptoms of general malaise.
• Never attempt to squeeze a boil because of the risk of pus entering the bloodstream. If boils or carbuncles are very painful, see your family doctor who may suggest lancing the boil.

Alternative treatments

If a boil develops it is perfectly appropriate to take the relevant remedy internally, while also applying a topical preparation to the skin.

Topical preparations

These include lotions, tinctures or creams that can be applied to the skin to soothe and heal. Choose from any of the following, but bear in mind that none of the substances mentioned for application to the skin should be taken by mouth.

Aromatherapy oils

Use laurel hydrolat to cleanse the affected area gently. Put one drop of niaouli (Melaleuca quinqueneriva) onto a cotton wool bud and apply gently to the boil.

Herbal preparations

• A warm, comforting poultice can be made from mixing slippery elm powder with water to make a paste. A few drops of lavender or eucalyptus oil can be added to the paste in order to guard against infection.

HOMOEOPATHIC MEDICINES

Type	General features	Worse	Better	Remedy
Early stage of inflammation with marked heat and redness of skin	Affected area is bright red and radiates heat. Sticking, throbbing, shooting pains develop rapidly, violently and intensely	Touch Jarring movement	Resting	Belladonna Used promptly, this remedy may prevent pus formation.
Extremely sensitive boils with thick, yellow pus	Slow-healing skin that becomes rapidly infected. Painful area is hypersensitive to cold draughts. Splintering, sharp pains in boils and abscesses.	Cold draughts Undressing Touch Lying on painful part At night	Warmth Wrapping up warmly Moist warmth	Hepar sulph Hepar sulph encourages 'drawing' process and speedy discharge of pus
Festering boils with thin, clear discharge	Slow-healing skin with a tendency for painful scars to remain behind. Violent, sharp, sticking pains in boils with tendency to formation of carbuncles	Contact with cold draughts Undressing Jarring Touch Pressure	Warmth Moist warmth	Silicea
Boils and abscesses that occur during menstruation	Recurrent boils and abscesses with thin, greenish or bloody pus. Extremely sensitive to stinging, burning pains and slightest change of temperature	At night Becoming heated Chill in bed	Rest Moderate temperatures	Mercurius

• Calendula cream or ointment can be applied to the boil or carbuncle after it has been lanced to discourage secondary infection from developing.

Home remedies
• A warm poultice made from soft, boiled, cooled onion placed on lint and bandaged in place can encourage resolution of a boil. Alternatively, a thin slice of lemon applied to the affected area can act as a natural antiseptic.
• Boils may be drawn to a head by applying a warm bread poultice to the inflamed area. Add a crumbled slice of bread to boiled water or milk, strain it, wrap in gauze and apply the poultice while it is still warm. This process may be continued at regular intervals until the boil has discharged.

Medicines intended for internal use
These ease pain, reduce inflammation and encourage a speedy resolution of the problem.

Anthroposophical medicines
Erysidoron I may be used to reduce redness and localized inflammation. Take five drops in water at two-hourly intervals while symptoms are acute, tailing off the dosage as symptoms improve. If there is a tendency to well-established, stubborn infection and inflammation, Erysidoron I may be taken in alternate doses with Carbo Betulae and Sulphur (formerly known as Erysidoron II) tablets at hourly intervals, until improvement begins. (These medicines should ideally be used under medical supervision due to the nature of the condition.)

Biochemic tissue salts
If a boil is developing, alternating doses of Ferr phos and Kali mur may stop inflammation and pus formation. Alternatively, if the boil has broken, but seems slow to heal, Combination D or tissue salt No. 3 are appropriate. If inflammation, pain and swelling are severe in the early stages, take three tablets at hourly intervals until the symptoms show initial signs of improvement. Once this occurs, dosage should be gradually reduced.

Herbal infusions
An appropriate herbal infusion can support the immune system in fighting infection so that boils and abscesses may be dealt with more speedily and efficiently. Suitable herbs for this purpose include the following: echinacea, wild indigo (not to be used in strong doses in order to avoid purgative or emetic effects), myrrh, burdock, dandelion root, garlic and thyme (to be avoided in pregnancy). Add 28g (1oz)

dried herb to 600ml (1 pint) boiling water. Leave to steep for fifteen minutes before straining.

If a tendency to develop boils or carbuncles has become a recurrent feature of life, it may be helpful to seek professional advice and treatment from a practitioner trained in any of the following therapies:
• Anthroposophical medicine
• Aromatherapy
• Ayurvedic medicine
• Biochemic tissue salts
• Homoeopathy
• Naturopathy
• Nutritional therapy
• Traditional Chinese medicine
• Western medical herbalism

Chilblains

Chilblains tend to affect people with poor circulation, especially when exposed to cold. Once chilblains appear they look like reddish-blue swellings on the skin, and are likely to feel maddeningly itchy or burning. Once they have been scratched, an itch-scratch-itch cycle can be set up that causes great misery and discomfort.

The areas most likely to be affected are the fingers and toes, but chilblains can erupt on the ears or other exposed areas of the body. Chilblains occur as a result of blood vessels becoming markedly shrunk, causing a great reduction in blood supply.

Practical self-help
• Try to improve generally sluggish circulation by taking up regular, rhythmic exercise. If you have a history of heart disease or are generally unfit, make sure the exercise is gentle, such as brisk walking.
• Always make sure that exposed areas of skin such as fingers and ears are well covered in cold, windy weather. Warm woollen socks and gloves are a must for those who suffer from chilblains.

• Never succumb to the temptation of putting cold hands or feet directly in front of a warm fire, since this can encourage a tendency to chilblain production, or can make existing chilblains worse. Instead, thaw cold fingers and toes out slowly and gently under warm, running water.

• Start the habit of gently massaging hands and feet each morning and night throughout the year to improve the circulation.

• Increase the amount of calcium-rich foods in your diet, such as fresh, green, leafy vegetables, almonds and dairy products, since these are thought to ease problems with chilblains.

SEEK PROFESSIONAL HELP

• If chilblains are widespread, severe or occur on a regular basis.

• If a tendency to chilblains is combined with symptoms of breathlessness, fatigue and chest pains on exertion.

Alternative treatments

For chilblains it is perfectly appropriate to take a remedy internally, while also applying a topical preparation to the skin in order to reduce irritation and discomfort.

Topical preparations

These include lotions, tinctures or creams that can be applied to the skin to soothe and heal.

Anthroposophical medicines

If coldness and poor circulation to the hands and feet is an established problem, copper ointment may be massaged in well twice a day. The ointment may leave marks on fabrics and clothing.

Aromatherapy oils

Add two drops each of lavender (Lavendula angustifolia) and tea tree (Melaleuca alternifolia) oils to one teaspoon of gel base and apply gently to the affected area if the skin is unbroken.

Herbal preparations

Tamus (black bryony) cream should be applied to chilblains that are cracked and painful, while Rhus tox (poison jury) may be more soothing when applied to inflamed and maddeningly itchy chilblains.

Home remedies

• If skin is irritated but the surface has not been broken, the juice of an onion may feel very soothing when applied to itchy areas. Alternatively, applying a warm poultice of onion to the affected area of skin each night may have a similarly positive effect.

• A very small amount of fresh garlic juice may be applied to inflamed, irritated areas of skin.

HOMOEOPATHIC MEDICINES

Type	General features	Worse	Better	Remedy
Burning, purple-coloured chilblains	Generally chapped, thickened, cracked skin with fingertips that split very readily. Burning, itching sensations with raw, bleeding skin	In winter Touch of clothing	Warm, dry weather	Petroleum
Intolerably itchy chilblains	Swollen, burning, red-tinged skin with awful itching. Itching moves location of scratching. Skin bruises very easily	Contact with cold air Freezing conditions Touch	Gentle movement	Agaricus
Burning, itching chilblains that are painfully sensitive to cold air	Dry, thickened, itchy sensitive skin with generally achy legs and feet. Warm bathing is soothing to irritated, inflamed skin	Exposure to damp, cold conditions Undressing Contact with cold draughts Becoming sweaty	Warm bathing Gentle rubbing Warm, dry weather	Rhus tox

Medicines intended for internal use

These ease pain and irritation, reduce inflammation and encourage a speedy resolution of the problem.

Biochemic tissue salts

Tissue salt No. 2 may be helpful where chilblains occur with signs of general circulatory problems. On the other hand, more localized symptoms of aching and discomfort in the hands and feet may respond to Combination Remedy P. In the initial stage of pain three tablets may be taken at hourly intervals. Reduce dosage as pain improves.

Herbal preparations

Copious drinks of buckwheat leaf tea will strengthen the tiny blood vessels.

Home remedies

Increase the amount of fresh garlic in your diet, as it has a beneficial effect on the circulatory system.

If a tendency to develop chilblains has become a recurrent feature of life, it may be helpful to seek professional advice and treatment from a practitioner trained in any of the following therapies:

- Acupressure
- Anthroposophical medicine
- Aromatherapy
- Homoeopathy
- Naturopathy
- Nutritional therapy
- Reflexology
- Traditional Chinese medicine
- Western medical herbalism

Eczema

Those who suffer from eczema will know that the symptoms can vary from mild dryness and itchiness that affect a small surface area of skin, to extreme itching, flaking, weeping or bleeding of large areas of the body. Although considered to be a relatively minor condition, it must be stressed that the distress, loss of confidence and sheer discomfort caused by a severe eruption of eczema can drastically reduce quality of life.

Although the severity of symptoms can vary greatly, the following are common features of eczema:

- Persistent irritation and itchiness of the skin.
- The appearance of small, itchy, fluid-filled blisters that ooze fluid after scratching.
- Crusty scabs that form once the weeping surface of the skin dries out. If these are dislodged by uncontrollable scratching (this may often happen unconsciously at night), the irritated area is likely to start weeping again. As a result, a vicious circle is set up, so that the skin becomes persistently inflamed and irritated.

Eczema often develops in babyhood or childhood, characteristically affecting the flexions (crooks of the elbows, backs of the knees and folds of skin behind the ears), and may often clear up spontaneously during, or after the teenage years. On the other hand, it may also develop in adulthood, remaining as a chronic problem that is subject to repeated flare-ups at regular intervals.

Eczema may be divided into two major types, which are categorized as atopic or contact eczema. The former usually develops in those who have a history of allergic problems, or whose relatives have suffered from asthma and/or hay fever, while the latter may be caused by contact with certain chemicals or metals such as detergents, bleaches, nickel or rubber.

Because an alternative medical approach to treatment regards skin problems as a superficial sign of a more deep-seated imbalance in the system as a whole, conditions of this kind are best treated by a trained practitioner. The practitioner will assess the case as a whole with a view to establishing optimum health and well-being for the patient on all levels, rather than concentrating on temporary alleviation of symptoms.

However, there are certain positive lifestyle changes that can minimize the distress of skin disorders or discourage severe flare-ups of the condition. These are listed below, in addition to suggestions of alternative medicines that may be used for short-term relief of mild symptoms of eczema. However, it must be stressed that long-term management of well-established or severe skin disorders should be handled by a trained practitioner for all the reasons given above.

Practical self-help

• If contact eczema is a problem, always wear thin cotton gloves when doing chores that involve coming into contact with substances that may cause problems. Gloves should be worn when peeling or chopping potatoes or citrus fruit and tomatoes. However, avoid wearing rubber gloves, since they can trigger an adverse reaction if you suffer from contact eczema.

• Be careful when using detergents, always selecting those that have been specially formulated for those who have sensitive or allergic skins. Most important of all, be sure to rinse items thoroughly after washing (rinsing twice over is a good rule to follow) to remove detergent residues from clothing, towels and bedclothes.

• Certain foods may aggravate eczema. Potential problem items may include:

  • Wheat (which may be in thickening agents and sauces, as well as the more obvious bread and pasta).
  • Convenience foods that include food colourings, additives and preservatives.
  • Potatoes and other foods that belong to the nightshade family, including tomatoes, aubergines and green peppers.
  • Dairy foods, and eggs.
  • Sugar.

If you suspect that one of these foods may be aggravating your problem, cut it out of your diet for a month. If you observe a change for the better while avoiding this item, reintroduce it, watching to see if there is any reaction. If an adverse reaction takes place (intensification or reappearance of the problem), avoid it again for a few weeks. If improvement occurs again with re-emergence of the problem once the offending food is reintroduced for a second time, the chances are that you have identified a food to which you are sensitive and should avoid until the condition can be dealt with at a deeper level (ideally, through alternative medical treatment).

• Although some eczema sufferers find that hot, sunny weather aggravates their condition, many find that carefully regulated, moderate exposure to sunlight improves it. However, great care should be taken to avoid overexposure to the sun, avoiding times of the day when it is at its strongest and most likely to cause damage to the skin. Use a sunscreen and always patch-test it first to check that it will not trigger off an adverse reaction. Apply the product to a very small area of skin for a few days, and wait to see if there is any reaction before using it on larger areas of the body.

• Always ensure that irritated, dry or itchy patches of eczema are kept well moisturized, especially after bathing or showering. It is also important to keep skin well lubricated and supple during the winter when weather conditions and centrally heated rooms are likely to have a dehydrating effect on the skin. Liberal use of emulsifying cream and ointment may be very helpful after bathing in keeping the drying effect of water on the skin to a minimum, but always check that any products you use are lanolin-free, since lanolin can trigger severe skin reactions in those who are allergic or sensitive to it.

• Take great care when using scented soaps, bubble baths or body creams and lotions. Where possible, use skin-care products and cosmetics that are hypoallergenic, and make sure that new products are patch-tested over a small area of skin for a few days before embarking on general use.

• Consider taking an oil of evening primrose supplement, which has a reputation for easing eczema. Oil of evening primrose may also be applied to irritated patches of skin in oil or cream form, after initially patch-testing it on a small area of skin.

SEEK PROFESSIONAL HELP

• Where eczema is causing great distress in young babies or the elderly.

• If eczema is well established, severe or widespread.

• If eczema has arisen as a result of a general atopic condition and is combined with hay fever and/or asthma.

• If there are any indications of infection having developed as a result of persistent scratching breaking the surface of the skin. Signs to look out for include heat and redness, swelling and pus formation.

Alternative treatments

Topical preparations

These include lotions, tinctures or creams that can be applied to the skin to soothe and heal. Choose from any of the following, bearing in mind that none of the substances mentioned for application to the skin should be taken by mouth.

HOMOEOPATHIC MEDICINES

Type	General features	Worse	Better	Remedy
Intensely itchy, blistery eczema that is especially distressing at night	Maddeningly irritating eczema that itches and burns, leading to great restlessness. Patches are initially blistered, rapidly becoming crusty and weepy. Skin is generally very sensitive to cold air	Damp, cold air Undressing Becoming hot and sweaty Resting in bed Lying on affected parts	Rubbing Continued movement Warm, dry weather Being wrapped up	Rhus tox
Dry, rough burning skin that is soothed by warmth	Eczema may alternate with asthma, and may be made worse by anxiety or stress. Blistery eruptions with violent burning after scratching. All symptoms are worse as the night goes on	Cold in any form Physical or mental stress Alcohol At night	Warm air Warm bathing Warm compresses Company	Arsenicum album
Weeping eczema affects areas where there are folds of skin	Thick, crusty eczema that weeps a honey-coloured fluid: all discharges are thick and sticky. Skin cracks easily around the nose, mouth, ears or nipples. Folds of skin feel raw: eruptions bleed easily	Before and after periods At night Scratching Becoming heated in bed	Contact with fresh air	Graphites
Eczema in folds of skin with weeping and bleeding after scratching	Rough, thickened skin that heals very slowly and festers easily. Nipples and fingertips become deeply cracked. Burning and itching eruptions with hard, thick crusting. Area feels cold after scratching	Cold weather Touch	Warm air Dry weather	Petroleum
Extremely itchy, red eczema that is very much more irritable for bathing	Dry, rough, scaly skin that feels much worse for becoming heated in bed at night. Burning after scratching with sensitivity to contact with air. Unhealthy skin that becomes quickly infected and heals slowly	Washing Becoming overheated in bed	Moderate temperatures	Sulphur

Aromatherapy oils

Many essential oils will help this condition, but you should seek advice from a qualified aromatherapist.

Flower remedies

Rescue Remedy cream may be applied to irritated areas of skin to soothe inflammation and ease itching.

Herbal preparations

• One teaspoon of marigold lotion (Calendula) may be added to a glass of boiled, cooled water and applied to irritated or weeping skin as a soothing compress. Alternatively, the lotion may be dabbed onto sensitive areas of skin at regular intervals to soothe inflamed skin.

• After applying marigold lotion (Calendula), cream or ointment may be applied to the affected area directly, or on a dry dressing. However, those who are sensitive to lanolin should be aware that the ointment includes lanolin as an ingredient.

Home remedies

• If skin feels dried out and papery, try an oatmeal bath to nourish the skin. Place a couple of tablespoons of oats in a muslin bag and place this beneath the hot tap as you run your bathwater. Oatmeal soap can also feel very calming and soothing to irritated skin.

• If the skin is inflamed, a poultice made from watercress and chickweed mixed with fine oatmeal may provide a great deal of relief. Wrap the herbs in thin gauze and apply to the affected area as often as necessary.

• Raw, grated carrots may be made into a poultice and applied to sensitive areas of skin.

• Wheatgerm, evening primrose or vitamin E oils may be applied to the skin to encourage healing.

Medicines intended for internal use

These ease pain, reduce inflammation and encourage a speedy resolution of the problem.

Biochemic tissue salts

Combination D may be helpful in easing the irritation and distress of an acute flare-up of eczema. Take four tablets three times daily until symptoms improve, tailing off the dosage accordingly. Alternatively the tablets may be made into a paste and applied to affected areas of skin: crush ten or twelve tablets to a powder (use a rolling pin) and mix to a paste with a little boiled, cooled water.

Herbal preparations

• Herbal teas that have a reputation for aiding skin conditions by nourishing and cooling the blood and skin include chamomile, red clover, nettle, chickweed and marigold (Calendula).

• Blue flag root compound (containing flag lily, burdock and sarsparilla) may be taken in tablet form to ease skin problems. The recommended dose is one tablet to be taken after meals three times daily. It should not be given to children under twelve years of age, and use is to be avoided in pregnancy.

• Skin tablets containing burdock root and wild pansy may ease the irritation and discomfort of dry eczema. The recommended daily dosage is two tablets to be taken three times daily with water. However, because of the risk of gastrointestinal upsets, the tablets should not be given to children, or used in pregnancy without the strict supervision of a herbal practitioner.

Home remedies

Eat raw carrots or fresh carrot juice in order to provide adequate supplies of beta-carotene, which is invaluable in maintaining the health and quality of the skin.

While the home prescriber can obtain short-term relief from the use of the remedies listed above, eczema is a chronic condition that should be treated by a professional alternative therapist in order for long-term, more established improvement to occur. Treatment may be sought from any of the following:

• Anthroposophical medicine
• Aromatherapy
• Ayurvedic medicine
• Homoeopathy
• Naturopathy
• Nutritional therapy
• Shiatsu
• Traditional Chinese medicine
• Western medical medicine

Nerve pain

See sections on neuralgia (page 129), shingles (pages 230-1), sciatica (pages 211-14) and multiple sclerosis (pages 340-1).

Psoriasis

Psoriasis is a distressing skin condition characterized by patches of red, thickened, scaly skin that often affects the elbows and knees. Some psoriasis sufferers find that their skin condition is extremely itchy, while others do not.

There appears to be a link between stress and psoriasis, with the condition either reappearing or becoming much more intense during or following times of stress or anxiety. It may also become more intense following a throat infection, or may be aggravated by prescription drugs for rheumatoid arthritis or malaria.

Symptoms rarely develop before the age of ten, most often developing between the ages of fifteen and thirty years of age. They include:
• Small red spots that merge together to form oval or round patches.
• Thickened nails that may grow away from the nail bed in severe cases.
• A form of arthritis in the joints of the knees, ankles and fingers, which does not affect all psoriasis sufferers.

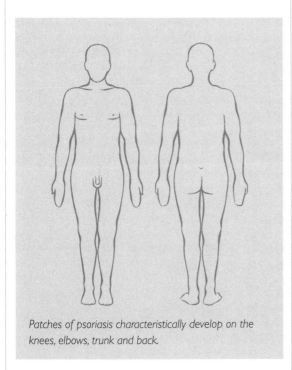

Patches of psoriasis characteristically develop on the knees, elbows, trunk and back.

Practical self-help
• It has been suggested that lecithin, which can be found in sunflower and soya oils, may ease symptoms of psoriasis.
• Moderate, careful exposure to sunlight can benefit psoriasis sufferers considerably. However, always ensure that fragile areas of skin are protected, and that exposure to direct sunlight is avoided during the times of day when the sun is at its strongest and likely to do the most damage.
• If stress, tension and anxiety are contributing to problems with psoriasis, make a concerted effort to find constructive ways of dealing with the situation.

Relaxation techniques, meditation and diaphragmatic breathing can help a great deal with long-term management of a stressful lifestyle. Systems of movement such as t'ai chi and yoga are also invaluable ways of combining meditation with movements that condition the body.
• Avoid drinks which act as circulatory stimulants such as alcohol, tea, coffee and caffeinated drinks. Opt instead for soft drinks that are free of added sugar and artificial sweeteners, filtered water, herb teas and caffeine-free coffee substitutes.
• Avoid red meat, animal fats and sugar where possible, increasing the proportion of fibre in the diet from whole grains, fruit, vegetables and pulses.
• Include regular helpings of oily fish in the diet, including herrings, mackerel and salmon.
• Oil of evening primrose may alleviate symptoms. Six 500mg capsules may be taken on a daily basis.

SEEK PROFESSIONAL HELP
• If psoriasis is well established, becoming increasingly severe, or spreading to new areas of the body.
• If joint pains are severe.

Alternative treatments
It is perfectly appropriate to take a remedy internally, while also applying a topical preparation to the skin in order to reduce dryness and scaling. However, it should be stressed that psoriasis is a chronic condition that should ideally be treated by a trained practitioner, rather than attempting home management of the situation (this is especially relevant with reference to homoeopathic prescribing).

Some of the following may be helpful in providing short-term relief of symptoms. If the skin shows any signs of increased sensitivity, stop self-treatment and seek professional alternative help.

Topical preparations
These include lotions, tinctures or creams, that can be applied to the skin to soothe and heal. Choose from any of the following, bearing in mind that none of the substances mentioned for application to the skin should be taken by mouth.

Herbal preparations
An infusion of yarrow may be soothing when added to the bathwater. Steep 50g (2oz) yarrow in 1l (1¾ pints) boiling water. Leave the liquid to soak for fifteen minutes before straining.
NB Yarrow should not be used during pregnancy.

Home remedies

• If skin is very dry, suspend a muslin bag filled with oatmeal beneath the hot tap while the water is running. Oatmeal soap will nourish and soothe dry, thickened areas of skin.

• Bathing in a solution of sea salt can also be extremely soothing to irritated skin.

• If patches of psoriasis are itchy and irritated, applying a compress made from plantain or dock leaf can be very soothing. Make the compress by soaking a clean, soft cloth in a cold infusion of the leaves mentioned above. Make the infusion by soaking one teaspoon of dried leaf in a cup of hot water. Strain after ten to fifteen minutes and allow to cool.

HOMOEOPATHIC MEDICINES

Type	General features	Worse	Better	Remedy
Psoriasis with burning of the skin that is eased by warmth	Rough, dry, scaly skin that may look dehydrated like parchment. Appearance of psoriasis may alternate with asthma, and may be much worse when anxious	Periodically Contact with cold or chill At night Stress or anxiety	Warmth Being distracted by company	Arsenicum album
Rough, scaly skin that chaps very easily	Pale, unhealthy skin that dries out and cracks frequently. Skin is cold, unhealthy and sweaty with a tendency to slow healing. Chilly, sluggish and easily exhausted from lack of stamina	Cold, winter weather Bathing Physical effort Stress and anxiety At puberty or during the menopause	Rubbing Scratching Summer weather When constipated	Calc carb
Dry, raw skin in folds that is worse for warmth	Extremely dry hands and soles of the feet. Skin disorders may be associated with urinary, liver or gastric problems. Anxious and inclined to get worked up about speaking in public	Warmth Pressure of clothes Eating Before a period	Cool compresses Movement Gentle exercise in the fresh air	Lycopodium
Psoriasis with thick, crusted skin on the elbows and joints	Blotchy, roughened, hard, cracked patches on skin with poor circulation. Folds of skin are especially affected. Depressed, apathetic and lethargic with skin problems. Whole system feels better for vigorous exercise in the fresh air	Contact with cold, raw air Before a period During pregnancy Touch Rubbing Scratching	Warmth Warm compresses Aerobic exercise	Sepia
Weeping, crusty patches of psoriasis that break easily	Dry, rough, irritable skin that becomes cracked and bleeds easily. Thickened skin exudes a honey-coloured discharge that rapidly forms a crust. Slow-healing, unhealthy skin	Warmth Contact with cold During and after periods Warmth of the bed At night	Touch Walking in the fresh air	Graphites

Medicines intended for internal use

These ease pain, reduce inflammation and encourage a speedy resolution of the problem.

Biochemic tissue salts

Combination D may be helpful in easing an acute flare-up of psoriasis. Take four tablets three times daily until symptoms improve, tailing off the dosage accordingly. Alternatively, the tablets may be made into a paste and applied to affected areas of skin. Crush ten or twelve tablets to a powder (use a rolling pin) and mix to a paste with a little boiled, cooled water.

Herbal preparations

• A combination of blue flag extract, burdock root, yellow dock, sarsparilla and buchu leaf may be obtained as an over-the-counter product, marketed under the name Skin Eruptions Mixture. The recommended dosage is one 5ml teaspoon to be taken three times a day. Because the active ingredients in this medicinal preparation encourage elimination of body fluids through urination and gentle purging, it should not be used by children, in pregnancy or when breastfeeding.

• Herbal teas that may ease symptoms of psoriasis include burdock, sarsparilla and yellow dock, especially if taken together.

Professional alternative medical help may be obtained from any of the following:
• Anthroposophical medicine
• Aromatherapy
• Ayurvedic medicine
• Homoeopathy
• Naturopathy
• Nutritional therapy
• Shiatsu
• Traditional Chinese medicine
• Western medical herbalism

Raynaud's disease

Raynaud's disease is a circulatory problem caused by the small arteries that supply the fingers and toes becoming oversensitive to cold. As a result of this overreaction, blood flow is reduced to the affected fingers and toes. In the early stages of the problem, once the chilled hand or foot becomes warm, normal circulation is restored quite quickly (within approximately fifteen minutes).

Common symptoms include:
• Pale or bluish-tinged skin that commonly affects the fingers, and sometimes the toes. This can often be triggered by cold, wintry conditions.
• Burning discomfort, or a tingling sensation in the affected area, although the problem is usually painless.

Once the spasm has passed, fresh blood should be able to flow into the affected part so that skin colour returns to normal.

Raynaud's disease is usually associated with another condition (such as rheumatoid arthritis, see page 341) or may occur as a side effect of some drugs, such as beta blockers. In addition, certain occupations can encourage this problem to develop, such as working on a regular basis with vibrating equipment (e.g. chainsaws or pneumatic drills).

Practical self-help

See advice given for chilblains (pages 221–3), and cramp (pages 202-4).

In addition, consider supplementing with vitamin E to reduce platelet stickiness and magnesium to reduce vascular spasm.

SEEK PROFESSIONAL HELP

• If episodes begin to occur on a frequent basis.
• If recovery time lengthens with each acute bout of the problem.
• If symptoms occur within the general context of circulatory problems.
• If there is any structural change in the fingers – for example, if they become thin and spindly.

Alternative treatments

See advice given for chilblains (pages 222-3) and cramp (pages 203-4).

Shingles

The misery of shingles tends to affect those who have previously had chickenpox and become run down or excessively physically and/or emotionally stressed.

As a result, the herpes zoster virus becomes activated and the symptoms of shingles appear.

These may include:
• Severe pain that usually develops on one side of the body, often affecting the chest or back.
• Excruciatingly sensitive and painful skin eruptions that may begin as a blistery rash, and can appear anywhere on the body, commonly affecting the face, chest, waist or back.

Although the rash should become crusty and clear up after a few weeks, severe residual pain can remain in the areas that were affected by the rash. This is called post-herpetic neuralgia and may remain for a lengthy period of time.

Practical self-help

• Wear loose-fitting clothing that is less likely to irritate the skin than restrictive or tight garments.
• Cool or warm bathing may ease the discomfort of the skin eruptions, depending on the individual.
• Since shingles may set in as a result of being run down or stressed, it is essential to make time for rest, relaxation and any activities that promote a sense of well-being once recovery is under way. It is important to treat symptoms as soon as they occur in order to minimize the risk of post-herpetic neuralgia developing, the pain of which can make a relaxed state almost impossible to achieve.
• Concentrate on boosting your immune system by improving your diet. During the acute phase of the illness you may consider taking a vitamin B complex supplement each day to support your immune and nervous system.
• Keep away from pregnant women, anyone who has leukaemia or whose immune system is compromised, for example, from chemotherapy.

Alternative treatments

In the case of shingles, it is quite appropriate to take the relevant remedy internally, while also applying a topical preparation to the skin. However, a professional opinion should be sought as soon as possible if any areas of the face are affected, or in severe cases of shingles.

Topical preparations

These include lotions, tinctures or creams that may be applied to the skin to soothe and ease inflammation and irritation. Choose from any of the following, bearing in mind that none of the substances mentioned for application to the skin should be taken by mouth.

Aromatherapy oils

Use five drops of ravensar (Ravensara aromatica) in one teaspoon of gel base and apply to the skin where the virus first appeared. This does not apply to shingles around the eye. Always work in conjunction with your family doctor.

Herbal preparations

• Cool compresses may be soothing when applied to the painful area. For maximum relief, soak the compress in diluted Hypericum tincture. One part of tincture should be dissolved in ten parts of water. The compress can be applied to the skin as often as necessary in order to provide relief.
• A soothing infusion may also be made from dried mullein, mallow and marsh mallow roots. Add 8g (1oz) of each to 3l (5¼ pints) water. Simmer for three minutes and strain. The liquid may be used on a compress as often as necessary.
• A mixture of Hypericum and Calendula cream or ointment can be applied to painful areas to provide pain relief and encourage healing. Either may be used in the early stages, but it is important to bear in mind that the ointment has a lanolin base which may result in a skin reaction in those who are sensitive to it.

Home remedies

Vitamin E oil may be applied to sensitive areas to relieve pain and irritation, while also discouraging the possibility of scarring.

Medicines intended for internal use

These ease pain, reduce inflammation and encourage a speedy resolution of the problem.

Professional alternative medical help may be obtained from any of the following:
- Anthroposophical medicine
- Aromatherapy
- Ayurvedic medicine
- Biochemic tissue salts
- Homoeopathy
- Naturopathy
- Nutritional therapy
- Reflexology
- Shiatsu
- Traditional Chinese medicine
- Western medical herbalism

Ulcers

See mouth ulcers (pages 134-6) and varicose ulcers (mentioned under varicose veins, pages 321-4).

HOMOEOPATHIC MEDICINES

Type	General features	Worse	Better	Remedy
Severe burning and stitch-like pains that bring tears to the eyes	Bluish-coloured skin eruptions that are much worse for the lightest touch and contact with air. Pains are characteristically shooting, stabbing or stitch-like. Neuralgic pains remain after eruptions have gone	Contact with damp, cold air Change of temperature Moving arms Breathing Touch	Sitting bending forwards	Ranunculus bulbosus
Shingles with digestive problems	Eruptions may be limited to the right side of the body. Neuralgic pains with persistent nausea, loss of appetite and sick headaches. Symptoms may appear or develop suddenly	Heat Early hours of the morning Mental effort	Gentle movement	Iris
Intense stitch-like pains at night that cause extreme restlessness	Pains may affect the left side or move from left to right. Severely itchy, burning, dry skin eruptions that are much worse for contact with cold draughts of air	Uncovering painful areas of skin Becoming chilled after sweating At night Jarring movements Resting in bed	Warm bathing Warmth Rubbing Changing position Gentle movement that does not exhaust	Rhus tox
Severe itching that changes places on scratching	Painful, itchy skin that becomes much more irritable by warm bathing. Thick, crusty eruptions that discharge gluey liquid. Burning, smarting pains on the skin with extreme sensitivity to contact with air	Warmth Cold draughts of air Movement Touch At night	Fresh air Wrapping up well Eating	Mezereum

Urticaria (hives)

Urticaria is characterized by the sudden appearance of itchy, red weals on the skin that may affect any area of the body, and can vary greatly in size. They may look like small red spots or large, blotchy patches that extend across a surface area of several inches. The length of time that they last can also vary a great deal from a few minutes' duration to several days. In some cases, urticaria may cause long-term distress by recurring at frequent intervals, often moving from one part of the body to another.

Triggers for an attack of urticaria may include any of the following:
• Stress.
• An allergic reaction to certain foods or additives. Potential problem foods may include fish, nuts or strawberries.
• Conventional drugs such as aspirin or codeine.
• Exposure to house dust mite, sunlight or pollen.

SEEK PROFESSIONAL HELP

• If there are signs of severe swelling around the lips, face or throat.
• If there is any indication that breathing or swallowing is becoming difficult.
• If itching and irritation of the skin are intense.

Alternative treatments

For urticaria it is quite appropriate to take a recommended remedy internally, while also applying a soothing topical preparation to the skin. Any of the measures suggested below should be effective in easing the short-term distress of urticaria, but home prescribing is not adequate to deal with the underlying imbalance in the body that leads to the tendency for the problem to recur, so if urticaria is a recurrent problem, consult a trained practitioner.

Topical preparations

These include lotions, tinctures or creams that can be applied to the skin to soothe and heal. Choose from any of the following, bearing in mind that none of the substances mentioned for application to the skin should be taken by mouth.

Flower remedies

Rescue Remedy cream may be added to irritated patches of skin to reduce heat and itching.

Herbal preparations

• If skin is stinging and burning with hives, diluted nettle (Urticadioica) tincture should ease the irritation. One part of tincture should be added to ten parts of boiled, cooled water.
• If diluted nettle (Urticadioica) tincture eases the situation temporarily, further relief may be gained by applying nettle cream to the affected areas.

Home remedies

• Parsley juice or honey may be applied to the skin to ease irritation.
• Dock leaves or plantain may be rubbed onto itchy areas of skin. However, this should not be done too frequently, since dock leaves may become irritant after excessive use.

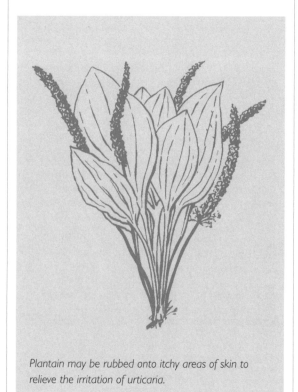

Plantain may be rubbed onto itchy areas of skin to relieve the irritation of urticaria.

HOMOEOPATHIC MEDICINES

Type	General features	Worse	Better	Remedy
Large, raised, blotchy weals that are awfully sensitive to heat	Hiving is rosy-pink and looks as though water is trapped beneath the surface of the skin. Any contact with warmth causes great distress. Affected areas such as the face feel taut and swollen	Warmth Resting Warm drinks Touch Pressure	Cool bathing Undressing Contact with cool air Movement	Apis
Small, blistery fluid-filled spots that are awfully itchy at night	Maddening itching of the skin causes awful restlessness at night. Hiving sets in after getting chilled and wet, with marked sensitivity of the skin to cold draughts of air. Depressed and despairing with irritation of the skin	Cold, draughty conditions Chill and damp air Uncovering Rest Excessive physical effort	Warmth Rubbing Continued movement Stretching Changing position	Rhus tox
Small, itchy spots that are soothed by warmth	Terribly irritated red spots that burn violently. Skin is generally soothed by contact with warmth, such as warm bathing or applying warm compresses to the affected area. Skin symptoms lead to extreme restlessness and anxiety	At night Cold or chilly conditions Lying on irritated areas Physical effort	Warmth Sitting propped up in bed Distraction Gentle movement	Arsenicum album
Recurring, long-standing urticaria with easily infected skin	Skin is generally extremely sensitive to cold air. Severe urticaria threatens to make breathing difficult through swelling of the throat, face and lips. Hypersensitive on physical and mental levels	Cold, dry air In the winter Exposure to cold winds Undressing or putting limbs out of bedclothes Touch At night	Wrapping up warmly Moist warmth Humid weather	Hepar sulph

Medicines intended for internal use

These ease discomfort, reduce inflammation and encourage a speedy resolution of the problem.

Professional alternative medical help may be obtained from any of the following:

- Anthroposophical medicine
- Biochemic tissue salts
- Homoeopathy
- Naturopathy
- Nutritional therapy
- Shiatsu
- Traditional Chinese medicine
- Western medical herbalism

Warts

Warts appear as a result of the presence of a virus in the body, and may affect the hands, feet (where they are called verrucas), the genital area or anywhere else on the body. They are potentially contagious, and may be spread from one person to another by physical contact. They may vary in size and shape, with some warts being quite tiny and others large and jagged, and may appear in clusters that nestle closely together or in isolation.

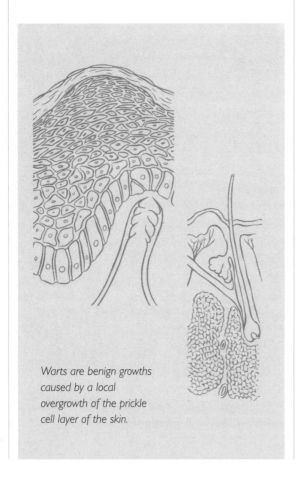

Warts are benign growths caused by a local overgrowth of the prickle cell layer of the skin.

Practical self-help

• Since warts are triggered by the presence of a virus, it is of great importance to do as much as possible to support the efficient functioning of the immune system. Avoid full-fat dairy products, additive-packed convenience foods, red meat, alcohol, tea and coffee, and follow the advice for healthy eating in the section on influenza (pages 154-6).

• Consider supplementing with vitamins C, E and B complex to help your immune system. A course of powdered garlic tablets may also be taken while the wart is healing.

SEEK PROFESSIONAL HELP

If you observe any changes in the texture, shape or sensation of your warts. For example, if a wart suddenly feels softer than usual, becomes uncharacteristically itchy or begins to bleed or exude a discharge, these would be appropriate reasons for seeking a medical opinion.

Alternative treatments

If warts are a long-established or recurrent problem the prescription of internal treatments is best left in the hands of an alternative therapist, who is likely to view the presence of a skin eruption as an indication of a deeper imbalance in the body as a whole. The selected medicine will be aimed at re-establishing health at a fundamental level, rather than merely providing symptomatic relief of the skin problem. However, some of the measures listed below may be helpful in cases where warts are a minor or infrequent problem.

Topical preparations

These include lotions, tinctures or creams that can be applied to the skin to speed up healing and resolution of the problem. Choose from any of the following, bearing in mind that none of the substances mentioned for application to the skin should be taken by mouth.

Herbal preparations

Diluted thuja tincture may be used to swab warts to encourage them to shrivel and fall away. One teaspoonful of tincture should be added to a cup of water, and the solution should be dabbed onto the wart each day for a ten-day period.

Home remedies

• Soak the rind of two lemons in cider vinegar for ten days and swab the wart with the solution until improvement is visible.

• The juice of an onion may also be painted on the wart in order to encourage shrivelling.

• Dandelion sap may help when applied directly to the wart twice or three times a day for a period of ten days.

• Once healing has been achieved and the wart has gone, wheatgerm oil should be applied to the affected area to discourage recurrence of the problem.

Medicines intended for internal use

These encourage the system as a whole to deal with the problem.

Biochemic tissue salts

Combination Remedy K may be used for minor or very infrequently developing warts. Take four tablets three times a day, tailing off as soon as improvement occurs.

Professional alternative medical help may be obtained from any of the following:

• Anthroposophical medicine
• Aromatherapy
• Homoeopathy
• Naturopathy
• Western medical herbalism

HOMOEOPATHIC MEDICINES

Type	General features	Worse	Better	Remedy
Moist, rapid-growing warts	Itchy, burning sensations in warts that feel worse for bathing in cool water. Brown spots on the skin with a tendency to hirsuteness (excess hair growth). Skin is generally greasy and dirty-looking	Cold, damp conditions Warmth of bed Exposure to sunlight	Sweating Wrapping up warmly Movement Rubbing	Thuja
Large warts that bleed from touch or washing	Cauliflower-shaped, dry warts with sharp, sticking pains. Skin is generally dry with coppery-coloured spots on the shins. Orifices of the body such as the mouth and nose look red, swollen and cracked	Touch Jarring Movement Cold, damp air Heat of bed Loss of sleep	Mild weather	Nit ac
Jagged, large warts that itch and bleed easily	Warts appear on the tips of the fingers, nose, brow and eyelids. Skin becomes cracked and ulcerated very easily with a tendency for soreness to develop in folds of skin. Warts emerge when run down or overstressed	Dry, raw air Physical effort Extreme temperatures	Humid conditions Washing Warmth Gentle movement	Causticum
Dry, fleshy, itching warts	Extreme skin sensitivity with sharp, biting pains. Skin problems alternate with discomfort in joints. Warty outgrowths may emerge on genital area	Touch Emotional stress Stretching At night	Warmth Rest	Staphysagria

PSYCHOLOGICAL AND STRESS-RELATED CONDITIONS

Addictions

Many people in the Western world find they need support from a chemical prop in order to keep up with the pace of living in a highly sophisticated, stressful society. This temporary help may come from using obvious crutches such as alcohol, cigarettes, coffee, tea, prescription or recreational drugs, or from more diverse complications such as sugar, chocolate, painkillers, exercise, gambling, dieting, shopping or work.

Although some of the items mentioned in the above list may be surprising, it is important to realize that it is possible to develop a dependence on or addiction to activities or substances that seem to be totally benign. It is also important to stress that not all dependencies are sinister or life-threatening: for instance, if you enjoy relaxing with a cup of tea after a hard day's work and the odd chocolate biscuit, this is hardly going to rank very high in the pecking order of addictions. However, once you reach the point of experiencing panic, severe anxiety or fear of being unable to cope without cigarettes, alcohol or prescription or recreational drugs, this is a more serious addiction.

Making the initial admission that the problem exists is usually the hardest hurdle to overcome. The first move is to seek help from an appropriate combination of any of the following: family doctor, support group, counsellor or alternative practitioner. The latter may play a particularly positive role in prescribing medicines that encourage emotional and physical resilience during withdrawal, and supporting us through what can often be a particularly distressing and traumatic time.

Because the subject of addiction and dependence is so complex, it is vital to appreciate that professional help must be sought. Do not attempt to cope with the problem alone, particularly during the withdrawal period, since objective, professional advice and support are invaluable at this time.

Practical self-help

• Although making the initial admission that you have an addiction can be extremely difficult, this makes the second step of seeking help from an appropriate support group easier. Sharing experiences with others who have gone through similar traumas can be especially therapeutic, since addiction can be an extremely isolating problem. Support groups can also provide invaluable practical advice regarding simple, effective strategies for coping at difficult times when it is tempting to give up the challenge.

• Counselling can be extremely helpful in coming to terms with the psychological issues that often underpin a tendency to addiction and dependency. Reliance on a substance, activity or co-dependent relationship is often a way of coming to terms with the stresses and strains that are part and parcel of everyday life. If a dependence reaches a point at which it is seriously compromising the day-to-day quality of our lives and relationships, it is vital that professional help should be sought in order to gain a sense of perspective on the factors that leave us vulnerable to a state of addiction. By exploring these issues with the help of a trained counsellor or psychotherapist, we stand a good chance of eventually coming to terms with our psychological problems. Although this process is very painful at times, the potential benefits considerably outweigh the drawbacks.

• Addictions to prescription or recreational drugs, alcohol, cigarettes or an eating disorder such as bulimia or anorexia nervosa (see pages 245-6) may lead to dietary deficiencies. As always, it is better to try to improve the nutritional value of your diet rather than developing an overreliance on nutritional supplements. For advice on healthy eating, see the section on weight gain, page 324.

• Useful supplements that may be helpful during withdrawal include vitamins A, C and D, B complex, manganese and potassium. For the sake of convenience, a good-quality multimineral and multivitamin may be more suitable.

• It can be very helpful when coming to terms with addiction to explore appropriate substitutes that ease some of the discomfort of withdrawal. To do this, identify the situations and times of day when cravings are strong and work out a positive strategy so that an acceptable alternative can be put in the place of the addictive substance. For example, if the early evening is a vulnerable time when there is a strong temptation to have a stiff drink and a cigarette, make a point of being otherwise enjoyably employed, or substitute an appealing non-alcoholic drink and a small, healthy snack.

• The depression or frustration that can develop after the withdrawal of an addictive substance or activity can be eased a great deal by taking up regular aerobic exercise, which makes the body release natural antidepressant chemicals called endorphins. Endorphins can play a major role in encouraging us to feel positive and dynamic at times when we might otherwise be feeling low. It is regularity of exercise that is most important, so it is better to aim for two or three half-hour sessions that occur on a regular basis, rather than leaving it for a week or two and overdoing it for an hour or so. It is also helpful to bear in mind that exercise itself can become addictive if things are allowed to get out of hand. See the section on burn-out on pages 239-42 for helpful advice on how to avoid this problem.

SEEK PROFESSIONAL HELP

• If there is any suspicion that it has become difficult or impossible to do without any of the following for even a short period of time, or if increasingly larger amounts are needed to achieve the same effect:
  • Alcohol
  • Prescription drugs
  • Recreational drugs
  • Painkillers
  • Cigarettes
  • Food that includes large amounts of potentially addictive substances such as coffee, tea, sugar and chocolate.
• If you have become dependent on a punishing exercise programme or strict dieting regime.

Professional alternative medical help may be obtained from any of the following:

• Anthroposophical medicine
• Aromatherapy
• Flower remedies
• Homoeopathy
• Massage therapy
• Naturopathy
• Nutritional therapy
• Shiatsu
• Traditional Chinese medicine
• Western medical herbalism

Anxiety

Anxiety is a diffuse condition that ranges from mild sensations of uneasiness and tension to full-blown, disabling panic attacks. When the latter occur for the first time, it can be a terrifying experience because of the intensity of the symptoms involved.

Common symptoms of severe or long-term anxiety may include any combination of the following:
• Tightness or pain in the chest.
• Trembling muscles.
• Rapid pulse and unpleasant awareness of rapid heartbeat (palpitations).
• Dry mouth with difficulty in swallowing.
• Hot flushes.
• Nausea.
• Diarrhoea.
• Indigestion.
• Stomach cramps.
• Vomiting.
• Reduced appetite.
• Lack of concentration.
• Poor memory.

Temporary anxiety is often the response to a stressful or demanding event, such as sitting an examination or speaking in public. Common symptoms of this form of transient anxiety may involve an uneasy sensation of 'butterflies' in the stomach accompanied by general sensations of muscular tension. However, this is generally a much less intense experience of anxiety than the symptoms experienced by those with long-term, chronic anxiety patterns. Long-term anxiety often leads to persistent problems such as tension headaches, irritable bowel syndrome, insomnia, general fatigue and burn-out.

Short-term anxiety may be effectively helped by making positive changes in lifestyle. More long-term problems of this nature do need help from a trained alternative practitioner in order to deal with the underlying predisposition to the problem. Additional help from a counsellor or psychotherapist may also help.

Practical self-help

• If general muscular tension is a problem as well as anxiety, relaxation or meditation techniques may help a great deal. Try inducing a meditative state by sitting in a straight-backed chair or lying flat on your back with your hands relaxed at your sides, and your head comfortably supported. Keep your spine straight but not stiff, and relax the limbs. If you are sitting in a chair make sure that your hands are resting gently open on your knees, while your feet are placed firmly on the floor. Wear loose, comfortable, warm clothes so that your mind is not encouraged to wander as a result of sensations of tightness, pressure or discomfort. Surroundings should also be pleasantly lit, peaceful and well ventilated with no hint of chilliness (always remember that your body temperature is likely to fall as you enter a deeply relaxed state). Close your eyes gently as you become aware of your breathing patterns. Observe the rhythm and depth of your breathing without altering anything at this stage. Begin slowly to regulate each breath, making it as steady and effortless as possible. As you breathe out, repeat a word or sound slowly to yourself; in time it should be possible to focus your mind exclusively on your breathing. Continue this process for as long as feels comfortable to you, making sure that you stop if there are any sensations of light-headedness, dizziness or disorientation.
• Diaphragmatic breathing techniques can also be an invaluable help. Most people instinctively respond to an anxious situation by tensing their muscles and taking rapid, shallow breaths from the upper chest. This has a powerful effect on the body, contributing to feelings of tension and panic as the ratio of oxygen to carbon dioxide is disrupted, inducing a sensation of helplessness. Positive breathing techniques can break

this vicious circle and restore equilibrium by promoting feelings of tranquillity and calmness.

To learn diaphragmatic breathing techniques lie flat on the floor with knees bent and feet flat on the floor (feet should be placed about a hip width apart). Lying in this position gives maximum opportunity for developing awareness of the motion of the diaphragm (the sheet of muscle that separates the chest cavity from the abdomen). A straight-backed sitting position can also be adopted. Induce a deliberate state of relaxation, bringing your attention to

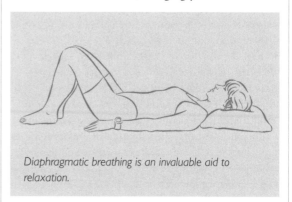

Diaphragmatic breathing is an invaluable aid to relaxation.

the movement of the breath entering and leaving your body. As you begin to gain awareness of this process, slowly and gently change the rhythm, making sure that your lungs fully inflate from the base to the tip as you breathe in, and that you exhale completely from the tip to the base of the lungs as you breathe out. If this seems difficult to establish, place your hand lightly on your abdomen at the level of your navel. As you inhale, your hand should rise gently upwards and outwards as your lungs fill with air. When you exhale, your hand should sink back to its original position as the breath is thoroughly expelled from the lungs. Make sure that you do not force the pace of each breath, and stop if dizziness, disorientation or light-headedness occur. Stop and start as you feel comfortable, making use of this technique whenever you feel tense or anxious.
• Regular exercise is an excellent way of burning up the excess adrenalin produced whenever we become anxious or fearful. Excess adrenalin leads to a state of arousal that can contribute to problems with high blood pressure, disturbed sleep patterns or digestive problems. Physical activity promotes a calmer, more clear-headed state of mind. Any aerobic activity is suitable, and bear in mind that regularity is more important than the length of time spent

on each session. For example, it is better to aim for three twenty-minute sessions of exercise each week, rather than a two-hour session every two or three weeks.

• The foods that are best avoided when feeling anxious are, paradoxically, those that we are most likely to reach for when in a low mental and emotional state. These include strong tea, coffee, any food or drink containing a lot of sugar, alcohol and chocolate. All of these have a strong tendency to make us feel even more tense, jittery and exhausted; anything containing caffeine or alcohol can exacerbate sleeping difficulties, which often accompany anxiety.

• Healthy alternatives include herbal teas or fruit-flavoured tisanes, grain or fig-based coffee substitutes, decaffeinated coffee (it is best to choose one that has been produced by a water-filtering process rather than using chemical solvents that may leave traces in the product) and fruit-flavoured, low-sugar, carbonated non-alcoholic drinks. Other advice on healthy eating can be found in the section on weight gain, page 324.

• If you feel overburdened by stressful factors in your life it is essential to find positive ways of managing these pressures. This may often be achieved by giving yourself plenty of time in which to relax and unwind before tackling a difficult problem, stressful event or professional confrontation. Creating this space avoids feeling harassed and rushed before a demanding experience. The day before an important engagement is an excellent time to make plans for ways of tackling the potentially stressful event. Make sure you have a refreshing, relaxed night's sleep by doing something deliberately relaxing or enjoyable before going to bed, for example, watching a favourite film, listening to music, spending the evening unwinding with a close friend or having a long walk in the fresh air. Avoid drinking coffee in the evening, eating late, and above all, make sure that work is put aside in the early evening. A sound sleep can also be encouraged by soaking in a warm bath (avoid hot baths because they can be overstimulating rather than relaxing), and sip a mug of warm chamomile tea before going to bed.

SEEK PROFESSIONAL HELP

• If anxiety symptoms are persistent, severe or interfering with the quality of life.
• If anxiety symptoms descend for no apparent reason.

• If anxiety-related problems have not responded to self-help measures within a short period of time.

Professional alternative medical help may be obtained from any of the following:
• Acupressure
• Anthroposophical medicine
• Aromatherapy
• Ayurvedic medicine
• Flower remedies
• Homoeopathy
• Massage therapy
• Naturopathy
• Nutritional therapy
• Shiatsu
• Traditional Chinese medicine
• Western medical herbalism

Burn-out

Burn-out can affect us both physically and emotionally, leaving us open to a range of problems including mood swings, difficulties with concentration, mental and physical exhaustion, poor digestion, muscle aches and headaches. It can arise because of excessive hours spent at work, too many late nights, burning the candle at both ends or an inability to learn the art of relaxation and switching off.

Unfortunately, many of us are misled into thinking that this problem is best dealt with by taking strenuous exercise in order to boost energy levels and reduce stress. However, although it is certainly true that regular, rhythmic, aerobic exercise conditions the heart and lungs, and aids stress reduction by channelling excess adrenalin, excessive or punishing training schedules create their own problems that effectively cancel out the positive benefits of exercising.

Those of us who feel most burnt out tend to experience a form of dependence on an activity such as work or exercise, often suffering great physical and emotional distress if the activity is withdrawn. This behaviour can become very problematic and irrational, and is simply illustrated by the example of an injured runner who is so addicted to the sport that he is unable to rest long and fully enough for his injury to heal properly. By returning to his punishing regime long before his body has had a chance to heal, he is likely to cause further damage.

If we take this example further, a vicious circle may be set up that ends in a state of physical and mental burn-out, including symptoms of fidgetiness, dissatisfaction, anxiety, disturbed sleep pattern and possible depression. Physical symptoms that may be associated with a burnt-out state include strains, sprains, aches, pains, dizziness and lack of co-ordination. If a substantial number of any of the following occur, professional help should be sought:

- Irritability.
- Mood swings.
- Unexplained anxiety.
- Introspection.
- Withdrawal from relationships.
- Frustration.
- Recurrent infections.
- Raised pulse rate.
- Lowered energy levels.

Emotional or physical pain is the body's way of telling us that something is amiss. As a result, if it is consistently ignored, the situation is likely to become steadily worse and increasingly incapacitating. Unfortunately, people who are most at risk of suffering burn-out because of a dynamic psychological make-up are least likely to be kind or patient with their bodies, pushing them to their limit or, sometimes, beyond.

If the first signs of burn-out appear, following some of the self-help suggestions listed below may be very helpful in easing the situation. However, if more developed symptoms have occurred it is very important to seek professional alternative medical help in order to obtain treatment that is most likely to steer things in a more positive direction.

Practical self-help

- Investigate ways of changing your working patterns so that there is always a break for lunch, rather than being tempted to work through the day without having any time to eat in a relaxed way. Taking a break means that time spent at work should also be more productive.

- Investigate forms of exercise and movement that encourage a state of balance and harmony between mind and body. Teachers of yoga and t'ai chi are likely to emphasize the important role body awareness plays in learning to relax through breathing techniques. Because these systems are non-competitive, strong emphasis is put on listening to your body and only going as far as feels comfortable. As a result, stress injuries are less likely to occur, while a sense of relaxation is likely to be enhanced. It may also be a revelation to discover that exercise systems of this kind are not a soft option, but require stamina, flexibility and co-ordination.

- Explore relaxation techniques and meditation as a way of unwinding and making essential space and time for yourself. There are increasing numbers of relaxation audio-cassette tapes on the market, and a reasonable choice of video tapes becoming available. Once you have mastered the skills of a relaxation technique, always make sure that you spend a little time each day consciously mentally relaxing and becoming aware of areas in your body that are holding tension. As you enter a relaxed state, let the

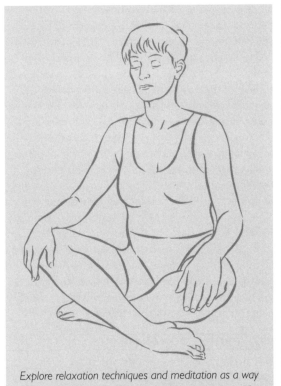

Explore relaxation techniques and meditation as a way of unwinding and making space and time for yourself.

tension melt from the taut parts of your body. If this is done on a regular basis it will be surprising to see how clarity of thought and physical and mental energy are increased. See the section on anxiety for advice on meditation and breathing techniques (page 238).

• Avoid the tendency to reach for 'quick fix' food and drink when feeling stressed or burnt out and try to stay well within or, ideally, below your recommended daily or weekly allowance of alcohol. For food and drink to avoid see the anxiety section, page 239, and for advice on healthy eating see the weight gain section, page 325.

• Physical burn-out often occurs in those who have taken up a sports activity to help overcome weight problems, body-image problems or an emotional trauma, such as the break-up of a relationship. While exercise can have very positive effects, if sustaining a demanding exercise regime is becoming more important than maintaining a lively social life, a rewarding job or time spent with other members of the family, the situation is becoming imbalanced and needs to be changed for the better. If this is difficult to do alone, counselling may be very helpful in confronting the tensions and emotional conflicts that may be masking an excessive attachment to exercise.

SEEK PROFESSIONAL HELP

• If depression or anxiety occur with symptoms of burn-out.
• If there are any signs of a growing sense of introversion or withdrawal occurring in someone who was previously outgoing and extrovert by nature.
• If there is preoccupation with weight loss or marked loss of appetite.
• If poor or incomplete recovery occurs after an infectious illness.
• If infections occur on a frequent or recurrent basis.

Alternative treatments

For burn-out it is perfectly appropriate to take the relevant internal remedy while also making use of an external application.

Topical preparations

These include essential oils, infusions and tinctures that can be used in massage, soothing baths or vaporized to encourage relaxation and revitalization. Choose from any of the following bearing in mind that none of the substances mentioned for application to the skin should be taken by mouth.

Herbal preparations

Make an infusion of any of the following and add to a warm bath to induce a reviving effect on mind and body, which can make clarity of thought a greater possibility: peppermint,* rosemary or rose petal. (Herbs marked with a * may interfere with the action of homoeopathic remedies.) Add three generous handfuls of your selected herb to a pan of cold water and leave to stand overnight. Bring to the boil the next day and strain when required. Add to a warm bath when needed.

Medicines intended for internal use

These ease tension, encourage detoxification and promote a speedy resolution of the problem.

Biochemic tissue salts

A general state of physical and mental burn-out where a general tonic is required may respond to Combination Remedy L. If symptoms have built up slowly over a period of time, four tablets may be taken three times a day until the situation improves. However, symptoms that appear rapidly and acutely may initially respond more effectively to tablets taken hourly for a short time.

Flower remedies

• Pine may be helpful for those who become burnt out and feel extreme guilt as well as a sense of failure. This may take the shape of taking blame for other's mistakes.
• Elm may be appropriate for anyone who has a tendency to take on an excessive workload and ends up feeling overwhelmed by the resulting responsibility and sheer volume of work.
• Beech may be indicated for those who have perfectionist tendencies that lead to intolerance of faults in others as well as themselves. As a result, irritability and oversensitivity may occur in response to mistakes made by others.

Once a treatment bottle has been made up, take four drops four times a day, holding the dose for a few moments in the mouth before swallowing. Alternatively, the treatment may be made up in a glass of water and sipped as often as needed throughout the day.

Herbal preparations

• Any of the following may be taken in tincture, capsule or infusion to act as a nervous restorative: wild oat, skullcap, ginseng or vervain.

• If a nervous relaxant is needed to encourage relaxation and ease digestive problems, the following may be appropriate: passionflower or valerian. (Valerian should be used with care since it may result in headaches, palpitations or muscular spasms with long use.)

Professional alternative medical help may be obtained from any of the following:
• Acupressure
• Anthroposophical medicine
• Aromatherapy
• Ayurvedic medicine
• Chiropractic
• Flower remedies
• Homoeopathy
• Massage therapy
• Naturopathy
• Nutritional therapy
• Osteopathy
• Reflexology
• Shiatsu
• Traditional Chinese medicine
• Western medical herbalism

HOMOEOPATHIC MEDICINES

Type	General features	Worse	Better	Remedy
Anxiety and digestive problems with burn-out	Bloating, rumbling and gurgling with alternating diarrhoea and constipation. Acidity with heartburn and indigestion. Poor muscular tone with strong determination and commitment to exercise	Chill or overheating Mental strain In the afternoon and evening Pressure of clothes	Distraction and occupation Gentle movement Warm drinks	Lycopodium
Burn-out with muscular aching and tenderness	The whole body is bruised, aching and sore. Inability to rest because of discomfort felt from lying on any surface however soft. Shifting pains move from joint to joint. Awful, overwhelming tiredness and exhaustion from muscle strain	Touch Movement Jarring, jolting movements After sleep	Resting with the head lower than the body	Arnica
Anxious mental and physical prostration in overachievers	Tense, nervous perfectionists who have marked anxiety about health and preoccupation and fear of illness. Extreme physical and mental restlessness with possible addiction to exercise or compulsion to neatness. Pushes beyond point of reasonable limits and goals and becomes exhausted as a result	At night Being chilled Exertion Cold food and drink Alcohol	Warm food and drink Warmth Warm compresses Company Contact with fresh air	Arsenicum album
Burn-out in over-stressed individuals who work and play to excess	Competitive high achievers who have difficulty switching off from stimulation. May become addicted to 'joggers' high'. Coffee and alcohol consumption increases because of exhaustion. Constipation, insomnia and recurrent headaches as a result of stress	Coffee Alcohol Disturbed sleep Noise In the morning	Later in the day Warmth Sound, uninterrupted sleep Rest	Nux vomica

Depression

Although many of us may complain from time to time about feeling depressed, it is important to realize that there are varying degrees of depression from deep-seated clinical depression to a transient 'low' state that may lift quite spontaneously. In the past, depressive states were divided into two separate, but related categories, reactive and endogenous depression, but these terms are generally no longer considered fashionable. However, because some therapists still use these terms, some insight into the differences is useful.

Reactive depression may occur as the result of a traumatic or distressing event that threatens identity and security. This may involve the breakdown of a long-term relationship, bereavement, severe financial problems or redundancy. Although the depressed feelings may be very intense and distressing, there is a good chance that they will gradually recede as the initial problem that sparked off the depression has resolved itself.

Endogenous depression, on the other hand, tends not to occur as a reaction to a specific upsetting event, but can descend for no obvious reason while life seems to be going very smoothly. As a result, endogenous depression can be extremely alarming and frightening, since there is no external factor that can be changed to improve matters. This often leaves the sufferer feeling helpless and powerless, as they are at a loss to know what they can do to rectify the situation.

Depression may occur during phases of life that involve major change, such as puberty, pregnancy and the post-natal period or the menopause. Certain illness may also give rise to depression, such as pre-menstrual syndrome, chronic fatigue syndrome (Myalgic encephalomyelitis or ME) or chronic pain.

Whether it is reactive or endogenous, the symptoms of depression are varied and may include any of the following:

• Abrupt or severe mood swings including feelings of despondency, despair, indifference, apathy, anxiety, hopelessness or sadness.
• Poor-quality sleep with a tendency to wake frequently.
• Early waking with powerful emotions of anxiety and/or despair.
• Poor memory.
• Inability to concentrate.
• Sexual problems with absent or lowered libido.
• Digestive problems including indigestion, stomach pain, loss of appetite, nausea, heartburn and alternation between diarrhoea and constipation.
• Poor eating patterns with total lack of interest in food or tendency to comfort eating.
• Palpitations and hyperventilation (a tendency to breathe quickly and shallowly).
• Lack of energy.
• Recurrent negative thought patterns.

When deciding whether alternative medical help is appropriate, it is important to differentiate between contained, short-term episodes of depression that are a reaction to stressful events and long-term problems. Long-term depression must be treated by a trained alternative practitioner; do not attempt to self-prescribe at home. An objective opinion should be sought about the most appropriate form of alternative treatment that may be of most help, rather than placing the responsibility of selecting treatments into the hands of someone caring for a depressed partner or relative.

However, if short-term, mild feelings of depression occur in reaction to a specific event which is already showing signs of resolving itself, some of the self-help measures suggested below may be of great value in alleviating the situation.

Practical self-help

• Poor eating patterns are often a result of feeling low. If this is the case, take a good-quality multi-vitamin/multimineral supplement for a few months in order to make up for any vitamin or mineral deficiencies. However, it is important to stress that this is not a long-term solution, since the best way of ensuring good-quality nutrition is to make strenuous efforts to improve the quality of food and drink taken on a regular basis. For advice on sensible healthy eating see the weight gain section, pages 324-6.

• Become aware of foods and drinks that may contribute to erratic or severe mood swings, including chocolate, anything containing a lot of sugar, 'junk foods' that contain a substantial amount of chemical additives, preservatives and artificial flavourings, alcohol, strong tea and coffee.

• Make sure that your diet includes a substantial amount of B vitamins, which are extremely important in times of emotional and physical stress because of their reputation for supporting the health and resilience of the nervous system. They include nuts, whole grains, green leafy vegetables, fish, yeast extract, soya flour, bananas and brown rice.

• Since depression often alternates with episodes of anxiety, see the advice given in the anxiety section (pages 238-9) for additional help.

• It is vital when feeling low to allow yourself sufficient space within which to recover. Although it may be terribly difficult to muster up sufficient motivation, doing things that you find relaxing, uplifting or rewarding at a time like this can help a great deal: finding the impetus to get going in the first place is usually the hardest part. The activity could be anything at all that you find pleasurable, such as walking, having a long, aromatic bath, listening to music, reading a novel, watching a favourite video, or spending time with a close, sympathetic friend.

• When you are depressed you need a safe space within which you can express your feelings. This could be achieved by talking frankly to a friend, relative or partner. However, it is important to bear in mind that those close to someone suffering from depression are often too emotionally involved to be able to listen uncritically to the feelings being expressed. It is also true that carers often find that their emotional resources are under such strain they are unable to provide the calm, listening ear that is needed at especially fraught times. As a result, it can be most helpful to talk frankly about emotional problems with a counsellor or psychotherapist, who will be able to take an objective stance and can interpret what is being said from a professional perspective, encouraging their client to explore issues that are likely to result in valuable emotional insights.

• It is an ironic fact that although regular aerobic exercise is extremely helpful in reducing the emotional distress of depression, this is probably the very last thing you feel like doing when at a low ebb. However, the benefits of regular exercise include:

• The increased secretion of endorphins, chemicals in our bodies that resemble natural antidepressants.

• An increase in self-esteem and confidence in your body: this can be especially important if you are subject to negative feelings about yourself.

• A boost to the processes of elimination and removal of toxic waste from our bodies caused by the deeper breathing necessary during exercise. Waste elimination is an important contributing factor to feeling alert and energized: feelings that often suffer greatly during periods of depression. It is not necessary to gasp for breath during exercise – you are exercising hard enough if you can carry on a conversation without a sense of strain or getting out of breath.

Once you have decided on an activity that appeals to you, make sure that you are not too ambitious and begin slowly, avoiding making unrealistic demands on yourself, and you will have a greater chance of continuing your exercise programme.

SEEK PROFESSIONAL HELP

• If there are any signs of a sense of unreality or feeling of isolation from others.

• If feelings of emotional numbness are present.

• If anxiety or panic arises in connection with issues that would normally cause few problems.

• If depressive feelings have descended for no obvious reason.

• If severe apathy or indifference develops.

• If there is any suspicion that suicide has become a possibility.

• If renewed depression occurs in someone who has previously suffered from the illness.

• If depression has become an established state and has not responded to self-help measures.

• If there is weight loss.

Professional alternative medical help may be obtained from any of the following:
• Anthroposophical medicine
• Aromatherapy
• Flower remedies
• Homoeopathy
• Massage therapy
• Naturopathy
• Nutritional therapy
• Shiatsu
• Traditional Chinese medicine
• Western medical herbalism

Eating disorders

Although eating disorders such as anorexia nervosa and bulimia nervosa primarily affect women, there is a growing awareness and acknowledgement that these are problems that can also affect men who are young, ambitious and eager to achieve. There appear to be strong links between the emergence of eating disorders and certain psychological stresses and strains that can leave vulnerable personalities open to this sort of self-punishing behaviour.

They may include any of the following:
• Generally speaking, children of overcompetitive, appearance-conscious parents who set extremely high or rigid standards of behaviour and achievement for their children may be vulnerable to problems with self-image and confidence. These problems may be expressed in a negative preoccupation with weight, especially if one or both parents exhibit an ambivalent attitude towards food and eating.
• If someone feels dissatisfied with or helpless about changing their emotional environment, this may lead to a preoccupation with strict weight control. Within this context, eating disorders may be seen as a reaction against feelings of helplessness, powerlessness and vulnerability in other areas of life.
• Traumatic, unsatisfactory or unwelcome early sexual encounters may also give rise to feelings of poor self-esteem, self-loathing or guilt that may be translated into eating disorders.
• Lack of emotional support, bereavement or shock at a critical phase in emotional and physical development may also lead to ambivalent feelings about self-image.

Although there are subtle differences between the symptoms of anorexia (self-induced starvation) when compared with those of bulimia (cycles of bingeing on food followed by self-induced vomiting and/or laxative abuse), there are identifiable features that run through the general category of eating disorders. These include:
• An unbalanced, obsessive relationship with food, especially with those items that are regarded as 'forbidden' because of their calorific value.
• Excessive monitoring of weight gain or loss, with readings sometimes being taken several times a day.
• Overconsideration of the calorific values of food in a desperate attempt to keep weight within or below rigid limits. These limits are often on a downward sliding scale, so that once a desired weight has been reached, the goalposts are moved to a lower weight that becomes the new bottom line.
• Strict limitation of the amount of food eaten (to the degree of items being weighed before they are consumed), or bingeing followed by self-induced vomiting and/or purging by taking laxatives on a regular basis.
• Unstable or fluctuating weight as a result of an erratic cycle of bingeing followed by periods of starvation.
• Irregular or absent periods in women due to body fat falling below an optimum level.
• Mood swings, depression and anxiety.
• Hormonal changes that may result in growth of extra body hair (lanugo), reduction in hip and breast contours and diminished sex drive.
• Long-term dental problems due to the teeth being repeatedly washed in stomach acid during vomiting.

If an eating disorder has reached a well-established or advanced state, hospitalization may be necessary to avoid severe malnutrition, permanent organ damage and even death. However, alternative treatment can play a very positive role in treating those who suffer from eating disorders.

When appropriate alternative measures are combined with empathetic counselling, psychological support and sound nutritional back-up, the patient will have the best chance of coming to terms with surfacing psychological insights. However, because of the complex issues surrounding well-established eating disorders, this is a situation that must be dealt with by a trained alternative practitioner, who should ideally also possess psychotherapeutic or counselling skills in order to guide that patient towards an improved state.

Practical self-help

• Admitting that a problem exists is often the most

difficult hurdle to overcome before recovery can begin. Once this acknowledgement has been made, appropriate help and support may be given in dealing with the problem.

• Writing a daily account of your feelings can be a positive way of helping you gain perspective on emotional fluctuations. In this way, a long-term perspective may be gained on how your psychological well-being and resilience affects the intensity of problems you may have in relation to food.

• Consider the reasons you may give for avoiding meals in the company of family and friends. Explore your feelings around this issue, taking into account how you really feel about eating in the company of others.

• Slowly add small, additional helpings of nutritious foods at mealtimes, or ensure you have healthy snacks readily available such as raw vegetables, pieces of fresh fruit, or rice cakes with savoury toppings.

• Check that you are not likely to be zinc deficient. There is a strong connection between low levels of zinc in the body and an increased susceptibility to develop eating disorders. The following foods are good sources of zinc: green vegetables, eggs, milk, whole grains, yeast, nuts, seeds and meat.

• Loneliness can encourage a problematic relationship with food and disrupted or erratic eating patterns. By preserving relationships with close friends and maintaining a healthy social life you are less likely to develop an obsessive relationship with food.

• For well-established, long-term emotional problems it is very helpful to seek the professional advice of a counsellor or psychotherapist. He or she will be trained to explore the psychological problems that often form the bedrock of difficulties with eating disorders.

SEEK PROFESSIONAL HELP

If symptoms of eating disorders are well established and severe.

Professional alternative medical help may be obtained from any of the following:
• Anthroposophical medicine
• Flower remedies
• Homoeopathy
• Naturopathy
• Nutritional therapy
• Shiatsu
• Traditional Chinese medicine
• Western medical herbalism

'Empty nest' syndrome

This is a problem that is most likely to hit women as they experience the menopause, especially if they have chosen to have children in their twenties. This can be a very difficult emotional situation to handle, especially for people who have sunk most of their creative energy into bringing up children and meeting the needs of a family. As a result, feelings of confusion, despondency and bereavement may surface as children become independent and no longer need the same degree of care and attention that they once did. Men can also experience a traumatic time during the transitory phase as they may be also having to come to terms with developing a fresh role and purpose for themselves as they face retirement.

'Empty nest' syndrome may give rise to a wide range of symptoms including:
• Severe or unpredictable mood swings.
• General, diffused feelings of sadness or anxiety that may be especially severe or noticeable on waking.
• Apathy or indifference.
• Lack of concentration.
• Reduced or absent libido.
• Disrupted appetite with lack of interest in food or desire to eat comfort foods frequently.
• General restlessness.
• Muscular tension and aches and pains.

A form of empty nest syndrome may also develop in people who have chosen a career in preference to a family, they may be hit very hard in their forties when the chance of having children has reduced greatly.

Alternative self-help measures may give sufficient support to get you through a difficult time. However, if symptoms are especially persistent, severe or having an adverse effect on the quality of your life, professional help should be sought.

Practical self-help

• As family demands and responsibilities lessen and change, it becomes possible to explore new challenges or to focus anew on interests that have been set to one side while family demands were dominant. By becoming involved in fresh physical or mental occupations such as joining a sports club, attending adult education classes or doing voluntary work, new horizons may open up at a time when they are least expected. This phase of life can be a positive fresh start rather than the beginning of a negative downward spiral. You are also likely to make new friends who may be in a similar situation, which is a positive antidote to feelings of loneliness and isolation.

• Allow yourself the opportunity to express your feelings in the company of someone with whom you feel sufficiently relaxed. This could be a close family member, good friend or family doctor. However, it is also important to speak frankly with your partner about your feelings, since it is sometimes easy to neglect speaking to the person most involved in the situation. By expressing feelings of insecurity, fear, anger or confusion about your children becoming independent, you can give your partner the opportunity to be equally honest about their own emotional reactions to the situation. This may be especially important if your partner is approaching retirement since this can be a time when feelings of insecurity or anxiety can be very apparent. By communicating with each other and forming a shared understanding of the situation at this important stage of your relationship, you may experience renewed closeness.

• Use the extra time available to you to explore fresh, healthy approaches to cooking. This is especially important at a time when you need as much support as possible from a nutritious diet. Steam or stir-fry foods to preserve vitamin content, freshness and crispness and avoid deep-frying, battering or boiling as cooking methods, always using small

quantities of cold-pressed virgin olive oil if fat is required. Experiment with home-made Indian dishes that combine pulses and rice with spices, or Chinese recipes that concentrate on stir-fried vegetables with small amounts of poultry, fish or seafood. Keep foods that contribute to mood swings to a minimum, such as chocolate, alcohol, anything containing a lot of sugar, strong tea or coffee, and additive-laden convenience foods. For further advice on healthy eating see the weight gain section, pages 324-6.

• If your confidence has suffered while feeling low, consider the importance of taking up an enjoyable and absorbing form of exercise that is appealing to you. Regular physical exercise can increase our overall fitness, improve our emotional well-being, boost confidence and discourage the onset of osteoporosis (brittle bones).

• If depression or anxiety related to empty nest syndrome does not respond to self-help measures alone, psychotherapy or counselling sessions can help you gain a more balanced, realistic perspective on your situation.

SEEK PROFESSIONAL HELP

• If symptoms are severe, persistent or do not respond to self-help measures.

• If the symptoms of empty nest syndrome occur in someone who has previously suffered from depression.

Alternative treatments

For empty nest syndrome it is quite appropriate to take the relevant internal remedy while also applying a topical preparation to the skin.

Topical preparations

These include essential oils that can be massaged on the skin to uplift the mood or induce relaxation. Choose from any of the following, bearing in mind that none of the substances mentioned for application to the skin should be taken by mouth.

Herbal preparations

During a period of emotional stress it may be very helpful to add an infusion of lavender or lemon balm to your bathwater. Soak three generous handfuls of either dried herb in a small pan of cold water. Leave overnight and bring slowly to the boil the following day. Strain the liquid and add to your bathwater.

HOMOEOPATHIC MEDICINES

Type	General features	Worse	Better	Remedy
Sweet on the surface with repressed anger at children for leaving	Anger is not expressed when upsetting events occur, leading to explosive outburst of temper in response to trivial, inconsequential triggers. Trembles and shakes with anger and tension	Early morning Emotional stress Touch Smoking	Rest Sleep Warmth After eating	Staphysagria
Tense and burnt out from throwing excessive energy into work	Classic picture of personal and professional overloading. Reacts to children becoming independent by taking on excessive workload. Stress-related symptoms of recurrent headaches, indigestion and constipation. Reliance on caffeine to keep going, alcohol to unwind, and prescription drugs to cope with stress	Waking Stress Noise Contact with cold draughts Smoking Coffee	Sound sleep By the evening and night Warmth Rest Peace and quiet	Nux vomica
Low, exhausted and depressed with indifference towards family	Black depression with indifference and lack of enthusiasm for anything. Quick-tempered and irritable with extreme reaction to emotional demands. Diminished or absent libido. Bouts of anxiety with fear of losing control or strong sense of being unable to cope	Sitting still Brooding Emotional stress or demands Skipping regular meals Before a period	Warmth Fresh air Aerobic exercise Brisk walking in the fresh air Sound sleep in a warm bed Eating small amounts often	Sepia
Severe or uncontrollable bouts of crying with grief at children leaving home	Sadness, distress and depression that do not resolve themselves with the passing of time. Alternating or contradictory moods: manic laughing fits alternate with episodes of uncontrollable weeping. Constant sighing or yawning when depressed. Tense and anxious with muscle tension and spasms	Stimulation Cold conditions Smoking Alcohol Coffee	Eating Distraction from sadness Warmth	Ignatia
Weepy and sad with a longing for sympathy and emotional comfort	Easily moved to tears in sympathetic company. Generally feels much better after a good cry. Changeable moods that move quickly from anxiety to irritability to depression. Wants to cling on to children when they need to be independent. Feels more positive and cheerful after gentle exercise in the fresh air	Solitude During the menopause In the evening At night Rest In bed Overheated, stuffy rooms	Gentle exercise Sympathy Contact with fresh, cool air Cool drinks and cool food After a good cry Sympathy and attention	Pulsatilla

Medicines intended for internal use

These ease tension and distress and promote a balanced perspective of the problem.

Flower remedies

- Honeysuckle may be helpful for those who cling too much to the past and who find it difficult to adapt to change.
- Wild rose may ease those who feel low, apathetic and resigned to their unhappy state.
- Willow may be indicated when emotional distress takes the form of resentment and bitterness towards others.
- Chicory may be of help to those who are inclined to be overpossessive of their family, with a resulting tendency to be overdemanding or inclined to self-pity.

Once a treatment bottle has been made up, take four drops four times a day, holding the dose for a few moments in the mouth before swallowing. Alternatively, the treatment may be made up in a glass of water and sipped as often as needed throughout the day.

Biochemic tissue salts

Tissue salt No. 6 may be helpful in easing symptoms of nervous debility and emotional strain, especially if there is any tendency towards insomnia. If symptoms are severe, take four tablets at hourly intervals until improvement sets in, or four tablets may be taken three times a day for lower-grade problems.

Herbal preparations

- An infusion of borage may be helpful in easing the distress of grief and sadness, due to its relaxing effect. Because of its reputation for supporting the adrenal glands, this plant can be especially helpful during the menopause, when these glands are brought into play to bolster oestrogen production. To make the infusion, add a cup of hot water to a teaspoonful of dried herb, cover and leave to stand for fifteen minutes. Strain, and sip as a warm, soothing tea.
- Low spirits and a general feeling of despondency may be eased by taking an infusion of rosemary. It can also ease digestive problems that are stress related. To make the infusion, follow the directions given above. **NB** Rosemary should not be taken for an extended period of time and its use should always be used with caution in pregnancy.

Home remedies

- A tablespoonful of apple cider vinegar taken in a small wineglass of warm water to which a little honey has been added may be very soothing when taken first thing in the morning and last thing at night.
- The following foods have a reputation for helping with general feelings of nervous debility and emotional lows. As a result they should be included as regular ingredients of the diet: wholewheat bread, brown rice, sesame seeds, sunflower seeds, buckwheat, millet, black grapes, broccoli, cabbage, watercress and beetroot.

Professional alternative medical help may be obtained from any of the following:
- Anthroposophical medicine
- Aromatherapy
- Biochemic tissue salts
- Flower remedies
- Homoeopathy
- Reflexology

Grief and bereavement

It is a sobering thought that we all must experience the pain of loss at some stage in our lives. Grief can be directly related to the death of a close relative, parent, child, partner or pet, as a result of the loss of a job or home, or in response to regret for loss of youth as our children are ready to leave home. From this perspective we can see that many of us may have needed to come to terms with a broad spectrum of grief experiences by the time we reach our middle years, which can make dealing with this challenging phase of life very difficult indeed.

However, it is possible to emerge from the experience of grief a wiser and stronger person. Coming to terms with grieving can be greatly helped by having some understanding of the stages we are likely to go through in response to a profound sense of loss. These may involve a combination of any of the following:

• An initial reaction of unreality, shock or numbness.

• Denial that loss has occurred.

• Guilt.

• Anger.

• Resentment towards the medical profession or other carers who were unable to prolong life of the person who has died.

It is quite common for the acute phase of grief to be followed by depression as implications of loss sink in, but despair and anguish are often a necessary part of the grieving process. Once this phase begins to lift, it becomes possible to take pleasure in life once again, even though episodes of sadness, depression or wistfulness may still occur at intervals. Once recovery is well under way these episodes should become briefer and feel less intense with the passing of time and as emotional resilience begins to grow.

Alternative approaches have a great deal to offer throughout the grieving process. As always, consult an alternative practitioner if you suspect you may be getting out of your depth using self-help measures, or if you do not seem to be responding positively.

Practical self-help

• If your sleep pattern is disturbed following the shock of grief and loss, see the advice given in the insomnia section (pages 252-5).

• Make a point of pacing yourself so that you have enough time and space to grieve. Rushing back to work in an attempt to re-establish a sense of normality can have an adverse effect if done too soon. Denying yourself sufficient emotional space can inhibit the natural course of grief, leading to emotional and physical problems further down the line.

• Be prepared for the reality that friends, relatives and colleagues are unlikely to be able to sustain the emotional support and help that they give in the initial stages of bereavement. You may find yourself lacking understanding and attention when you need it most. If this occurs, sensitive bereavement counselling can be of immense benefit, providing vital contact with someone who has the capacity to be objective about an extremely emotionally charged situation.

• It is not uncommon for anxiety, panic attacks and/or depression to follow the initial shock and trauma of bereavement. If this is the case, consult the general advice given in the anxiety and depression sections on pages 237 and 243.

SEEK PROFESSIONAL HELP

• If there are any signs of lingering depression (see the depression section on page 243).

• If the grieving process is not resolving itself or diminishing within a reasonable period of time.

Alternative treatments

For grief and bereavement it is perfectly appropriate to take the relevant internal remedy while also making use of external applications.

Topical preparations

These include essential oils that can be vaporized or used in aromatic baths to uplift or relax the mind and body. Choose from any of the following, bearing in mind that none of the substances mentioned for external application should be taken by mouth.

Home remedies

Bathe the face with orange blossom or rose water for their natural relaxing and uplifting properties. Alternatively, dilute one of these with water and pour into a spray bottle. If this is carried in your bag it can be used to spray the face and neck as often as needed.

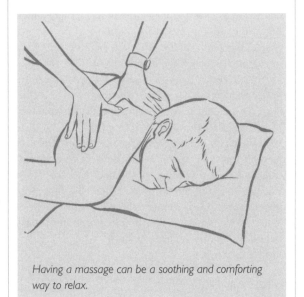

Having a massage can be a soothing and comforting way to relax.

HOMOEOPATHIC MEDICINES

Type	General features	Worse	Better	Remedy
Panic attacks and episodes of fear in response to bereavement	Required in first stages of bereavement, if bad news has come unexpectedly or suddenly. Needed if traumatic event was witnessed, such as an accident. Severe symptoms of anxiety, restlessness, agitation and fear set in very abruptly	Noise Touch During the night	Rest Moderate warmth Contact with fresh air	Aconite
Unresolved grief with severe mood swings and bouts of hysterics	Alternating spasmodic bouts of weeping with uncontrollable laughter. Uncontrollable, involuntary sighing, hiccuping or muscle twitching. Desperate sense of being unable to cope. Often needed for unresolved grief that has lingered too long	Touch Cold, open air Fright Shock Coffee Smoking Yawning	Eating Warmth Being left alone Taking regular, deep breaths Firm pressure	Ignatia
Suppressed grief with aversion to sympathy and attention	Becomes withdrawn in order to bottle up emotions and keep a stiff upper lip. Avoids understanding company because of the risk of bursting into tears, which makes everything worse. Feels humiliated and diminished by displays of emotion	Sympathy Comfort and affection Touch Weeping Being in company Noise Becoming overheated	Resting Peace and quiet Being undisturbed Cool, fresh air Cool bathing	Natrum mur
Anger and resentment with established experience of grief	Often needed where natural expression of emotion has been denied, resulting in anger and resentment being expressed towards the person who has died. Hostility may be mixed with guilt and self-reproach because of not having done enough. Physical and mental oversensitivity	Stress Stimulation Becoming chilled During the night	Warmth Rest After breakfast	Staphysagria
Established phase of grief with great need for sympathy, comfort and attention	Very weepy and clingy with craving for sympathetic company. Always feels worse when isolated and alone. Frequent episodes of weeping and expressions of emotional release in supportive company help a great deal	Being alone Resting In bed Evening and night Stuffy, overheated surroundings	Sympathy and attention Displays of physical affection After a good cry Gentle exercise Being in the fresh air Cool surroundings	Pulsatilla

Medicines intended for internal use

These help the system come to terms with shock, and support the mind and body in moving through the stages of grieving.

Biochemic tissue salts

The pain and shock of bereavement may benefit from a combination formula called Nervone. In the initial phase of shock tablets may need to be taken hourly, tailing off the dosage as symptoms improve. More established symptoms may respond better to four tablets taken three times a day until symptoms improve.

Flower remedies

Rescue Remedy may be of great help in easing symptoms of agitation, distress and general shock. Place a couple of drops directly on the tongue as often as needed, or add to a small glass of cold water and sip at frequent intervals. As with biochemic tissue salts and homoeopathic remedies, once relief has been obtained it is best to tail off the dosage.

Herbal preparations

• The following infusions may be very helpful in easing the initial symptoms of shock accompanying bereavement: chamomile, lemon balm and skullcap. The latter may also be helpful in aiding withdrawal if tranquillizers or antidepressants have been used on a short-term basis and are about to be slowly discontinued under medical supervision. To make the infusion, use 28g (1oz) dried herb or 50g (2oz) fresh herbs to 600ml (1 pint) boiling water. Cover and leave to stand for ten minutes before straining.

• An infusion of borage may also be helpful in easing palpitations, anxiety and feelings of tension connected to grief and sadness.

• Exhaustion following bereavement may be eased by taking a tincture of wild oats diluted in water daily. Eight drops of the tincture may be dissolved in a small glass of water taken each day until energy levels and well-being improve. This may also help with withdrawal from antidepressants and tranquillizers or provide an important aid in promoting sound sleep and relaxation.

Home remedies

Make sure that you do not neglect to eat foods containing the spectrum of B vitamins that have a reputation for supporting the system in times of stress. These include nuts, whole grains, green, leafy vegetables, fish, yeast extract, soya flour, bananas and brown rice.

Professional alternative medical help may be obtained from any of the following:
• Anthroposophical medicine
• Aromatherapy
• Flower remedies
• Homoeopathy
• Massage therapy
• Shiatsu
• Traditional Chinese medicine
• Western medical herbalism

Insomnia

Although very few people suffer from true insomnia, many are unable to switch off at night and enjoy a refreshing, uninterrupted, sound sleep. Although by morning you may feel that you have watched the clock all the night, chances are that you have snatched some brief phases of sleep, however unsatisfying they may have been. Before going any further, it is worth mentioning that as we get older our sleep needs decrease.

There are specific circumstances that may lead us to experience sleep problems, including:
• Going through a period of severe or extended stress.
• Caring for a young baby or elderly relative through the night for a lengthy period of time.
• An ongoing tendency to anxiety.
• Chronic depression.
• A traumatic experience such as shock or bereavement.
• The menopause.
• Pre-menstrual syndrome.

The nature of sleep problems can vary a great deal. Some people find that the depth or quality of sleep is poor, while others have difficulty falling asleep, or find that they wake at regular intervals during the night due to light or fitful sleep patterns. Some people seem to be very happy with four hours

or less of good-quality, refreshing sleep, but others suffer greatly when deprived of a good eight hours' uninterrupted rest. Being deprived of sleep can lead to the following symptoms:
• A tendency to suffer recurrent infections such as colds, coughs and sore throats due to impaired functioning of the immune system.
• Problems with memory and concentration.
• Excitability.
• Irritability.

If sleep disruption develops in anticipation of a specific stressful event or if it occurs on a mild or infrequent basis, adopting the following self-help measures may play a very positive part in relieving the situation. However, if severe symptoms arise for no apparent reason, or if sleep disturbance is a well-established problem, it is vital to seek professional alternative advice in order to deal most effectively with the problem. The self-help measures below are intended for short-term use only, and should not be used routinely over a lengthy period of time.

Practical self-help
• Always make sure that your bedroom incorporates the essential features that contribute to a good night's sleep. Your room should be airy and well-ventilated, and neither too chilly nor too hot. Blinds or curtains should block out early-morning light adequately, but the room should not be so dark that it is difficult to wake in the morning. If traffic noise is a problem, consider having double-glazing installed in order to cut down on the amount of noise that drifts into the room in the early hours.
• Make sure you have a comfortable bed as well as a comfortable bedroom.
• Examine your diet in order to establish if you are inadvertently contributing to sleep problems by taking foods or drinks that contribute to persistent wakefulness or restlessness at night. Caffeine is the main culprit, and is present in tea, coffee, colas and chocolate. If you take a large amount of any of these, reduce the amount taken slowly rather than cutting them out abruptly in order to avoid unpleasant symptoms of caffeine withdrawal.
• Make a conscious effort to relax and 'switch off' for an hour or two before going to bed, making sure that you avoid anything that is mentally or physically stimulating. Above all, avoid the temptation to continue working until the very last moment before retiring, since this is a major culprit in making it difficult to

unwind. This is due to the mind mulling over problems at the very time it needs to be relaxed and preparing itself for rest.
• Positive ways of inducing a relaxed frame of mind before bed include soaking in a warm, scented bath, listening to the radio, listening to a favourite piece of music or an audio book, going through a guided relaxation exercise, reading or sipping a soothing, warm drink.
• It is important to avoid eating a heavy or indigestible meal late at night since this can be responsible for bouts of indigestion that lead to fitful, disturbed or poor-quality sleep.
• Make a point of taking regular aerobic exercise three or four times a week. If this is enjoyed in the fresh air it can play a major role in encouraging sound, restful sleep patterns on a regular basis.
• If muscular tension and discomfort are making a good night's rest rather elusive, consider investing in a regular full-body massage. When a relaxing massage is combined with skilled use of aromatherapy oils sleep problems may be reduced.

SEEK PROFESSIONAL HELP
• If disturbed sleep is becoming a well-established problem.
• If sleep problems are not substantially improved by using alternative self-help measures.
• If sleep disturbance is associated with anxiety or depression.
• If you rely on drugs or alcohol to deal with the sleep problem.

Alternative treatments
For insomnia it is quite appropriate to take the relevant remedy internally while also applying a topical preparation to the skin.

Topical preparations
These include essential oils or tinctures that can be used externally to induce a restful night's sleep. Choose from any of the following, bearing in mind that none of the substances mentioned for application to the skin should be taken by mouth.
Aromatherapy oils
A blend of lavender (high esta), Roman chamomile (Chamaemelum nobile) and mandarin (Citrus reticulata), using three drops of each in two teaspoons of carrier oil, used as a body rub at bedtime can be remarkably helpful (do not use on children).

Herbal preparations

• The following herbs may be placed in a muslin bag and suspended beneath the hot-water tap while your bath is running: lavender, limeflower, chamomile or passionflower. Soak in the warm, scented bathwater as long as feels comfortable to induce relaxation and a sound night's sleep.

• Alternatively, an infusion of any of the herbs mentioned above may be made by placing three generous handfuls of your selected herb in a small pan of cold water. Leave to stand overnight, bring to the boil, strain and add to a warm bath.

• A warm footbath including a strong infusion of chamomile tea before bed may help induce relaxation and encourage a good night's rest.

Medicines intended for internal use

These encourage relaxation and rest.

Anthroposophical medicines

Avena Sativa comp. may be useful in cases of insomnia that are related to nervous restlessness. This tincture contains valerian, passionflower, hops, oats and a high homoeopathic potency of coffee. Twenty or thirty drops should be taken in a small glass of cold water half an hour before retiring.

Flower remedies

• Rescue Remedy may ease insomnia that follows a period of trauma or stress. Place a few drops directly on the tongue as required, or dilute in a small glass of cold water and sip at regular intervals.

• White chestnut may ease insomnia related to an inability to switch off from worrying or distressing thoughts.

• Star of Bethlehem may be appropriate where insomnia follows a traumatic experience, such as experiencing (or witnessing) an accident, loss of a loved partner or shock.

Once a treatment bottle has been made up, take four drops four times a day, holding the dose for a few moments in the mouth before swallowing. Alternatively, the treatment may be made up in a glass of water and sipped as often as needed throughout the day.

Biochemic tissue salts

Sleep problems that are associated with a tendency towards anxiety and nervousness, may respond to a formulation called Nervone. Take four tablets three times a day until improvement sets in, when the dosage should be tailed off. Alternatively, if sleep problems date from the interruption of sleep pattern by a long or severe illness, tissue salt No. 6 may be most appropriate. For dosage instructions see above.

Herbal preparations

• Valerian compound tablets (containing hops, passionflower, valerian, wild lettuce, Jamaican dogwood and skullcap) may help short-term insomnia. Take two tablets in the early evening followed by two tablets before retiring.

NB Caution should be used, since the tablets may cause drowsiness during the day. They should not be given to children under twelve, or taken during pregnancy or when breastfeeding.

• An infusion of any of the following may ease insomnia: chamomile, limeflower or passionflower. Add a cup of boiling water to a teaspoon of your selected herb. Cover, leave to stand for fifteen minutes and strain off the warm liquid. Sip as a warm drink early in the evening and half an hour before retiring.

Home remedies

• Lettuce tea has a reputation for improving poor-quality sleep and encouraging relaxation. Infuse a generous amount of chopped lettuce leaves in a cup and a half of boiling water. Strain and sip the warm liquid as a relaxing drink.

• Mix the juice of two freshly squeezed oranges with a little warm water and honey and drink before retiring.

• Alternatively, try mixing two teaspoonfuls of cider vinegar and one teaspoonful of honey with a small cup of hot water for a warm drink that has a reputation for encouraging a sound night's sleep.

Professional alternative medical help may be obtained from any of the following:

• Acupressure
• Aromatherapy
• Biochemic tissue salts
• Flower remedies
• Homoeopathy
• Massage therapy
• Naturopathy
• Nutritional therapy
• Reflexology
• Shiatsu
• Traditional Chinese medicine
• Western medical herbalism

HOMOEOPATHIC MEDICINES

Type	General features	Worse	Better	Remedy
Awful restlessness and anxiety at night with a tendency to wake after midnight	Chilly and mentally and physically restless with problems in achieving a sound night's sleep. May fall asleep without a problem, but wakes in the early hours of the morning, around 2am. Symptoms are soothed by warmth and sips of warm drinks	As night descends Becoming cold In the dark When alone Physical over-exertion Alcohol	Getting up and pottering about Company Warmth Regular sips of warm drinks	Arsenicum album
Poor sleep pattern after 'burning the candle at both ends'	Severe problems with mentally switching off at night. Feels awful in the morning: improves steadily as the day goes on. Tosses and turns until the early morning and falls into a deep sleep once it's time to get up. Sleep difficulties may be made worse by coffee addiction. Irritable, grouchy and antisocial on waking	Noise Stress Overworking Coffee Cigarettes Alcohol Cold, draughty conditions	Peaceful, quiet surroundings Warmth Solitude Sound sleep	Nux vomica
Insomnia that follows shock, bad news or trauma	Awful restlessness with anxiety and possible panic attacks. Restless sleep may be dream-ridden with nightmares or disturbing dreams. Tosses and turns constantly while trying to get into a comfortable position in bed	Chill or over-heating Shock In bed During the night	Rest Moderate temperatures Fresh air	Aconite
Sleep problems that date from bereavement and grief	Terrible difficulties in getting to sleep with persistent yawning and/or muscular twitching. Unpleasant sensation of jerking awake on falling asleep. Recurring nightmares and unpleasant dreams. Lack of sleep aggravates emotional instability and abrupt mood swings	Emotional stress Bad news Yawning Anxiety Becoming chilled Coffee Cigarettes	Solitude Regular, deep breaths Warmth Movement	Ignatia
Terrible insomnia with fear or dislike of going to bed	Dreads going to sleep because of feeling awful on waking. Also finds it difficult to drift off peacefully to sleep because of fear of not waking up. Unpleasant sensation of falling or suffocation on falling asleep. Alert and buzzing with ideas when it's time to go to bed	In the morning Waking from sleep Pressure of clothes During the menopause Before a period Becoming overheated	Fresh air Loose clothes	Lachesis

Panic attacks

See advice given for anxiety on pages 237-9.

Phobias

Phobias are irrational fears, the most common of which include:
- Open spaces (agoraphobia)
- Closed spaces (claustrophobia)
- Illness (including specific diseases such as cancer or heart disease)
- Germs
- Vomiting
- Insects and spiders
- Birds
- Mice
- Travelling by plane, car or train
- Heights.

Some phobia sufferers cope with their lives quite easily, especially if the phobia arises in connection with an activity that occurs fairly infrequently (such as travelling by air). However, others may feel extremely hemmed in and trapped – for example, if they suffer from agoraphobia and are unable to leave the house without a great deal of support. If the problem has escalated to these proportions it is essential to seek professional advice, such as counselling or psychotherapy.

Practical self-help

See the 'Practical self-help' section for anxiety on pages 238-9.

Alternative treatments

Any of the following may be helpful in providing additional medical help and support:
- Acupressure
- Anthroposophical medicine
- Aromatherapy
- Biochemic tissue salts
- Flower remedies
- Homoeopathy
- Relaxation techniques
- Shiatsu
- Western medical herbalism

Relationship break-up

The emotional trauma and turmoil that follow the breakdown of a relationship can be devastating in their intensity, at whatever stage in life the emotions are experienced. In many ways, the nature of the emotional reaction closely resembles that following bereavement, with phases of shock, anger, guilt and depression.

Alternative treatments can be of immense help in speeding up the process and helping us to come to terms with a series of reactions that would happen at a natural pace given enough time and space. Sensitive and responsible use of appropriate alternative self-help measures can also enable us to move on after the initial stage of the grieving process has passed. However, do not feel compelled to use alternative measures if you are coping well with expected reactions to separations. On the other hand, if you are clearly in need of extra help and support, or if grieving is holding you back from moving on with your life, short-term alternative help can be immensely valuable.

Practical self-help

- Above all else, avoid taking a 'stiff upper lip' approach, which tends to prolong sadness and often contributes to extra problems in the long run. Talking frankly about emotional reactions to a friend or counsellor can be enormously valuable.
- Be as open as possible with close friends about your feelings, since they are likely to have gone through very similar emotions themselves. While you may need to spend time alone in the initial phase of a break-up, it is also essential not to lose touch with close friends. Re-establishing a healthy social life at the appropriate time can be one of the most important factors in helping you move on emotionally.
- Taking regular aerobic exercise can do a great deal to help with emotional stress and trauma on a long-term basis, as exercise releases endorphins (a form of natural antidepressant) in the body.

• Make sure that you eat well and have an adequate supply of essential vitamins and minerals from your diet. Grieving over the end of a relationship can often result in erratic or poor eating habits. If this situation continues for too long, it can leave you feeling run down and vulnerable to recurrent problems such as minor infections. Consider using a vitamin B complex supplement which has a particularly positive role to play in maintaining the health and resilience of the nervous system.

• See the additional self-help measures suggested in the depression section (pages 243-4).

SEEK PROFESSIONAL HELP

If symptoms show signs of becoming severe, persistent or well established.

Alternative treatments

After the break-up of a relationship it is quite appropriate to take the relevant internal remedy while also applying a topical preparation to the skin.

Topical preparations

These include tinctures and essential oils that can be absorbed through the skin to soothe or uplift the spirits. Choose from any of the following, bearing in mind that none of the substances mentioned for application to the skin should be taken by mouth.

Herbal preparations

• When feeling stressed, an infusion of lemon balm or lavender may be extremely soothing when added to a warm bath. Add three handfuls of herb to a small pan of cold water. Leave to steep overnight and bring slowly to the boil the next morning. Strain, and add the fragrant liquid to your bathwater as required.

• Alternatively, try adding an infusion of chamomile or valerian to your bath to reduce feelings of tension.

Home remedies

See suggestions given in the grief and bereavement section on page 250.

Medicines intended for internal use

These reduce distress and despondency.

Flower remedies

• Rock Rose may be of help where a fearful reaction has occurred in response to the breakdown of a relationship, especially if it is combined with panic attacks, poor sleep pattern and a tendency to nightmares.

• Honeysuckle may be valuable if there is a tendency to be unable to let go of the past, combined with a severe feeling of nostalgia for what cannot be recaptured.

• If a poor or destructive relationship has been going on for a lengthy period of time before it eventually breaks down, olive may ease mental and physical weariness and exhaustion.

• Agrimony may be suitable for those who respond to emotional stress by keeping a stiff upper lip and insisting that they are fine. Relief from emotional pain may be sought by drinking alcohol or using drugs in private.

Once a treatment bottle has been made up, take four drops four times a day, holding the dose for a few moments in the mouth before swallowing. Alternatively, the treatment may be made up in a glass of water and sipped as often as needed throughout the day.

Biochemic tissue salts

The initial shock following the trauma of separation may be eased by tissue salt No. 6, which helps symptoms of panic alternating with hysterical weeping and extreme distress. Tablets may be taken hourly for severe symptoms, or three times daily until the situation improves.

Herbal preparations

• Tincture of wild oats (Avena Stativa) can be an effective aid in strengthening and supporting the nervous system, especially if someone has undergone the strain of an unhappy or unstable relationship that ends in a distressing way. Eight drops of tincture may be dissolved in a small glass of spring water and taken daily.

• If temporary or intermittent feelings of depression follow the break-up of a long-term or well-established relationship, Hypericum may be of help. It can be obtained in tablet form or taken as an infusion. To make an infusion, use one teaspoonful of dried herb in each cupful of hot water. Warm a teapot, add the herbs and fill the pot with boiling water. Cover, leave to stand for fifteen minutes, strain, and sip as a warm drink. Take three times a day.

• Feelings of stress and tension may be eased by an infusion of limeflower, which has a reputation for relaxing the nervous system. It may also ease stress-related recurrent tension headaches and insomnia. To make the infusion, follow the directions given above.

HOMOEOPATHIC MEDICINES

Type	General features	Worse	Better	Remedy
Initial tearful reaction to emotional trauma	Violent, spasmodic bouts of crying alternating with sudden laughing fits. Unable to cope without emotional support and help. Unresolved agitation, distress and tearfulness. Constant sighing with possible muscle trembling and twitching	Touch Cold Contact with open air	Being alone Warmth Breathing deeply Eating	Ignatia
Weepiness and depression that are greatly relieved by being in sympathetic company	Constant tendency to tearfulness that is worse for being alone and better for being in contact with supporting company. Distressed and weepy, but positively relieved after crying. Anxious and fearful of being left alone. Generally changeable moods	Rest When alone Feeling neglected or overlooked Evening Night Stuffy, badly ventilated rooms Eating	After a good cry Sympathy and attention Physical displays of affection Gentle exercise in the open air Cool, fresh air	Pulsatilla
Severe anxiety and panic attacks following emotional shock or trauma	Fearful reaction to prospect of breaking up of relationship. Extreme insecurity with panic attacks and fear of dying. Severe agitation: feels on the edge of collapse. Strongly indicated for initial emotional reactions to shock rather than lingering problems	Noise Night Touch Chill Overheating	Open, fresh air Rest Moderate temperatures	Aconite
Inward grief at break-up of relationship that cannot be expressed	Extremely negative reaction on physical or verbal comfort and sympathy. Keeps a stiff upper lip to avoid the humiliation of expressing emotions in public. Needs to be left alone when feeling low because of dislike of crying other than in private	After crying Company Sympathy and consolation Noisy or disruptive surroundings	Skipping meals Being alone Peace and quiet Rest Cool, fresh air	Natrum mur
Suppressed anger after relationship break-up	Extreme mental and physical oversensitivity following emotional trauma. Outwardly calm, but seethes inside with suppressed anger and humiliation. Angry and reproachful about breakdown of relationship. Especially appropriate in situations where natural expression of anger has been denied	At night Emotional strain Stimulation Chill	Warmth Rest Eating	Staphysagria

Professional alternative medical help may be obtained from any of the following:
- Acupressure
- Anthroposophical medicine
- Aromatherapy
- Flower remedies
- Homoeopathy
- Massage therapy
- Shiatsu
- Traditional Chinese medicine
- Western medical herbalism

PROBLEMS OF PREGNANCY AND CHILDBIRTH

Heartburn

Many mothers discover that the discomfort of heartburn is a common problem during the last few months of pregnancy. Heartburn occurs because digestive juices rise into the throat due to relaxation of the muscle that shuts off the upper end of the stomach from the gullet. This is made even more intense by the pressure exerted on the stomach by the growing foetus in the last few months of pregnancy. (Also see section on hiatus hernia, pages 171-2.)

Common symptoms of heartburn may include any of the following:
- An unpleasant taste in the mouth.
- A burning, acid sensation rising into the gullet.
- 'Repeating' of food eaten hours previously.
- Burning in the stomach and/or centre of the chest.

The symptoms of heartburn can often be considerably relieved by simple changes in lifestyle and diet, as well as becoming aware of the impact of posture on the problem. Appropriate alternative medical measures can do a great deal to ease the discomfort of heartburn, even if it cannot be eradicated completely. As always, it is important to bear in mind that a professional opinion should always be sought if symptoms of heartburn are especially severe or persistent.

Practical self-help

- If heartburn is worse at night, avoid eating heavy or large meals immediately before going to bed. Because bodily functions (including digestion) slow down at night, food cannot be broken down as efficiently during resting hours, which means that heavy meals take a longer time to digest than they would during waking hours. It is far better to concentrate on eating a regular, small number of nutritious and easily digestible meals during the day, and having a light snack and/or warm drink before bedtime.
- To ease heartburn at night sleep propped up on two or three pillows, which discourages the reflux of acid from the stomach, while also making breathing easier. However, it is best not to adopt this position when sleeping if you have any problems with swollen ankles.
- Heartburn may be eased considerably if foods or drinks that have a reputation for irritating the stomach lining are avoided. These include strong tea, coffee, alcohol, and highly spiced foods. Also avoid foods that take a long time to digest, such as full-fat cheeses, deep-fried foods, roasted nuts, potato crisps, cream, red meat and rich sauces. Additional items that may aggravate heartburn include acidic fruits such as grapefruit or oranges, raw peppers or onions, tomatoes, cabbage, sprouts, pulses and cigarettes.
- Meals should be kept small, light and as easy on the stomach as possible. Concentrate on fresh vegetable broths and soups, grilled or poached fish and poultry, stir-fried dishes and lightly steamed vegetables or fruit. Although fresh fruit and vegetables are usually best eaten raw in order to preserve as much of their vitamin content as possible, remember that they can aggravate symptoms of heartburn and indigestion. As a result, light steaming will preserve much of the vitamin content, while also making them easier to digest.
- If muesli-type cereals are a favourite, they can be made much more easily digestible by an overnight soaking in milk, fruit juice or water, which allows the starch to be broken down into sugar before

HOMOEOPATHIC MEDICINES

Type	General features	Worse	Better	Remedy
Heartburn that comes on after, or is aggravated by eating	Awful sensitivity to water during pregnancy: even the thought or sight of water brings on nausea and sickness. Anxiety with digestive discomfort with distressing, empty, sinking feeling in stomach	Eating salty foods Lack of fluid Lying too flat Warm food and drink Distress, emotional upset or anxiety	Sound sleep Cool drinks before they have a chance to be warmed in the stomach Reassuring company Massage	Phosphorus
Heartburn that is more intense at night	Burning pains and acidity of the stomach that are eased by sips of warm drinks. Restless, chilly and very anxious with nausea and heartburn. Fussy and fidgety when feeling unwell	During the night and early hours of the morning Becoming cold Cold food or drinks Physical exertion Solitude	Lying propped up in a warm bed Warm surroundings Frequent sips of warm drinks Company and distraction	Arsenicum album
Heartburn with acid that readily travels into the throat	Burning and discomfort extend from the stomach to the throat. Repeated burping with a little acid rising into the gullet each time. Becomes rapidly full when sitting down to a meal. Lots of gurgling, flatulence and rumbling in stomach and abdomen	Tight clothing Overeating Too much fibre in diet Becoming too hot or too cold In the afternoons Stress and anticipatory anxiety	Loosening clothing Moderate temperatures Contact with fresh air Small portions of warm food and drinks Activity and distraction Gentle exercise in the open air	Lycopodium
Severe nausea and heartburn follow eating meals that are rich or fatty	Heartburn may be sparked off by a diet that is too high in red meat, cheese, cream, rich sauces or rich puddings. Indigestion with dry mouth and no thirst. Taste of food eaten hours before when burping. Tearful and depressed when feeling unwell	Stuffy, overheated surroundings Lack of fresh air During the evening and night Heavy clothing or bedcovers Warm food and drinks Resting	Cool, well-ventilated surroundings Gentle exercise in the fresh, cool air Undressing or loosening clothes After a good cry	Pulsatilla

eating. Cooked cereals such as porridge may also be preferable since they are easier on the stomach.

SEEK PROFESSIONAL HELP

• If symptoms refuse to respond to self-help measures.

• If symptoms of heartburn are causing severe distress and discomfort.

• If food sticks or there is any difficulty swallowing.

• If there is any associated weight loss.

Alternative treatments

Medicines intended for internal use
These ease pain and discomfort and encourage a speedy resolution of the acute phase of the problem.
Biochemic tissue salts
The discomfort of heartburn may respond to tissue salt No. 8, while heartburn accompanied by acidity may respond more effectively to Combination Remedy C. Take four tablets three times daily until symptoms improve.
Herbal preparations
• Powdered slippery elm mixed with hot milk or water may be taken as a soothing drink before bed or on waking. One heaped teaspoonful should be mixed to a smooth paste with a little milk or water before slowly adding a cupful of hot liquid, stirring all the time to prevent the drink becoming lumpy. Malt-flavoured slippery elm is now available, or the unflavoured variety may be made less bland by the addition of cinnamon, nutmeg or honey.

• Steep a teaspoonful of finely grated fresh ginger root in a cup of boiling water for ten minutes. Strain off the liquid and sip at frequent intervals while still warm.

• Peppermint* tea often eases digestive pain and discomfort, while chamomile tea is an excellent soother of crampy, colicky digestive uneasiness that may be aggravated by feeling stressed. (Items with a * may interfere with the action of homoeopathic remedies.)
Home remedies
• A teaspoonful of lemon juice or cider vinegar dissolved in a cup of hot water and sipped every fifteen minutes is a recommended way of easing the discomfort of acidity and heartburn.

• If heartburn and digestive uneasiness is a recurrent feature during pregnancy, eating natural live yoghurt can do a great deal to soothe the digestive tract.

• If flatulence accompanies heartburn, chewing cardamom seeds makes the wind easier to expel.

• Eating regular helpings of grated carrot and apple is thought to ease heartburn and indigestion.

If heartburn occurs as part of a generally difficult pregnancy, treatment may be considered from any of the practitioners in any of the following therapies:
• Anthroposophical medicine
• Homoeopathy
• Naturopathy
• Nutritional therapy
• Traditional Chinese medicine
• Western medical herbalism

Labour and childbirth

When alternative medical measures are used appropriately during and following labour and delivery, they can offer a great deal of support in reducing anxiety, stimulating flagging energy levels, easing nausea, reducing pain, and speeding up physical and emotional recovery.

Many mothers who use alternative measures following childbirth have discovered the very positive role that these medicines can play in reducing the pain and sensitivity of bruised or lacerated tissues, and assisting the whole system to come to terms with the shock, excitement and trauma of childbirth.

The alternative approach can also be of tremendous value for those who had planned a natural childbirth, but discovered that a high-tech birth such as a Caesarean was necessary due to complications. In such a situation, judicious use of alternative medicines may do a great deal to enable the mother to come to terms with the disappointment and resentment that often follow a birth where medical intervention was necessary, as well as easing pain and speeding up healing of damaged tissue.

Although midwives are generally much more aware of the availability of alternative medicines than they used to be, it can still be very difficult to obtain

HOMOEOPATHIC MEDICINES

Type	General features	Worse	Better	Remedy
Feeble labour pains that are slow to start, or keep stopping	Often needed where baby is in a difficult, or breech position. Intermittent, weak labour pains that keep changing their character. Discomfort and distress is made more intense by becoming overheated. Exhausted, weepy and depressed in labour	Stuffy surroundings Heat Keeping still Warm compresses Lack of fresh air	Opening a window Undressing Gentle movement Cool compresses Attention, emotional support and sympathy	Pulsatilla
Long, slow arduous labour with insufficient dilation of cervix	Feeble contractions with pains that seem to fly about in all directions. Chilly, shivery and trembly but craves fresh air. Weary and bad tempered in labour	Becoming over-chilled Exhaustion	Fresh air that does not chill	Caulophyllum
Violent, fast labour with extreme terror and anxiety	Labour pains feel unbearable and intolerable, causing extreme restlessness and distress. Awful anxiety at onset or during second stage of labour. Fear of death, or desire to die with intense pain	Examination Touch Extreme heat or chill	Fresh air Undressing	Aconite
Awful nausea and vomiting with contractions	Persistent, violent retching during labour with great difficulty in raising vomit. Severe straining with sensation as though about to pass a stool. Exhausting, aching, bruised pains during labour. Abusive, quick tempered and extremely irritable when in pain	Cold draughts of air Becoming chilled Undressing Touch Noisy surroundings	Warmth Peace and quiet	Nux vomica
'Backache labour' with slow dilation of cervix and unproductive contractions	Severe pains in the lower back during labour drive to distraction. Mother feels she wants to give up and can't go through with birth. Frustration and fury with labour pains lead to outbursts of verbal abuse and anger	Overheating Contact with fresh air	Undressing or loosening clothes Sweating Moderate temperatures Warm compresses and application	Chamomilla

alternative treatment from a qualified midwife. Some mothers ask their alternative medical practitioner to be present during labour to provide appropriate treatment, while others are satisfied with discussing suitable alternative treatments with their practitioner beforehand. While this can be effective for some, it does have the disadvantage that often the mother and her partner are so involved and overwhelmed by the experience of childbirth that they are unable objectively to decide on the best alternative measures appropriate at that moment. For this reason alone, having the support and experience of a trained practitioner can do a great deal to take additional pressure off the mother and her partner.

Whatever you decide to do as far as alternative medicine is concerned, raise the issue as soon as possible with your consultant, who is likely to want to communicate with your practitioner, or talk to your midwife and family doctor if you plan to have a home delivery.

In the following section you will find an overview of the possible alternative medical support that may be of help during labour and delivery. However, it is important to stress that this is not intended to be a substitute for professional alternative medical support, and is provided primarily in order to give a broad idea of the potential help that alternative measures may provide.

Alternative treatments

Topical preparations
Choose from any of the following, bearing in mind that none of the substances mentioned for application to the skin should be taken by mouth.

Herbal preparations
• A soothing hot compress may be made from a strong infusion of any of the following: lemon verbena, chamomile, Calendula or lavender. Soak a soft, clean cloth in the infusion and apply it to the area just above the pubic bone to encourage pain relief and relaxation. Once the compress cools down it should be changed for a fresh one.
• A compress or footbath of black cohosh may be useful in promoting regular and speedy contractions.

Medicines intended for internal use
These ease pain, stimulate energy levels and assist contractions.

Herbal preparations
• Sipping an infusion of chamomile tea may be helpful where backache is severe, leading to extreme irritability and tension in response to pain.
• An infusion of black cohosh may be of help where panic and anxiety are inhibiting regular, productive contractions. It can also lessen the pain of contractions by assisting relaxation.
• If tension in the uterus is inhibiting progress of regular and fruitful contractions, an infusion of cramp bark may assist in easing the pain of over-strong contractions. It is also specifically indicated for cramping, spasmodic pains that lodge in the back and radiate down the thighs.

Professional help may be obtained from any of the following:
• Anthroposophical medicine
• Aromatherapy
• Homoeopathy
• Massage therapy
• Shiatsu
• Traditional Chinese medicine
• Western medical herbalism

Mastitis

Mastitis is a painful condition that arises if a duct in the breast becomes blocked due to milk leaking from the ducts into the breast tissue in a mother who is breastfeeding or, shortly after delivery, before milk production is suppressed in a mother who bottle feeds, resulting in the formation of a breast abscess. This can appear very like infective mastitis and should always be checked by a professional.

Early warning signs include any of the following symptoms:
• Pain, discomfort and a lumpy sensation in the affected breast.

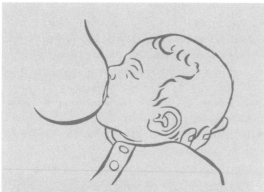

Fig.1 The baby is sucking on the nipple only. This does not allow proper suckling and is painful for the mother.

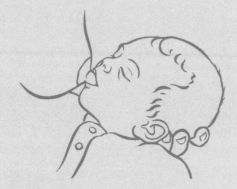

Fig.2 The baby is correctly sucking on the whole nipple and areola. This results in efficient feeding and should be comfortable for the mother.

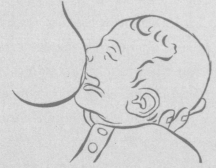

Fig.3 In this correct position the nipple is at the back of the baby's throat and he/she can use the tongue for suckling.

Cracked nipples can be avoided by ensuring the baby sucks on the nipple and the areola (fig. 1), not just the nipple (fig. 2). The nipple is then positioned at the back of the baby's throat and he/she can use the tongue for suckling (fig. 3).

• Redness and inflammation of the area immediately above the lump.

Feverishness and high temperature indicate that the problem is likely to have developed into mastitis and that prompt medical advice is needed.

Practical self-help

• Cracked nipples can predispose a breastfeeding mother to mastitis, and these can be avoided in two ways. Firstly, by making sure the baby is put to the breast properly, so that it sucks on the nipple and areola, not just the nipple. Secondly, by breaking the suction from the baby by putting your finger into its mouth before taking it off the breast so that the baby does not strip the skin off the nipple.

• The following simple hydrotherapy technique can be used if a blocked milk duct is suspected. Soak a flannel in hot water, wring it out thoroughly and apply it to the affected breast until it cools down. In the meantime, soak another flannel in cold water and apply this to the same breast once the cooled hot flannel has been removed. Keep this process up for an hour or so, alternating hot and cold flannels in turn.

• Keep liquid intake up by taking regular, long drinks of water.

• Put your baby to the affected breast first when breastfeeding, making sure that this breast is thoroughly drained at each feed. Also, position your baby in such a way that the force of gravity encourages draining of the blocked duct. This can be done by making sure that your baby feeds in such a way that the painful area of the breast is uppermost.

• If you have a baby who is not keen to feed regularly, make use of a breast pump if your breasts feel full and uncomfortable between feeds.

• Massage your breasts gently but firmly in the direction of the nipple during and between feeds. Also swing your arms regularly to encourage circulation.

• Check that your bra is the right fit and is not too small or constricting.

• Taking bed rest at the first signs of symptoms can do a great deal to improve the situation, especially if the problem has come on after a period of feeling run down and exhausted. Asking for extra help from relatives, neighbours or friends can often give you time to recover, especially if domestic pressure seems too much to cope with.

HOMOEOPATHIC MEDICINES

Type	General features	Worse	Better	Remedy
Mastitis with general aching and sore, sensitive glands	General feeling of aching and unwellness with shooting pains that radiate over the body. Terribly tender, swollen breasts that look a deep, purple-red in colour. Shooting pains radiate from breasts to armpits. Nipples become cracked and sore. Shivery, tired and feverish when unwell	Chill Becoming too hot Touch Pressure to the right side During the night	Moderate warmth Lying on the left side Lying on the stomach	Phytolacca
Hard, inflamed breasts with severely cracked, sensitive nipples	Left-sided symptoms with extremely painful nipples that cause great distress. Generally feverish with chilly extremities and hot, flushed head and face. Difficulty resting at night with the pain, with drowsiness and tiredness during the day	Pressure to the left side Becoming chilled Overheating During the night Damp	Contact with fresh air Wrapping up cosily Resting	Graphites
Mastitis with extreme sensitivity to, and intolerance of movement	Agonizingly painful breasts that feel much worse for the slightest touch, but improved by firm pressure to the painful area. Hard, sensitive breasts with generally dehydrated state. Antisocial and bad tempered when feeling under the weather	Jarring movement Exertion Light touch Warmth Becoming too hot	Resting Keeping in one position Lying on the painful side Cool drinks Peace and quiet	Bryonia
Severe pain and inflammation that set in abruptly	Area around the affected duct feels extremely hot to the touch. Bright red streaks radiate from the nipple along the surface of the breast. Pains are intensified by lying flat, touch or jarring. Quick tempered and very irritable when in pain	Sudden movement Pressure to the painful side Being disturbed Touch	Being left in peace and quiet Sitting semi-erect in bed Moderate warmth	Belladonna

SEEK PROFESSIONAL HELP

- If a high temperature or general state of feeling unwell has developed.
- If there has been no favourable response to self-help measures within twenty-four hours, or if symptoms have become more severe.

Alternative treatments

For mastitis it is quite appropriate to take the indicated remedy internally, while also applying a topical preparation to the skin.

Topical preparations

These include tinctures that can be applied to the skin to reduce discomfort and inflammation. Choose from any of the following, bearing in mind that none of the substances mentioned for application to the skin should be taken by mouth.

Herbal preparations

- Effective warm poultices may be made from cooked bran, linseed or slippery elm powder. Mix to a paste with warm water, spread onto a piece of clean gauze and apply warm to the affected breast.

• Add a strong infusion of chamomile to a footbath to reduce feverishness. Bathe the feet every couple of hours until there is a reduction in temperature.

Medicines intended for internal use

These ease pain, reduce inflammation and encourage a speedy resolution of the problem.

Biochemic tissue salts

Tissue salt No. 5 may be helpful in reducing inflammation. When symptoms are acute, take four tablets at hourly intervals, tailing off the dosage gradually as symptoms improve.

Herbal preparations

As well as being an excellent way of incorporating extra fluid into the diet, herbal teas have anti-inflammatory properties. Marigold (Calendula), yarrow and elderflower teas will help discourage feverishness and inflammation, while also encouraging the body to eliminate toxic matter more efficiently.

Home remedies

• Eat as much fresh garlic as possible to reduce the chance of infection, or use powdered garlic in tablet form as a useful supplement while symptoms persist.

• Inflammation and discomfort may be reduced by gently massaging distilled witch hazel or buttermilk into the affected breast.

Professional help and advice may be sought from practitioners trained in any of the following therapies:

• Anthroposophical medicine
• Homoeopathy
• Naturopathy
• Shiatsu
• Traditional Chinese medicine
• Western medical herbalism

Morning sickness

Although termed morning sickness, the nausea and vomiting that develop in pregnancy can occur at any point during the day, or in some unfortunate mothers, last late into the night. However, as a rule, bouts of vomiting and nausea are limited to the first twelve weeks of pregnancy (the first trimester), with symptoms often spontaneously resolving themselves around the end of the third month.

Fortunately, not every pregnant woman finds herself going through the misery of morning sickness, and many expectant mothers suffer no more than the odd bout of queasiness or indigestion, while others seem to experience very few digestive symptoms until they move into the last months of pregnancy, when heartburn may become a problem.

Morning sickness is unpleasant, but is harmless to the developing baby in the absence of maternal dehydration or severe weight loss. The developing baby acts as a sponge for any nutrients it needs, so only the mother is deprived unless the morning sickness is very severe. It is important to point out that the distress of morning sickness can be eased considerably by making simple but effective adjustments in lifestyle that can reduce nausea and general feelings of sickness. These are listed in the 'Practical self-help' section below. In fact, following this advice may be all that is needed to improve the situation considerably.

However, if symptoms refuse to respond to these measures, or if they are very severe, it is essential to seek help from a qualified alternative medical practitioner, rather than attempting to self-prescribe. This is partly due to the fact that great caution should be exercised with regard to any medicines used during pregnancy (especially within the first three months), but also because a trained practitioner will have a much more objective perspective on the symptoms, and will be able to place these within the context of the patient's overall state of health.

Homoeopathic medicines have been used for some time in treating women during pregnancy and labour, and no known adverse effects have been reported. In fact, skilled homoeopathic prescribing used within this context appears to have a beneficial effect on the mother, and possibly also on her baby. The same has also been suggested of herbal treatments and additional therapies such as massage.

Practical self-help

• Avoid taking any drugs in the first three months, as this is when the developing baby is most vulnerable.

HOMOEOPATHIC MEDICINES

Type	General features	Worse	Better	Remedy
Extreme, persistent nausea that is not relieved by vomiting	Distressing, difficult bouts of vomiting with empty retching. Mouth is full of watery saliva. Nausea which is made much more intense by the slightest movement, but is not in the least relieved by eating. Pale, exhausted, hot or clammy with vomiting and nausea	Vomiting Stooping Motion Strong smells Eating	Resting Fresh air Keeping as still as possible	Ipecac
Morning sickness with extreme anxiety and restlessness	Exhausted, chilly and fidgety with vomiting and nausea. Stomach is soothed by frequent sips of warm drinks while alcohol, coffee and cold food aggravate matters. Persistent, strong fear on part of the mother about her own health and that of her baby	Solitude Becoming chilled Eating Cold food or drinks Being too ill to tidy up surroundings	Company and distraction Warmth Frequent sips of warm drinks Resting propped up in bed Being wrapped up snuggly with fresh air to head and face	Arsenicum album
Nausea and morning sickness that are aggravated by cooking smells	Symptoms are eased considerably by eating small amounts at regular intervals. Unpleasant sensation of dizziness and headache with empty feeling in stomach. Desire for tart, sour flavours when hungry. Indifferent, depressed, irritable and weary	Empty stomach Smell of food or cooking Thinking of food Skipping meals Chill Emotional ties and demands	Eating small amounts of food at regular intervals	Sepia
Severe difficult bouts of vomiting with morning sickness	Nausea is relieved considerably once vomiting has occurred. Great difficulty in expelling vomit from stomach with lots of distressing gagging and retching. General state of physical and emotional burn-out with difficulty in meeting too many demands	Stress On waking Being chilled Lack of, or poor-quality sleep Spicy foods Coffee, alcohol and cigarettes	Later in the day and evening Resting Peace and quiet Warmth Sound sleep	Nux vomica
Morning sickness that occurs in the morning, evening or night	Symptoms are aggravated by eating too many rich, fatty foods such as cream, pork or cheese. Generally chilly, but feels much worse for being in overheated or stuffy surroundings. Prone to bouts of depression and weepiness	Lack of fresh air Overheated surroundings Rest In the morning and evening	Fresh, cool conditions Cool applications Gentle exercise in the fresh air A good cry Sympathy	Pulsatilla

• Avoid going for long periods of time without eating if queasiness and sickness are a problem. Although it may sound peculiar, nausea in pregnancy can often be eased by eating small amounts of appetizing food at regular intervals. This prevents blood-sugar levels falling too low. When blood-sugar levels plummet, the symptoms that may arise include any of the following:

• Disorientation
• Extreme nausea
• Dizziness and unsteadiness
• Fuzzy-headedness.

Eat something small every couple of hours, and ensure that you do not skip main meals. Most important of all, avoid sugary snacks, since these can lead to an initial boost of sugar in the bloodstream that is quickly reduced by the secretion of insulin by the body, causing even lower blood-sugar levels than before. Items to avoid include cakes, biscuits, chocolate and any kind of sweetened drink. Foods that encourage stable blood-sugar levels include chopped raw vegetables, fresh fruit, unsweetened fruit juices and rice cakes with toppings of low-fat cheeses or vegetarian pâté. Since dehydration can also aggravate the symptoms of morning sickness, always make sure to drink six to eight large glasses of filtered or still mineral water during the day.

• Avoid the additional problem of indigestion by making the effect to chew food thoroughly and to relax as much as possible during mealtimes, even though there may be a general shortage of time because of demands made by family and children.

• Because dairy foods are high in fat and generally difficult to digest, they should be eaten in small quantities if nausea is severe. Keep calcium intake up by eating whole grains, dark green, leafy vegetables such as spinach, and almonds. Vegetarians should ensure that iron intake is kept at a reasonable level by eating regular helpings of seeds, nuts and pulses.

• Many women who feel nauseous during pregnancy instinctively dislike the taste of tea, coffee, alcohol and cigarettes. This is quite helpful since these items are known to aggravate nausea by irritating the lining of the stomach. Drinking alcohol and smoking cigarettes can also increase the risk of miscarriage and low birth weight. Studies have suggested that caffeine (which occurs in tea, coffee and cola) can increase the likelihood of sudden infant death syndrome (also known as cot death). Opt instead for caffeine-free, grain-based coffee substitutes, mixed varieties of herbal teas or carbonated, fruit-flavoured, alcohol-free drinks.

• Occasionally there can also be a psychological aspect to morning sickness, especially when a mother feels anxiety or uneasiness about being pregnant. However much a pregnancy has been planned and looked forward to with anticipation, the most unexpected emotions can often come to the surface during pregnancy. It is vital to accept that this is quite common, and that it can be very valuable to talk about these feelings with an appropriate person with whom there is a rapport. This could be a relative, close friend, counsellor or general practitioner.

SEEK PROFESSIONAL HELP

• If symptoms of morning sickness are extremely severe, persistent or long lasting.
• If simple self-help measures do not yield positive results.
• If there are any indications of dehydration developing as a result of severe or protracted morning sickness.

Alternative treatments

Home remedies

• Since morning sickness is often worse on rising in the morning (hence its name), it is a good idea to keep some plain biscuits and a drink at the side of the bed. These can be taken as soon as you move from a horizontal to an upright position in order to keep sickness and nausea that are aggravated by having an empty stomach at bay. By sitting up very slowly and taking time to get out of bed, dizziness and disorientation are also likely to be less of a problem.

• Munching sesame seeds helps ease symptoms of morning sickness that are due to overacidity of the system.

Herbal preparations

• Sipping chamomile, limeflower or peppermint tea may be very helpful in easing nausea and digestive uneasiness.

• An infusion of fresh ginger root may also ease the distress and discomfort of morning sickness. In order to make this soothing drink, grate a 5cm (2in) piece of fresh ginger and add to a cupful of freshly boiled water. Cover and leave to stand until all of the juices of the ginger have been absorbed by the water. Strain and drink warm.

Professional help may be obtained from any of the following:

- Anthroposophical medicine
- Homoeopathy
- Naturopathy
- Nutritional therapy
- Shiatsu
- Traditional Chinese medicine
- Western medical herbalism

Pain and bruising after childbirth

The excitement and euphoria following birth can be rather clouded over by the pain and discomfort that arise from bruising, tearing or incision (an episiotomy) of the perineum (the area between the vagina and anus). When this area is damaged as a result of the delivery, it can feel extremely tender and sore when moving about, sitting down, passing water or opening the bowels.

The perineum can be prepared for childbirth by gently massaging olive oil into this area at regular intervals during the last few months of pregnancy to discourage tearing during delivery. However, if bruising and damage have occurred, the following measures will be helpful in aiding pain relief and speeding up the healing process.

Alternative treatments

For bruising and pain following childbirth, it is quite appropriate to take the relevant remedy internally while also applying a topical preparation to the skin.

Topical preparations

Tinctures, creams and essential oils can be applied to the skin in order to soothe and speed up the healing process. Choose from any of the following, bearing in mind that none of the substances mentioned for application to the skin should be taken by mouth.

Aromatherapy oils

Add four tablespoons of crystal sea salt to every bath for a month. Three drops of any, or all, of the following essential oils may be added to the bath: tea tree (Melaleuca alternifolia), lavender (Lavendula angustifolia), rosewood and/or Hydrosol helichrysum. Use Hydrosol helichrysum on the bruised area at the top of the legs.

Herbal preparations

- Many mothers have benefited from the soothing and healing properties of diluted Calendula tincture after childbirth. One part of tincture should be diluted in ten parts of water and applied to the perineum in the form of a compress. This may be done simply by soaking a sanitary towel in a solution of the diluted tincture and applying it to the painful area.

- If pain is very severe, consider using a combination of Hypericum and Calendula tincture instead. This herbal tincture combines the antiseptic properties of Calendula with the pain-relieving properties of Hypericum. The latter is particularly effective in easing pains in parts that are rich in nerve endings, or sharp, shooting pains from incisions. The diluted tincture may be used as a compress as directed above or added to the bathwater or when using the bidet.

Home remedies

- A tablespoonful of sea salt may be added to the bathwater to discourage infection, reduce inflammation and encourage healing.

- Make an infusion of chamomile tea and add it to the bathwater to soothe and ease pain, or apply it to the perineum in the form of a warm or cool compress (depending on which feels most soothing and comfortable).

- Swelling, inflammation and bruising may be eased by adding a teaspoonful of witch hazel to the bathwater, or gently apply it to the painful area on some soft cotton wool.

Medicines intended for internal use

These ease pain, promote re-absorption of blood and encourage a speedy resolution of the problem.

HOMOEOPATHIC MEDICINES

Type	General features	Worse	Better	Remedy
Bruising, aching, soreness and swelling following delivery	Restlessness and difficulty in finding a comfortable spot as a result of soreness and bruising. Arnica is the first remedy to be considered for the physical and emotional trauma of childbirth. For best results, use in the days immediately following delivery	Examination Touch Motion Jarring movements	Rest	Arnica
Extremely sensitive, slow-healing tear or episiotomy	Use calendula externally in the form of diluted tincture and/or cream. Effective in discouraging infection and speeding up the healing process. Ten drops of tincture should be added to bathwater or the bidet. Also use as a soothing compress. Cream should be applied after bathing	Chill	Gentle movement Rest	Calendula
Deep bruising that has not been completely resolved byArnica	Terribly sensitive, sore bruising that is initially relieved by Arnica, but the improvement does not hold. Pains are aching, squeezing or throbbing, leading to extreme tiredness and exhaustion	Warmth of bed Warm bathing Cool bathing Touch Examination	Cool compresses Gentle, continued movement	Bellis perennis
Lingering pains after epidural or forceps delivery	Tearing, shooting pains that remain in torn area or episiotomy. Extremely sensitive wounds or residual pain in episiotomy scar. Shooting pains in back from epidural	Jarring movements Touch Physical effort Following forceps delivery	Lying on stomach Massage	Hypericum
Sharp, stitch-like pains following Caesarean section or episiotomy	Sharp, stinging pains in and around wound that is extremely sensitive to touch. Often required after upsetting birth experience where there is a sense of having been cheated out of natural birth experience. Physical and mental stress linked to guilt, suppressed anger and resentment	Touch Stress Urinating At night Pressure of bedcovers	Warmth Rest	Staphysagria

Post-natal depression

The immediate weeks following the birth of a baby can be an emotional roller-coaster ride of tremendous highs and lows. These peaks and troughs are usually intimately linked with the powerful physical and emotional tiredness that occur in response to meeting the seemingly innumerable demands of a small baby. As a result, transient feelings of weariness, ambivalence about the role of motherhood and sadness can be a common response to this major life event shared by many mothers.

These feelings are quite normal, and are commonly termed the 'baby blues'. If such emotions are especially intense, persistent, or seem to escalate in severity as time goes by, you may be developing true post-natal depression, a serious illness that needs professional help from your family doctor, or a counsellor or alternative health practitioner.

Common symptoms of post-natal depression may include:

• Involuntary bouts of tearfulness, despair and depression that descend violently, without warning, and for no obvious reason.

• A pervading and persistent sense of emotional numbness, indifference or apathy.

• An overwhelming feeling of physical, mental and emotional tiredness that is resistant to improvement by periods of rest and relaxation.

• Feeling unable to cope with the pressure of domestic tasks or pressures of work.

• Reduced levels of self-confidence and self-esteem.

• Extreme or unrelieved anxiety about the health and well-being of the new baby.

Appropriate alternative medical measures can be of enormous help and support to mothers who are unhappy about resorting to the use of conventional medication such as antidepressants. When an appropriate form of alternative medicine is used in conjunction with some of the practical self-help suggestions listed below, it may be possible to establish emotional equilibrium with the minimum amount of stress and trauma. However, if symptoms are resistant to self-help measures, professional advice must be sought. Do not attempt to soldier on alone.

Practical self-help

• When unresolved emotions about the experience of birth are contributing to the baby blues, it can be immensely helpful to talk to a trained counsellor. Alternatively, talking freely about feelings associated with the birth with someone with whom there is a strong rapport and sense of mutual trust can also be therapeutic. This could be your family doctor, a close friend, alternative practitioner or family member. Unburdening yourself helps you come to terms with the powerful emotional conflicts that often surface in the weeks following childbirth. It also helps you to avoid falling into the emotional trap of feeling the need to keep a stiff upper lip, which can cause more long-term problems associated with repressed or stifled emotions.

• Ask for help in order to organize some time spent apart from your baby. This should be a strong priority, since it is all too easy to experience a profound sense of loss of identity when caring for a young baby. This need not be an immensely long break from the daily routine of feeding, changing and bathing, just enough to break the monotony and re-establish a sense of meeting needs of one's own for a change. Make a point of doing something enjoyable in the free time, such as taking a long walk, meeting a friend for a coffee in a favourite café, or having a pampering treatment such as a massage or facial.

• Make a point of keeping contact with some of the friends you met at relaxation or parenting classes, and try to meet up regularly after the birth. Even if it is only possible to chat occasionally on the phone, it can be enormously helpful, reassuring and therapeutic to have the opportunity of exchanging feelings, insecurities and frustrations with someone who is going through a similar situation at roughly the same time.

• Try to make sure that your diet is as nutritious as possible, ideally avoiding the items that can make mood swings and depression worse. These may include alcohol, strong tea and coffee, sweets and chocolate, carbonated drinks that contain sugar and caffeine, and refined foods of most kinds. Consider

HOMOEOPATHIC MEDICINES

Type	General features	Worse	Better	Remedy
Severe mood swings with depression	Moods move abruptly between silence and withdrawal and extreme excitability and chattiness. Anxiety about losing reason or doing harm to the baby. Frequent sighing with black, deep depression. Jittery and fidgety with foreboding that something awful will happen	Becoming cold or chilled	Movement Fresh air Warmth	Cimicifuga
Withdrawn and depressed with marked aversion to sympathy	Depression springs from suppressed feelings of grief and pain. Distress is made worse by expressions of affection and concern by others because of humiliation of being seen to cry in public. Unable to weep or releases tears only when alone	Company Physical expressions of affection Physical exertion Weeping Warmth Eating	Peace and quiet Privacy Rest Cool, fresh air Missing meals	Natrum mur
Mentally and physically exhausted, indifferent and stressed by demands of the new baby	Difficulty bonding with baby because of extreme sense of apathy, weariness or irritability. Feels wrung out with fear of being totally unable to cope or going out of control. Low libido after pregnancy	Sitting still Missing meals Domestic demands Touch	Sound sleep Warm bed Eating small meals regularly Brisk exercise in the fresh air	Sepia
Depression and resentment following a 'high tech' birth	Required where the process of childbirth has felt like a violation due to the need for invasive medical procedures. Especially helpful for emotional and physical pain following an unplanned Caesarean. Extremely sensitive stitches or scars that cause great distress	Touch Sexual contact Contact of clothes or bedcovers Stress or emotional demands	Rest After breakfast Warmth	Staphysagria

vitamin B complex, vitamin C, magnesium, calcium and zinc supplements.

• If periods of emotional numbness alternate with episodes of violent anger.

• If depression becomes persistent and severe and does not respond to self-help approaches.

• If feelings of extreme anxiety or fear occur when setting about everyday tasks that previously were automatic.

• If there is any sense of losing touch with reality or feeling uncharacteristically separated from others.

• If there are any suicidal thoughts or thoughts of harming the baby.

Alternative treatments

Topical preparations

These include essential oils, infusions and tinctures that may be used in aromatic baths or in other external ways. Choose from any of the following, bearing in mind that none of the substances mentioned for application to the skin should be taken by mouth.

Aromatherapy oils

Make an aromatic rub by adding four drops each of Roman chamomile (Chamaemelum nobile), lavender (Lavendula angustifolia), rosewood and ginger to four teaspoons of carrier oil. Massage the body morning and evening.

Medicines intended for internal use

These help re-establish emotional equilibrium and harmony.

Herbal preparations

• Try a soothing cup of rosemary herb tea with a pinch of valerian added in order to lift the spirits.

• Alternatively, an infusion of lemon balm, Hypericum or vervain may also ease transient feelings of depression.

Alternative medical treatment may be helpful from any of the following:

• Anthroposophical medicine
• Aromatherapy
• Biochemic tissue salts
• Flower remedies
• Homoeopathy
• Massage therapy
• Naturopathy
• Nutritional therapy
• Shiatsu
• Traditional Chinese medicine
• Western medical herbalism

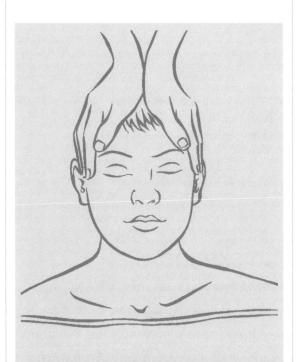

Face and scalp massage can comfort and help to ease tension during periods of stress.

CHILDHOOD PROBLEMS

Bed-wetting (enuresis)

Bed-wetting tends to occur as a result of a child's nervous system being unable to exert sufficient control over his or her bladder. This can sometimes be due to an infection of the bladder, or occasionally as a result of a mechanical problem, such as an anatomical abnormality of the kidney. Alternatively, a psychological perspective can also be worth exploring, since stress can contribute to bed-wetting continuing beyond the usual timescale within which it might be expected to clear up.

In general, approximately 10 per cent of children continue to wet the bed by the age of five, while some may continue to have problems until they are sixteen. However, it may be helpful to bear in mind that most three-year-olds are dry by night and day.

If a child of four or over shows signs of difficulty in gaining bladder control during both day and night, it is worthwhile consulting a medical opinion. This can be helpful in ruling out any anatomical problems or residual infections that might be contributing to the problem.

Practical self-help

• Bear in mind that most children outgrow bed-wetting and that it is something that should not be allowed to cause undue anxiety or distress. Above all, try to avoid making a child feel guilty about the problem, since this can lead to increased emotional stress and tension that can make matters worse.
• It can be a great help to leave dry sheets and night clothes readily to hand for older children so that they can change damp items for themselves, with the minimum amount of fuss and disruption. This can also be helpful in giving them a sense of being somewhat in control.

• 'Lifting' a child during the night or withholding drinks before bed is regarded by some medical sources as being of questionable value.
• Counselling appears to be of benefit to some children, while others may also respond well to mechanical devices that work on a behavioural level, such as using a pad and buzzer.

SEEK PROFESSIONAL HELP

If a child over the age of four has problems with incontinence during the day and/or night, or if a child has been dry at night and starts bedwetting.

Alternative treatments

If bed-wetting has become an established problem in an older child, it is best to seek professional help from an alternative medical practitioner. However, some of the following simple measures may be of initial help.

Medicines intended for internal use
Flower remedies
Cherry plum may be helpful in easing some of the psychological stress that can be caused by this problem.

Alternative help, treatment and advice may be obtained from practitioners of any of the following therapies:
• Acupressure
• Anthroposophical medicine
• Biochemic tissue salts
• Homoeopathy
• Shiatsu
• Traditional Chinese medicine
• Western medical herbalism

Chickenpox

Chickenpox is a viral infection that has a rather long incubation period lasting anything between one and three weeks. It begins with a generally unwell phase that may involve symptoms of feverishness and flu-type lethargy, shivering and listlessness. The emerging rash is likely to begin as red, blistery spots that appear to have fluid trapped beneath the surface. Chickenpox spots are characteristically itchy and rapidly spread over the body from the trunk to the back, arms, legs, head and face.

The rash is likely to remain extremely irritable until the individual spots have dried out. Once this phase has been reached your child has passed the infectious stage of illness.

Practical self-help
• During the feverish stage of illness it is likely that your child will not be very keen to eat. Although it may be counterproductive to eat at this stage, it is essential that your child drinks plenty of fluid to discourage the fever from rising further. Once an interest in food develops, make sure that you offer foods that are as light and easy on the digestion as possible. Broths, purées or steamed, fresh fruit are all suitable.
• Make a point of trimming your child's fingernails as short as possible so that they are not as likely to dislodge the crusts from spots when scratching. It is also helpful to get older children to rub itchy areas rather than scratching them, so that the crusty tops of spots are left intact. By following this advice, there is less of a chance that the spots might become infected and scar. The risk of infection can also be reduced by using some of the tinctures, creams and other topical preparations listed below.
• Once spots have become crusty it is important to take care when drying your child after a bath. If you rub at the skin with a towel it is very easy to inadvertently knock the heads of the spots off. However, if you gently pat the skin dry there is a reduced chance of this problem occurring.
• Avoid giving your child hot baths when they are in the early stage of illness as the spots are emerging, since this can contribute to their feeling enervated and more unwell. Sponge your child down instead, making sure that the room is kept comfortably warm.
• Avoid giving aspirin to your child when feverish in an effort to bring the temperature down and never give aspirin to a child under twelve. It is worth checking the labels of products sold for pain and fever to ensure that they do not contain it. Aspirin is best avoided in this situation because of the risk of Reye's syndrome developing. This is a potentially serious illness that can cause drowsiness, high temperature, vomiting, loss of consciousness and convulsions.

SEEK PROFESSIONAL HELP
• If you are pregnant and have been exposed to someone with chickenpox, but have not had it yourself.
• If a persistent or severe headache occurs, especially if it is combined with a stiff neck.
• If extreme lethargy or weakness develops.
• If there are any indications of bleeding beneath the skin, pus formation or general inflammation around the spots, suggesting that infection may be developing.
• If there are signs of breathing problems, including rapid, shallow or laboured breathing.
• If vomiting or convulsions occur.

Professional medical help and advice should always be sought if chickenpox occurs in a child who is less than a year old.

Alternative treatments
It is worth noting that for chickenpox it is quite appropriate to give the indicated internal remedy while also applying a topical preparation to the skin.

If there are any signs that you may be getting out of your depth with self-help measures, do not hesitate to seek advice from a trained practitioner.

Topical preparations
Lotions, creams or essential oils can be applied to the skin to soothe and heal. Choose from any of the following, bearing in mind that none of the substances mentioned for application to the skin should be taken by mouth.
Aromatherapy oils
• Make an aromatic rub by adding five drops of ravensar (Ravensara aromatica) to two teaspoons of carrier oil. Paint the affected areas with the balm, avoiding broken skin.
• A warm-water bath using five drops of lavender (Lavendula angustifolia), well dispersed, is comforting. But do not use for children under three.

Herbal preparations

• If skin is maddeningly itchy, add Urtica dioica (stinging nettle) tincture to the bathwater to soothe irritated skin. The diluted tincture may also be used to bathe itchy areas as often as required. (One part of tincture should be diluted in ten parts of boiled, cooled water and applied with soft cotton wool pads.)
• If the spots are proving painful as well as itchy, your child may respond better to a mixture of Hypericum and Calendula tincture. This combination has the advantage of promoting pain relief, while also encouraging rapid healing of the skin and discouraging secondary infection.
• Once the rash has been bathed with the appropriate diluted tincture, your child may be made comfortable by the application of marigold cream.

HOMOEOPATHIC MEDICINES

Type	General features	Worse	Better	Remedy
Early feverish stage of illness with abrupt onset of symptoms	High temperature with bright red, dry skin that radiates extreme heat to the touch. Extreme irritability with intolerance of bright light, loud noise and movement	Chill Jarring Noise Disturbance	Lying semi-erect in warm bed Peace and quiet Darkened rooms	Belladonna
Sudden onset of symptoms with extreme restlessness and anxiety	Rapid onset of feverishness with thirst and dry skin. Pain-sensitive and fearful when unwell. Aconite is often needed for the feverish stage before the rash has come out	Extreme changes of temperature During the night	Perspiring Sound sleep Contact with fresh air (provided it doesn't chill)	Aconite
Slow-emerging rash with persistent cough	Unpleasant coating on the tongue with severe chesty, rattling cough. Large, bluish-tinged spots that leave a red mark. Illness results in child becoming very irritable and bad tempered	Bathing Overheating Heat In the evening Lying down	Loosening and bringing up phlegm Cool conditions	Ant tart
Terribly itchy rash with chickenpox that leads to great restlessness at night	Child constantly tosses and turns in bed at night from irritation of skin. Moist, crusty spots that are especially sensitive to contact with cold, damp air	Scratching During the night Resting Lying still Contact with cold damp air Undressing	Changing position Rubbing Stretching Warm, dry surroundings	Rhus tox
Later stage of chickenpox with ongoing, slight feverishness	Rash may be slow to emerge, or may linger longer than expected. Chilly, but feels more unwell for becoming heated. Dry mouth without thirst with craving for contact with cool, fresh air. Normally independent child becomes weepy and clingy when unwell	Resting In the evening and at night Overheating Badly ventilated surroundings Feeling neglected	Gentle movement Contact with cool, fresh air Cool compresses Cool drinks and food Sympathy and attention	Pulsatilla

Although this formulation can also be obtained as an ointment, it is preferable to choose the cream, since this is less moisturizing and less likely to keep the spots moist. This cream is especially useful if the skin has been broken by scratching, and it is necessary to take steps to guard against infection setting in.

Home remedies

• Once the spots have emerged, itchy skin can be effectively soothed by letting your child soak in an

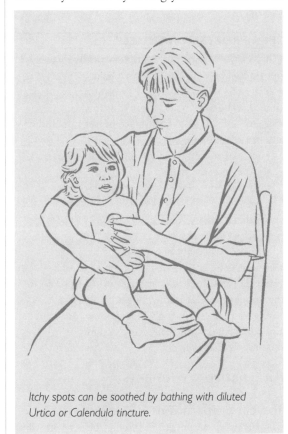

Itchy spots can be soothed by bathing with diluted Urtica or Calendula tincture.

oatmeal bath. Put a generous handful of oats in a bag of fine-textured gauze or muslin and suspend it under the hot-water tap while the bath is filling. However, test the temperature of the bathwater in order to make sure that it is comfortably warm rather than too hot.

• Irritation and itching may be eased by soaking in a very dilute solution of cider vinegar: for the correct proportion add one cup of cider vinegar to a generous bathful of warm water.

• Scarring from chickenpox spots can be discouraged by applying vitamin E oil to areas that have become scarred or discoloured.

• Skin condition in general can also be improved by encouraging your child to take foods seasoned by garlic and parsley.

Medicines intended for internal use

These ease discomfort, reduce inflammation and irritation, and encourage a speedy resolution of the problem with the minimum amount of complications.

Herbal preparations

A fractious, restless and generally overwrought child may be soothed by sips of warm, soothing herbal teas such as chamomile, vervain or lemon balm. The teas may be made generally more appetizing by adding a little honey, cinnamon or lemon juice (making sure that you avoid the latter if your child has sore spots in his mouth). Note that honey should not be given to babies under one year old.

Colic

Although a relatively common problem, severe baby colic can cause great distress to mother and baby, often leaving the former very disturbed at the intensity of the symptoms in her baby. Colic commonly occurs any time after birth up to three months. Some babies characteristically cry in the evenings, while others may be distressed after a feed at any time of day or night.

Symptoms include:
• Bouts of screaming and weeping in response to pain and discomfort with a flushed face.
• The child's knees may be drawn up to the chest in an effort to ease the pain.

When these symptoms first appear you should consult the doctor to ensure that your baby is not suffering from something more serious.

Practical self-help

• If you suspect that your baby is suffering from colic it is worth omitting certain items from your diet that may aggravate colicky pains in breastfed babies. These include strong tea and coffee, alcohol, raw onions, raw peppers, cabbage, cauliflower, Brussels sprouts, dairy foods, chocolate, citrus fruit, grapes, cucumber, beans, garlic, tomatoes, sugar, wheat, corn, spicy foods such as chillies or curries.

If you suspect some of these items may be causing a problem for your baby, omit them in turn for a week or so, reintroducing each one and monitoring the reaction. If your baby seems happier while the offending item is omitted, but has an adverse reaction once it is reintroduced, the chances are that this food or drink is best avoided while breastfeeding. Also take care with these foods when introducing your child to solids, since he may have a sensitivity to them.

• Check that your baby isn't constipated, which can aggravate or contribute to colic. Make sure that your baby takes plenty of fluid (especially in hot weather when dehydration can encourage constipation), massage the abdomen gently in a clockwise direction to encourage easier bowel movements, and include mashed apricots and prunes in your baby's diet once they have been introduced to solids.

• If excess wind is a contributory problem, try gently massaging your baby's back or abdomen. This may be done with or without the essential oils suggested below. Apart from releasing wind, massaging in this way is also extremely soothing and relaxing for your baby.

• When breastfeeding, always ensure that your baby is well locked on to your nipple, so that he or she can gain maximum benefit from the feed. Positioning your baby well while breastfeeding can also have an important part to play in discouraging the development of sore nipples.

• If you have chosen to bottle-feed it is important to check that the teat on your baby's bottle is the correct size. If it is the wrong size, there is a good chance that air will be swallowed along with the feed. If this occurs on a regular basis, your baby may be habitually in discomfort from trapped wind.

• Formula-fed babies may also suffer from feeds that are made up to the wrong proportions, so the crying you attribute to colic may be because of this. Too concentrated a formula may lead to severe thirst, because of the high proportion of salt, while a feed that is too weak can lead to episodes of distress and weeping due to unsatisfied hunger pangs.

• If you are at your wits' end trying to deal with a colicky baby and nothing you try seems to help, it can be extremely helpful to hand your baby over for a short time to someone who is feeling less stressed. This can be an important strategy for relieving the problem temporarily, since babies often pick up feelings from their mothers. As a result, tension, anxiety or frustration can make your baby more distressed, leading to a vicious circle of insecurity and pent-up feelings that can be passed from one to another.

SEEK PROFESSIONAL HELP

• If your baby seems uncharacteristically distressed or you feel he or she is in severe pain.
• If distress is accompanied by vomiting, constipation, diarrhoea or scanty flow of urine.
• If any signs of dehydration are present, including any of the following:
  • Drowsiness (the earliest sign to develop).
  • Concentrated urine.
  • Sunken fontanelle (soft spot at the crown of the head).
  • Sunken eyes.
  • Dry eyes or mouth.
  • Loss of elasticity of the skin.
• If your baby is restless and shows signs of being in general discomfort, it is important not to jump to the conclusion that it may be baby colic. If you suspect a more serious problem, or you are generally concerned about your baby's condition, always seek medical advice.

Alternative treatments

Topical preparations
Choose from any of the following, bearing in mind that none of the substances suggested for application to the skin should be taken by mouth.

Herbal preparations
An infusion of any of the following herbs may be added to your baby's bathwater, or applied as a warm (not hot) compress to the abdomen. Suitable herbs include chamomile, linden blossom, lemon balm, hops or catmint. To make the infusion add half a teaspoon of the selected herb to 100ml (3½fl oz) boiling water. Leave to stand for fifteen minutes, strain and allow to cool before use.

Medicines intended for internal use
These ease pain, release wind and encourage a

speedy resolution of the problem.

Anthroposophical medicines

A homoeopathic potency of chamomile root can be used to soothe the discomfort and distress of baby colic. A tablet may be crushed and dissolved in water and given at hourly intervals for up to three doses or until improvement sets in.

Biochemic tissue salts

General colicky pains may be eased by a few doses of Combination Remedy E. Alternatively, baby colic that is aggravated by touch and cold, and soothed by bending the legs, warmth and firm pressure may respond better to tissue salt No. 8. For acute symptoms, tablets may be taken hourly, tailing off the dosage as symptoms improve. In less pressing circumstances, four tablets may be taken three times a day until improvement is observed.

Herbal preparations

• A teaspoonful of any of the following herb teas may be given warm in order to ease the pain and discomfort of colic: chamomile, catmint or dill.

• Alternatively, try simmering half a teaspoonful of

HOMOEOPATHIC MEDICINES

Type	General features	Worse	Better	Remedy
Colicky pains with diarrhoea that does not resolve	Colic occurs in breastfeeding babies whose mothers drink a lot of strong tea. Severe pains are located around the navel and are eased by stretching or arching backwards	Pressing knees against the chest At night Feeding Lying down	Firm pressure Stretching Bending backwards	Dioscorea
Colicky pains that are associated with teething	Excessive amounts of wind with colic that is sometimes helped when released downwards. Baby lies crying with knees pressed to the belly. Good response to massage and a warm hand placed on the painful area	Tight clothes around the waist or abdomen Cold drinks At night Becoming chilled	Pressure to painful part Warmth Rubbing sensitive part Pressing knees to belly	Mag phos
Colicky pains that are associated with persistent constipation	Cramping pains in breastfeeding babies whose mothers may eat too many spicy foods or drink a lot of coffee. Colic is most intense when waking from sleep, leading to frustration with pain and irritability. Lots of unproductive urging with constipation and colic	Becoming chilled Disturbed sleep Pressure or touch Eating After waking	Sound, uninterrupted sleep Warmth After passing a stool Peace and quiet	Nux vomica
Colic that comes on, or is more intense in the afternoon	Severe rumbling, gurgling, excess wind and distension with colicky pains. Colic in breastfeeding babies whose mothers may have too much fibre in their diet from eating beans, cabbage and whole grains	Afternoon and early evening Feeding Pressure of clothes around waist After waking Overheating or becoming chilled	Fresh air Breaking wind Loose clothes Warm drinks	Lycopodium

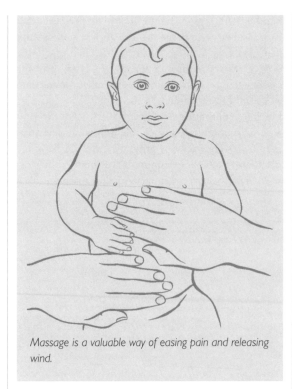

Massage is a valuable way of easing pain and releasing wind.

caraway, angelica or fennel seeds in a small cupful of boiling water for five minutes, leave to stand for ten minutes, and strain the seeds away. A few drops of the liquid can be given to your baby as required to soothe colicky pains.

Alternative help, treatment and advice may be obtained from practitioners of any of the following therapies:

- Acupressure
- Anthroposophical medicine
- Homoeopathy
- Nutritional therapy
- Traditional Chinese medicine
- Western medical herbalism

Cradle cap

This skin condition can occur any time between the first three months after birth and the age of three, commonly affecting the area around the scalp and hairline. Rarely, it may also affect the eyebrows or

ears, making them look as though they are encrusted with a thick dandruff. When cradle cap occurs, a baby's scalp may be covered with a thick, brownish-yellow crust or the irritation may spread to the face in the form of small pimples or blotches. The latter may become especially noticeable if your baby becomes overheated or distressed.

Since cradle cap, in common with other skin conditions, can be an indication of a more deep-seated problem, it is important to consult an alternative practitioner if symptoms are well established, severe or refuse to respond to the self-help measures listed below. Your baby's lack of reaction to these suggestions need not mean that he is unresponsive to an alternative approach, but it may indicate that a more objective professional opinion is needed to treat the underlying predisposition to the problem.

Practical self-help

- Avoid washing your baby's hair too frequently, since this can aggravate the problem by encouraging increased production of oil or sebum.
- It is best to avoid picking off any crusts or scales that are not loose, since this can result in soreness, bleeding and possible infection. Scales that are already loose can be gently and carefully removed with a soft brush or clean fingernail.
- Rub a softening liquid such as almond or olive oil into your baby's scalp and leave it overnight. Gently comb the scalp the next day, detaching the loosened crusts with great care and without pulling or tugging. Then wash the scalp gently with a pH-balanced shampoo, making sure that all traces of detergent are thoroughly rinsed away.

SEEK PROFESSIONAL HELP

- If there are any signs of soreness, severe itchiness or inflammation.
- If there is any suspicion of infection. Common signs include redness, pus formation or weeping.
- If the surface area affected seems to be spreading or if symptoms are gathering in intensity.
- If there is no improvement in response to self-help measures within a few days.

Alternative treatments

It is worth bearing in mind that in the case of cradle cap, it is quite appropriate to give your baby an internal remedy while also applying a topical preparation to the skin.

Topical preparations

Infusions, tinctures, creams or lotions can be applied to the skin to soothe and heal. Choose from any of the following, bearing in mind that none of the substances mentioned for application to the skin should be taken by mouth.

HOMOEOPATHIC MEDICINES

Type	General features	Worse	Better	Remedy
Moist cradle cap that may have an unpleasant odour	Thick, scaly or cracked cradle cap that becomes easily moist and sweaty. General tendency to cracked, dry skin in other places such as folds or flexions of skin. Restless at night and lethargic during the day	Contact with cold air Becoming over-heated in bed Washing Motion	Rest Contact with cool things	Graphites
Cradle cap that is especially severe around the margins of the hair	Cradle cap with extremely dry, cracked skin that is worse for hot, sunny weather. Very flaky skin in general with especially dry lips that crack in the corners or in the middle of the lower lip	Being comforted or cuddled Sunshine Becoming too hot Summer weather Touch	Rubbing Shady, cool conditions Fresh, cool air Sweating	Natrum mur
Cradle cap that is made more irritable by being covered	Thick, scaly, brown-coloured cradle cap with generally dry skin. Chapped skin in flexions and folds of skin. Irritation and sensitivity of the skin is aggravated by clothing and eased by exposure to the air. Irritable and bad tempered waking from sleep	In the afternoons Clothed or covered areas Overheating Waking from sleep	Contact with fresh air Moderate temperatures Motion Being distracted	Lycopodium
Cradle cap with a tendency to sour-smelling sweats on the head	Cradle cap in chilly, sweaty, large babies that tend towards constipation. Walking, talking and teething happen later than expected. Cutting teeth, in particular, causes great distress	Washing Becoming chilled or overheated When constipated	Touch Undressing when overheated	Calc carb
Intensely itchy cradle cap that leads to extreme restlessness at night	Itching and burning of scalp when exposed to warmth. Compulsive scratching and rubbing of scalp. Thick, crusty, moist cradle cap causes immense distress at night in bed: baby constantly tosses and turns in frustration	At night At rest Becoming chilled	Movement Warm rooms	Rhus tox

Aromatherapy oils

Add five drops of rosewood to 50ml (1¾fl oz) jojoba oil and 'paint' the baby's scalp gently with the blend. When washing the baby's head, use shampoo on the scalp *before* rinsing off gently with water.

Herbal preparations

• After shampooing, rinse the scalp with an infusion of meadowsweet, burdock or Indian tea. The equivalent of a teaspoon of herbs should be added to a teapot of hot water.

• Mild cradle cap may respond well to the application of Calendula cream or ointment morning and evening. The cream and ointment provide lubrication for the scalp while discouraging infection and inflammation. However, avoid using the ointment if your child is sensitive to lanolin, since it may provoke a skin reaction.

Medicines intended for internal use

These ease discomfort and itching and reduce inflammation.

Biochemic tissue salts

Mild cases of cradle cap may be eased by Combination Remedy D. Give four tablets three times a day, tailing off the remedy as symptoms improve. When giving the remedy to babies, the tablets may be crushed into a powder or dissolved in water for easier administration. If there is no change in symptoms after a few days, consider an alternative approach rather than continuing routinely with the remedy.

Alternative help, treatment and advice may be obtained from practitioners of any of the following therapies:

• Anthroposophical medicine
• Homoeopathy
• Traditional Chinese medicine
• Western medical herbalism

Croup

Croup is simply laryngitis in a child, but gets its name as the small larynx of a child leads to stridor, the noise of croup. It is an extremely distressing condition that commonly affects babies and children under the age of five. Small children may show an increased tendency to develop this problem in the winter months, when they are likely to be more generally susceptible to coughs and colds.

The symptoms of croup can be very alarming for both parents and children, especially when they arise for the first time.

Common symptoms may involve any of the following which may vary in intensity, depending on the severity of the attack:

• A hoarse, rasping sound that occurs when breathing in, caused by a child's air passages becoming swollen or inflamed.
• Sensitivity of the throat.
• Pain or discomfort in the chest.
• A hollow, metallic-sounding or barking cough.
• Severe attacks that need immediate medical attention are characterized by a child developing pale, clammy, blue-tinged skin, especially around the mouth.

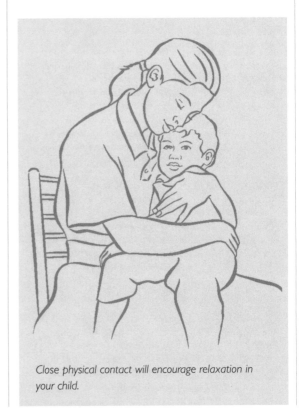

Close physical contact will encourage relaxation in your child.

The frightening nature of croup is often made more intense by the way it characteristically develops, or becomes more severe at night. This may be linked to the way feeling unwell during the hours of darkness can often feel more upsetting than suffering the same illness during daylight hours.

If your child has mild croup, he or she may respond very well to the following advice. However, if severe bouts of croup occur on a recurrent basis, alternative medical help should be consulted in order to deal with your child's predisposition to the problem.

Practical self-help

• Although you may be alarmed at your child's symptoms, try to be as reassuring as possible in order to prevent him or her panicking and tensing up further, which can make breathing problems more difficult. Speak as calmly and softly as possible and keep close physical contact through cuddling and stroking.

HOMOEOPATHIC MEDICINES

Type	General features	Worse	Better	Remedy
Severe cough with laboured breathing wakes child from sleep	Harsh, dry, rasping coughing spasms: distressing sensation of breathing through a dry sponge. Breathing problems on falling asleep. Cough makes a sound resembling a saw being drawn through dry wood	Sugary foods or drinks Talking Excitement Touch Cold drinks Inhaling	Warm drinks	Spongia
Croup that comes on, or gets more intense after midnight	Bouts of croupy coughing that come on immediately after lying down. Croup develops after measles. Distress and discomfort from intensity of coughing spasms leads child to hold his sides. Hoarseness with retching and vomiting with cough	After midnight Lying down Talking Stooping Warmth Cool drinks	Holding sides Firm pressure Fresh air	Drosera
Attacks of croup develop suddenly after exposure to dry, cold winds	Abrupt, violent emergence of symptoms: child wakes from sleep in great distress. Hoarse, dry cough that makes breathing very difficult. Extreme panic, restlessness and anxiety with croup	After midnight Exposure to dry, cold winds Cool drinks Smoky atmospheres Becoming over-heated	Contact with fresh air Moderate temperatures Perspiring	Aconite
Cough with stringy mucus that is coughed up with great difficulty	Breathlessness, retching and gagging with coughing spasms. Child must make a great effort to loosen sticky, yellow-coloured phlegm. Chest pains radiate from below breastbone to back and shoulders	Cold, damp weather On waking Stooping Undressing Sitting In the morning	Warmth Movement	Kali bich

• Move your child to a steamy atmosphere to enable him to breathe more easily. The ideal environment can be created in your bathroom by filling the bath with hot water while also running a hot shower. Shut the bathroom doors and windows to keep as much steam in the room as possible. Sit with your child on your lap, encouraging him to breathe as slowly and evenly as possible to benefit from the steamy atmosphere.

NB Always make sure that your child is not left unattended while the hot tap is running in case he accidentally becomes burned or scalded. Also avoid leaving a small child unattended if the bath has been filled with hot water.

• Some children will respond better to being taken outside into cool/cold air – it is thought that this works by reducing vocal-cord swelling and thereby relieving the obstruction to the airflow that causes stridor.

SEEK PROFESSIONAL HELP

• If there is any suspicion that the child has swallowed a foreign body (e.g. a small toy), but on no account try to look into the child's throat yourself.
• If stridor (see above) occurs in a child who is not suffering from a cold or cough.
• If croup occurs in a baby or child under five years of age.
• If pallor, drooling or blueness around the mouth occur.
• If there are any signs of severe distress or pain.
• If your child has severe croup with laboured, difficult breathing.
• If your child has not responded to self-help approaches within twenty minutes.

Alternative treatments

It is worth bearing in mind that in the case of croup, it is quite appropriate to apply a topical preparation to the chest, while also giving the relevant internal remedy.

Medicines intended for internal use

These ease anxiety and discomfort, reduce inflammation and encourage a speedy resolution of the problem.
Herbal preparations
• Children above the age of three may benefit from an infusion of vervain and coltsfoot. A teaspoonful of each should be steeped in a cup of hot water. Strain

after ten minutes and give a teaspoonful as needed, checking the temperature beforehand to make sure it is not too hot.
• An elecampane infusion may be made by pouring a cup of cold water onto a teaspoonful of the shredded root. Leave it to stand overnight, strain and give it as a warm drink to soothe an inflamed larynx and loosen mucus.

If bouts of croup are beginning to occur on a recurrent basis, alternative help, treatment and advice may be obtained from practitioners of any of the following therapies:
• Anthroposophical medicine
• Homoeopathy
• Naturopathy
• Traditional Chinese medicine
• Western medical herbalism

Earache

Although earache is by no means a problem that is restricted to the childhood years, there is no doubt that it is a condition that children are generally more susceptible to than adults. This is because the Eustachian tube (that joins the back of the nose and the cavity of the ear) is longer in adults than in children. Consequently, infections can be rapidly conveyed from the passages of the nose to the ears in children. Because children also have a greater likelihood to develop inflamed adenoids, ear, nose and throat problems tend to be a common feature of juvenile illness.

Common symptoms of ear infections may include any of the following:
• Sharp, stabbing pains in the ear.
• Muffled hearing or a sensation of fullness in the painful ear.

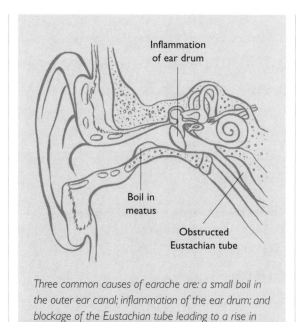

Inflammation
of ear drum

Boil in
meatus

Obstructed
Eustachian tube

*Three common causes of earache are: a small boil in
the outer ear canal; inflammation of the ear drum; and
blockage of the Eustachian tube leading to a rise in
pressure in the middle ear from retained secretions.*

• A general sense of unwellness, dizziness or feverishness.
• Pulling or rubbing the ear is often a tell-tale sign
in small babies that earache may be developing.
• If an ear infection is neglected, there is a possibility of a build-up of pus occurring, which may perfo-
rate the eardrum and trickle out of the ear in the
form of a discharge.

If earache is caught in its early stages, there is a
good chance that self-help measures plus an appropriate alternative medical approach can do a great
deal to resolve the problem without complications.
However, if your child does not respond to these
measures promptly, or if there is a tendency for
repeated ear infections to occur, it is very important
to seek professional help to deal with the problem
effectively.

Practical self-help

• Warm compresses can be extremely soothing to
painful ears, feeling comforting and easing the pain.
The simplest can be made by wrapping a hot-water
bottle with a very soft cloth and putting it against
the painful area. Alternatively, immerse a clean
flannel in hot water, wring it out well and place it
against the painful area until it cools down, when the
process can be repeated.
• If your child has a tendency to develop recurrent

ear infections, always make sure that his or her ears
are covered well in cold, windy weather by making
use of a hat or ear muffs (in an older child).
• If your child shows signs of feverishness, make
sure that they are given plenty of fluids to drink. If
they are suffering from a sore throat and swollen
glands in addition to earache, it is best to avoid
acidic drinks such as citrus juices, which can make
the throat more sensitive. Also avoid the temptation
to give frequent milky drinks, which can contribute
towards excess mucus production, making ear and
chest infections more severe. Concentrate instead
on plain water, which is the best fluid to reduce
feverishness and discourage dehydration.
• Never insert foreign objects too far into a painful
ear (such as a cotton wool bud), thereby inadvertently making the problem worse. If applying soothing oil on a wad of cotton wool to the ear, always
make sure it is possible to retrieve it easily. However,
if a foreign object does disappear into your child's
ear, take him straightaway to the accident and emergency department of your local hospital in order to
have the item removed professionally.
• Always prevent your child's ears coming into
contact with water if an ear infection is diagnosed.

SEEK PROFESSIONAL HELP

• If your child suffers from repeated or recurrent
earaches.
• If there is any sign of swelling, redness or sensitivity of the bony area behind your child's ear.
• If there is any sign of a discharge running from
the ear, especially if it is blood-streaked, has pus in
it or gives off an offensive smell.
• If earache is combined with feverishness, leading
to potential problems with dehydration in small
babies (see page 278 for signs of dehydration).
• If your baby has not responded to self-help measures within a few hours, or if symptoms appear to
be increasing in intensity.

Alternative treatments

In the case of earache, it is quite appropriate to give
the relevant internal remedy while also applying a
topical preparation to the painful area.

Topical preparations

Oils, tinctures and compresses can be applied to the
painful area to soothe and heal. Choose from any of
the following, bearing in mind that none of the

HOMOEOPATHIC MEDICINES

Type	General features	Worse	Better	Remedy
Earache with associated teething problems	Feverish with one pale and one flushed cheek. Painful sensitivity to cold or noise. Sticking pains in the ears with stuffed-up sensation. Baby screams and howls with pain, throws toys about the room and cannot be pacified	At night Touch Exposure to cold, damp air or cold winds Becoming too hot	Being driven in a car Rocking Warm compresses to the painful side	Chamomilla
Initial stage of earache with rapid onset of high temperature	Violent, abrupt onset of pain with ear that looks bright red and feels hot to the touch. Skin looks generally flushed and dry. Associated sore throat and swollen glands with right-sided earache. Normally good-tempered baby becomes extremely irritable and restless	Movement Jarring Loud noise Becoming chilled Stimulation	Warmth Warm compresses to the painful ear Resting in a dark room	Belladonna
Earache that develops rapidly after exposure to dry, cold winds	Symptoms develop with violence and intensity with child waking from sleep in great pain. Thirsty and feverish with cool body and hot head. Fearful, restless and extremely anxious with earache	Becoming chilled or overheated Lying on painful side At night Exposure to cold winds Loud noise Bright light	Moderate warmth Fresh air Perspiring	Aconite
Persistent earache and swollen glands with thick, yellow discharge	Sharp, splinter-like pains in ears with offensive smell from mouth or discharge. Extremely chilly with aversion to cold draughts; becomes distressed if a hand or foot is left out of bedcovers. Great dislike of being touched with uncharacteristic irritability and short temper	Exposure to cold air During the winter Undressing Lying on painful side At night	Warmth Wrapping head up well Humid heat	Hepar sulph
Early stage of earache with itching in ear	Rapid onset of symptoms that are less violent than those requiring aconite or belladonna. Left-sided ear pain, or symptoms that are more intense on the left than on the right side. Alternates between being pale and flushed	At night Movement Jarring Contact with cold air Touch	Resting Cool compresses	Ferrum phos

substances mentioned for application to the skin should be taken by mouth.

Herbal preparations

• Hypericum oil may be used to ease inflammation and pain in the ear.

• A warm compress of chamomile can also be extremely soothing to painful ears. Make an infusion by steeping the fresh heads of the flowers in hot water and straining off the liquid, or use chamomile tea bags. Soak a clean cloth or flannel in the warm, strained infusion and apply warm to the painful area. Once it has cooled down, repeat the process.

Home remedies

• Warmed vitamin E oil can be very soothing to painful, inflamed ears. Pierce a capsule of the oil with a sterilized pin and squeeze a few drops of the oil onto a warmed spoon. Once the oil is comfortably warm, apply a drop or two to the painful ear.

Medicines intended for internal use

These ease pain, reduce inflammation and encourage a speedy resolution of the problem.

Anthroposophical medicines

The distress of earache may be eased by using a combination formula of Apis mellifica and Levisticum officinalis. Give up to five pills every two to three hours, tailing off the treatment as symptoms improve. For babies, crush the tablets between two teaspoons into a fine powder, dissolve in water and administer with a teaspoon.

Biochemic tissue salts

Earache that sets in or is worse during warm weather may respond to tissue salt No. 7. Alternatively, if earache occurs in autumn and winter, and is accompanied by a cold and congestion of the chest, it may respond better to Combination Remedy J. Crush one tablet into a powder and give six times a day until symptoms improve. However, if improvement is not forthcoming reasonably swiftly, consider another alternative approach.

Herbal preparations

If your baby is fractious and finding it difficult while suffering from earache, a few teaspoons of warm chamomile tea may help a great deal in settling them down.

If bouts of earache are beginning to occur on a recurrent basis, alternative help, treatment and advice may be obtained from practitioners of any of the following therapies:

• Anthroposophical medicine
• Ayurvedic medicine
• Cranial osteopathy
• Homoeopathy
• Naturopathy
• Traditional Chinese medicine
• Western medical herbalism

Fever

The onset of a high temperature is usually regarded as a sign that the body is mobilizing its resources to fight infection. Normal body temperature is approximately 37°C (98.6°F), although there can be individual variations of a degree or so either way. In children a rise in temperature often heralds the onset of a childhood infection, with the temperature moving rapidly up to around 40°C (102°F). Adults, on the other hand, tend not to experience as much of an abrupt rise in temperature when they become ill.

Common symptoms of fever may include:
• Shivering.
• Marked thirst.
• Raised temperature.
• Restlessness.
• Flushed, hot skin.
• Rapid pulse.

Apart from the onset of an acute illness, a fever can develop after exposure to extreme heat or cold, or following the shock of a traumatic experience.

Practical self-help

• It is vitally important to keep fluid intake up when a fever has developed. Water is the best choice, and additional drinks of lemon and honey will provide energy and extra vitamin C. However, avoid acidic ingredients such as lemon juice in illnesses such as mumps, where glandular pain and sensitivity are present.

• Do not encourage someone who is recovering from a high temperature to eat too soon, since the effort of eating can cause a renewed increase in fever. However, make sure that fluid intake is not allowed to drop.

• Once appetite returns and the fever has gone, give plenty of home-made vegetable soups, fresh fruit juices and natural yoghurt.

• Young children may benefit from a tepid bath with the water poured over the head. The head acts as a big radiator to get rid of body heat, so cooling it in this way is effective. A child will hate it, but will feel much better once he has cooled down.

• Strip off clothes totally, unless this causes goose bumps, in which case a layer should be put back on, as shivering causes yet more heat production.

• The child can be taken outside to help cool down, provided this does not cause goose bumps.

• Do not cover a child up or put them near a fire when they have a fever, as this can lead to febrile convulsions from too high a temperature.

SEEK PROFESSIONAL HELP

• If delirious.

• If the temperature reaches 40°C (102°F).

• If any symptoms develop that suggest a febrile convulsion may be about to occur. These include drowsiness, confusion, restlessness and muscular jerking and twitching. Although febrile convulsions need not be dangerous, they can cause distress when they occur unexpectedly. It is essential to get swift medical help if a febrile convulsion occurs.

HOMOEOPATHIC MEDICINES

Type	General features	Worse	Better	Remedy
Abrupt, violent onset of fever with dry, hot skin	Rapid development of symptoms with extreme restlessness and irritability. Skin is so bright red and dry it radiates heat. Pupils are dilated and pulse is rapid and pounding	Cold draughts Becoming chilled Light Noise Jarring movement Touch	Being lightly covered Resting propped up in bed Peace and quiet	Belladonna
Rapidly developing high fever after chill from dry, cold winds	Terrible restlessness and anxiety with fever that often develops overnight. Fever may also set in as a result of emotional shock or trauma. Pulsating pains with headache and fever	Emotional stress Becoming chilled Noise Bright light At night	Sound sleep Fresh air	Aconite
Early stage of inflammation that is less violent than belladonna or aconite	Great exhaustion and prostration with feverishness. Chilly and sore with burning pains in chest, shoulders and muscles in general	At night Jarring movement Cold drinks Touch Suppressed sweat	Cold compresses Lying down	Ferrum phos
Slow-developing low-grade fever with aches and pains	Tired, weary and weak. Shivers up and down the spine. Apathetic and lethargic: wants to be left alone in peace. Dizziness with feverishness and severe headache	Movement Stress Cold, damp conditions	Sweating In the afternoon Resting with head elevated	Gelsemium

• If there is any sign of rigor developing (characterized by severe shivering, shaking or chattering of teeth).

• If a stiff neck develops, especially if it is accompanied by a severe headache, nausea and vomiting.

Alternative treatments

The following suggestions are made for use in situations of mild feverishness. However, if the temperature does not reduce within a short period of time, do not hesitate to seek the advice of a practitioner.

Medicines intended for internal use
Biochemic tissue salts
Tissue salt No. 4 may be helpful in the initial stages of fever where inflammation and chills are present. Shivering and aches and pains with high temperature may respond to tissue salt No. 8. In acute stages of fever, tablets may be needed at hourly intervals until symptoms show signs of improvement.

Herbal preparations
• Hibiscus tea can be drunk warm or iced with lemon as a long, refreshing drink.
• Elderflower, lemon balm, peppermint or vervain tea are soothing, warm drinks that may be taken at the first sign of feverishness.

Home remedies
A very small amount of cayenne pepper may be added to warm water, tea or hot milk. However, bear in mind that cows' milk products should be avoided if there is any sign of bronchial congestion or inflammation of the sinuses as well as feverishness.

German measles (rubella)

This is a generally mild viral illness with an incubation period of three weeks. It should result in little more distress than a general sense of being under the weather, and the emergence of a slight rash.

Symptoms may include the following:
• A raised temperature.
• Enlarged glands at the back of the neck and behind the ears.

• A small, flat, reddish-pink rash that usually emerges initially on the face, moving rapidly to the rest of the body.

The rash should not cause undue distress and may have cleared up by the end of the first week of illness.

SEEK PROFESSIONAL HELP

• If symptoms are accompanied by extreme distress or fatigue.
• If there are any signs of lingering headache, stiffness of the neck, nausea and/or vomiting.
• If bleeding occurs under the skin.
• If your child experiences problems when breathing.

WARNING

Although German measles is a relatively minor infectious illness, it is important that children suffering from this disease should be kept apart from pregnant women, as the German measles virus can lead to birth defects in the unborn child. As a result, always make sure you tell any friends, colleagues or family members if you suspect your child may be incubating or in the early stages of German measles. They will then be aware that they should remain out of contact with your child until he or she has made a full recovery.

German measles often appears as a non-specific rash, and a great many other viruses have similar

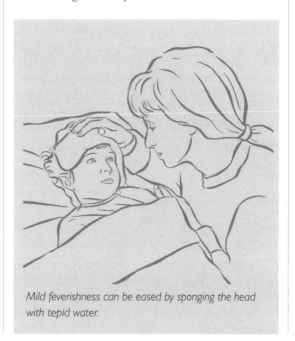

Mild feverishness can be eased by sponging the head with tepid water.

symptoms. It is not possible to diagnose German measles without doing virology blood tests.

For information on general self-help and alternative treatments, see the advice given in the measles section, which is also appropriate for treating German measles.

Measles

Measles is a highly contagious viral infection that has an incubation period of roughly ten days to two weeks. It begins with a period of general unwellness, lethargy and feverishness. There may also be signs of a dry cough, sore eyes and runny nose. Once the feverishness subsides, it is usually followed by the appearance of small ulcers inside the mouth that look like grains of salt. The temperature is likely to rise again with the emergence of a raised, red rash that spreads from behind the ears to the forehead, and eventually over the trunk. The spots should get larger as they emerge over the body, gradually joining together. However, once the rash has fully emerged, the temperature should subside and the patient should begin to feel better.

Additional symptoms are:
• Earache.
• Swollen glands.
• Sensitivity to light.
• Diarrhoea.

The following suggestions can do a great deal to make your child more comfortable and less distressed when suffering from measles. However, if there is any suggestion of eye complications occurring, or if your child appears unduly unwell (especially if he or she is less than a year old) it is essential to seek professional medical help.

Practical self-help

• Never force your child to eat during the feverish stage of illness since this can result in a further increase in temperature and possible nausea. It is far more important instead to ensure that plenty of liquids are taken that will encourage the feverishness to subside and discourage dehydration. If your child is not keen to drink water, offer a variety of drinks that may be more appealing such as diluted fresh fruit juices or lollipops made from fruit-flavoured juices. However, avoid milky drinks, since these can encourage mucus production, making congestion in the nose and chest more distressing. Once the feverishness has subsided introduce light, easily digestible foods such as soups, broths and cooked cereals.
• If your child finds exposure to bright light uncomfortable ensure that his or her room is dimly lit and that curtains are kept closed in daylight hours.

SEEK PROFESSIONAL HELP

• If there is any sign of marked light sensitivity and eye infection.
• If vomiting occurs with severe, or persistent, headache and/or stiffness of the neck.
• If coughing is severe and leads to laboured, difficult breathing.
• If the temperature remains high after the rash has fully emerged, or if the condition of your child does not improve at this stage.
• If there are signs of persistent marked weakness or severe lethargy with high temperature.
• If an ear infection is suspected.
• If bleeding occurs from any orifice or is visible under the skin.

Alternative treatments

For measles it is quite appropriate to give a suitable internal remedy while also applying a soothing topical preparation to the skin. However, if symptoms are severe, do not hesitate to seek advice from an alternative practitioner who is trained in any of the therapies mentioned below.

Topical preparations

Lotions, tinctures or creams can be applied to the skin to soothe and heal. Choose from any of the following,

HOMOEOPATHIC MEDICINES

Type	General features	Worse	Better	Remedy
Sudden emergence of symptoms with extreme restless anxiety	Feverishness sets in abruptly and violently. Eyes become rapidly sensitive and tender with harsh, croupy cough and running nose. Temperature peaks rapidly with extreme distress, oversensitivity to pain and fearfulness.	Extreme changes of temperature from hot to cold During the night	Refreshing sleep Moderate temperatures Cool air that does not chill	Aconite Aconite is most often needed in the first 24–48 hours of illness
Initial onset of symptoms with extremely high temperature and hot, red skin	Symptoms develop with extreme violence and rapidity. Bright red, hot, dry skin that radiates heat when touched. Rapid pulse with glassy looking eyes and dilated pupils. Light sensitive with severe throbbing headache. Normally placid child becomes awfully irritable and bad tempered when feverish.	Jarring movement Bright light Noise Disturbance Becoming chilled	Warmth Lying quietly semi-erect in bed Darkened rooms Peace and quiet	Belladonna Belladonna is most often needed in the first 24–48 hours of illness
Slow emergence of symptoms with deep red, flushed skin	Feverish state develops slowly with severe headache that is severely aggravated by the slightest movement. Severe dry, irritating cough with tickling in the throat and thirst for long, cold drinks. Child becomes withdrawn and irritable when disturbed	Warmth Slightest movement Eating Interruption and disturbance	Lying still Cool temperatures Contact with fresh air Long, cool drinks Firm pressure to painful parts	Bryonia
Measles symptoms with marked sensitivity of the eyes	Extremely painful, watery, burning eyes. Running nose with bland nasal discharge. Eye and nose symptoms respond well to fresh air. Hoarse, dry cough	Onset of evening Contact with warmth Bright light	Wiping the eyes Contact with fresh, cool air	Euphrasia
Later stage of measles with catarrhal problems	Often indicated once the rash has fully developed. Dry mouth without thirst and persistent cough that is dry at night and loose in the morning. Thick, greenish-yellow mucus from nose and chest. Normally contented child becomes very clingy, demanding and weepy	Warm food or drinks Contact with heat in any form Lying in bed Stuffy, badly ventilated rooms In the evening or at night	Cool food or drinks Contact with harsh, open air Gentle movement Sympathy, attention and affection	Pulsatilla

bearing in mind that none of the substances mentioned for application to the skin should be taken by mouth.

Aromatherapy oils
Gently sponge affected areas with hydrosol of chamomile to relieve itching. Seek advice from a qualified aromatherapist.

Herbal preparations
• Diluted Hypericum and Calendula tincture can do a great deal to ease the discomfort of the rash when added to the bathwater or used to swab the spots as often as required. Use one part of tincture to ten parts of boiled, cooled water and apply to the spots as often as needed on a clean, soft, cotton wool pad.
• After bathing with the tincture, Calendula cream may be applied to the skin as often as required to reduce discomfort and inflammation.

Home remedies
• Sore eyes may be soothed by applying cool compresses of cotton wool soaked in cold water to the closed eyelids.
• Alternatively, cool tea bags can also be extremely soothing to sore eyes when applied to closed eyelids.
• Irritated skin may be soothed by the application of cool water in which fresh peas have been cooked.
• Alternatively, a solution of apple cider vinegar diluted in water may also do a great deal to reduce inflammation and discomfort. Half a teaspoonful of vinegar should be diluted in 150ml (5fl oz) water.
• Although calamine lotion has a reputation for drying out spots, it unfortunately tends to have a very short-lived effect, leaving the skin rapidly irritated once again.

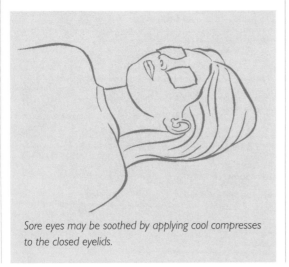
Sore eyes may be soothed by applying cool compresses to the closed eyelids.

Medicines intended for internal use
These ease irritation, reduce inflammation and discourage complications by encouraging a speedy resolution of the problem.

Herbal preparations
Children who are fractious and restless may be soothed by frequent sips of warm chamomile or vervain tea, especially if they have a stomach upset in addition to general symptoms such as a sore throat and sore eyes.

Mumps
Mumps is an extremely uncomfortable viral illness that has an incubation period of between two to four weeks. It usually involves initial symptoms of vague unwellness, combined with feverishness. As the illness progresses, the parotid glands positioned beneath the ears become painful and enlarged, while the salivary glands located under the tongue and the jaw may also become sensitive and swollen. This is likely to make swallowing and using the jaw very painful and difficult. The swelling and pain may be limited to one side of the face and neck, or may affect both sides equally.

It is important to make sure that children suffering from mumps do not come into contact with adults who have not acquired immunity in childhood, since this childhood illness can give rise to very unpleasant symptoms in adults. Women may be subject to a condition called oophoritis that involves inflammation of the ovaries, while adult males may develop orchitis, a painful swelling and inflammation of the testicles that may, in rare cases, render them sterile.

Practical self-help
• Warmth can be very soothing when applied to

inflamed, painful areas of the face. Wrap a hot-water bottle in a soft towel or cloth and hold it to the swollen parts. However, make sure that the hot-water bottle is not too hot, so that there is no danger of a small child becoming burned by accidental contact with the hot rubber. A flannel immersed in warm water and wrung out well can also make an effective, simple warm compress at short notice.

• Although your child may not show much interest in food during the early stage of the illness, make sure he or she drinks frequently to reduce feverishness and discourage dehydration and constipation. Although fruit juices can be refreshing, it is best to avoid citrus-flavoured drinks, since they can aggravate pain in the salivary glands. Use your imagination in encouraging your child to drink by making freshly squeezed juices, or giving him plenty of fruit with a high water content, such as watermelon.

• Because your child may have difficulty in opening his or her mouth during a severe attack of mumps, drinks are best given through a straw, and foods should be passed through a blender. Soups and broths are also easier on the jaws than solid food, in addition to being more readily digestible.

SEEK PROFESSIONAL HELP

• If convulsions, a stiff neck or very severe headache develop.

• If vomiting occurs, especially if accompanied by pains in the abdomen.

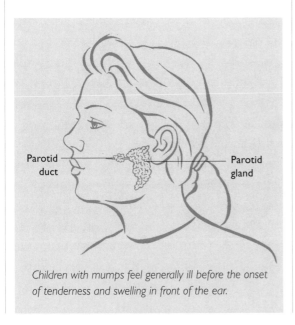

Children with mumps feel generally ill before the onset of tenderness and swelling in front of the ear.

Parotid duct

Parotid gland

• If there are any signs of visual disturbance or hearing problems.

• If your child seems severely unwell, weak or lethargic.

Alternative treatments

In cases of mumps it is quite appropriate to give the appropriate remedy to be taken internally, in addition to applying a topical preparation to the skin. However, if symptoms do not respond to self-help measures within a short space of time, or if you feel out of your depth, do not hesitate to seek the advice of a trained alternative practitioner.

Topical preparations

Tinctures, lotions or essential oils can be applied in compress form to ease inflammation and pain. Choose from any of the following, bearing in mind that none of the substances mentioned for application to the skin should be taken by mouth.

Aromatherapy oils

Using a warm flannel, apply hydrosol of chamomile or hydrosol of lavender to the affected area three times a day.

Herbal preparations

• A soothing compress may be made by saturating a soft cloth in warmed Hypericum oil and applying it to stiff, swollen and painful parts of the face.

• If chamomile tea is more readily available, this can also be used to make an effective warm compress. Steep the dried flower heads or a couple of chamomile tea bags in hot water. Leave for thirty minutes, strain and leave to cool until the liquid reaches a comfortably warm temperature. Soak a soft cloth in this solution and use as suggested above.

Medicines intended for internal use

These ease discomfort, reduce swelling and encourage a speedy resolution of the problem.

Herbal preparations

If your child is fractious and irritable when unwell, a few sips of soothing, warm chamomile and marsh mallow tea may help. Steep 28g (1oz) of each in 300ml (10fl oz) boiling water for ten minutes. Strain, cool slightly, and give a few sips to your child as often as required. To make the tea more palatable, try adding a little nutmeg, cinnamon or ginger as well as a teaspoonful of honey. (Honey should not be given to babies under one year old). If marsh mallow is not easily available, make the tea using chamomile alone.

HOMOEOPATHIC MEDICINES

Type	General features	Worse	Better	Remedy
Rapidly developing, severe symptoms with high temperature	Dry, bright red skin that radiates extreme heat. Severely sensitive, painful throat with badly inflamed glands that are worse on the right side. Extreme distress when swallowing: child has to bend forward when drinking. Irritability and bad temper when unwell	Jarring movement Being disturbed Becoming chilled Stooping Bright light Loud noise	Moderate warmth Sitting semi-erect in bed Peaceful surroundings	Belladonna
Slow onset of symptoms with general state of ill health	Terribly thirsty with dry skin, mouth and lips. Pain and swelling of glands made worse by movement of the slightest kind. Generally fractious, headachy and constipated with extreme drowsiness and lethargy	Becoming heated Sitting up Movement Making an effort	Perspiring Lying completely still Long, cool drinks Cool environment	Bryonia
Mumps with terrible stiffness and inflammation of the glands	Great difficulty in moving the jaw due to painful, enlarged glands: eating, drinking and talking cause great distress. Severe swelling and pain in the tonsils: irritating dryness at the back of the throat. Flushed and feverish with marked thirst. Jaborandi is suitable for complications of mumps in adult males	On the left side Perspiring Cold		Jaborandi
Stony, tense glands beneath the ear and jaw with mumps	Stiffness and tension in glands of the face and jaw make swallowing very distressing. Additional problem of dryness in throat also causes problems when eating or talking. Puffy, swollen appearance of uvula and tonsils	Warm drinks Warmth in general Cold and chill During the night	Moderate, stable warmth	Phytolacca
Lingering stage of mumps once fever has subsided	Strong, unpleasant metallic taste in mouth with excess saliva and enlarged tongue: child drools at night. Heavy sweats have an offensive odour: breath is also very smelly. Extreme discomfort, restlessness and anxiety at night	Sweating During the night Extreme fluctuations in temperature Becoming over-heated or chilled	Rest Moderate, stable temperatures	Mercurius

Nappy rash

Nappy rash can be the bane of a mother's and baby's life, since it may prove to be an extremely persistent problem. Generally speaking, it is best to treat nappy rash in its earliest stages in order to avoid the complication of a secondary infection setting in, which can make the condition much more intense. It is also sensible to try to get to grips with the problem when it is in its initial stages, since a well-established skin rash is always harder to treat than one that has recently emerged in a mild form.

Nappy rash can appear as a mild or extremely inflamed spotty rash that may cover the buttocks, thighs and genital area. A severe case can lead to the formation of raised red patches that become raw and sore during or after urinating or passing a stool. If white patches appear inside the mouth on the cheeks and/or the tongue, this suggests that your baby has developed oral thrush, which can spread throughout the digestive tract, leading to or aggravating nappy rash.

A mild bout of nappy rash may respond very well to the measures suggested below, but a well-established or severe episode of the problem is likely to require professional help and advice from a trained alternative practitioner. This is especially the case if your baby has a tendency to develop thrush or secondary infections.

Practical self-help

• Bathe or wash the infant regularly.
• Use a barrier cream on the affected area (any unscented moisture cream).
• Make a point of changing damp or soiled nappies frequently to avoid urine and faeces increasing sensitivity of the skin, making it feel extremely raw and sore.
• Allow the air to come into contact with the affected area by leaving your baby's nappies off at regular intervals. Although this can be inconvenient,

since some accidents are inevitable, it does encourage healing to take place by keeping the rash dry and aired. For the same reason, it is best to avoid putting plastic pants on your baby, since they can make the problem worse by keeping moisture in. It is best to try a variety of different combinations of disposable nappies and terry nappies with liners to discover the most comfortable combination. It is important to also dry the spotty area thoroughly after bathing and changing nappies.
• If you use washable nappies, always ensure that they are thoroughly rinsed after washing, so that no residue of soap powder is left that can irritate your baby's skin. Avoid using biological formulations that can aggravate sensitivity of the skin.
• If you have a thirsty baby, it is best not to rely too much on sweetened fruit juices. Apart from the general health problems associated with sugary drinks such as dental decay, sweetened citrus drinks are very acid-forming and can irritate an already sensitive skin.

SEEK PROFESSIONAL HELP

• If you suspect that a secondary infection has set in.
• If there are white patches in your baby's mouth.
• If severe nappy rash has led to the formation of sores or shallow ulcers.
• If your baby has not responded positively to self-help measures within a few days, or if he is subject to recurrent episodes of the problem.

Alternative treatments

For nappy rash it is quite appropriate to give the relevant internal remedy while also applying a soothing preparation to the skin.

Topical preparations

Tinctures, lotions, creams or ointments can be applied to the skin to soothe and heal. Choose from any of the following, bearing in mind that none of the substances mentioned for application to the skin should be taken by mouth.

Herbal preparations

• After each nappy change, bathe the inflamed area with an infusion of chamomile, thyme or lavender. Once the skin is quite dry, apply Calendula cream to soothe the area and promote healing. For dried herbs use 15g (½oz) to 600ml (1 pint) of water, for fresh herbs use 45g (1½oz) to 600ml (1 pint) of water.
• If you suspect your baby may also be suffering from thrush (see page 299), bathe the affected area

with a weak solution of cider vinegar and warm water. Alternatively, use an infusion of rosemary.

Home remedies

• Mild nappy rash may be eased by applying egg white to the affected area and leaving it to dry by exposing that part to the fresh air. By doing this, a protective covering may be formed that allows the skin to heal more rapidly.

• Distilled witch hazel can be soothing to irritated skin when applied with soft cotton wool.

• If thrush is an added complication, cool natural yoghurt may be applied to the skin to soothe and ease irritation. For maximum effect, this should be applied after swabbing the affected area with a dilute solution of cider vinegar and water. Use half a teaspoon of vinegar to a large cup of water.

Medicines intended for internal use

These reduce irritation, discomfort and inflammation.

Anthroposophical medicines

Calendula lotion can be very soothing when applied to nappy rash that is sore, inflamed or irritated. One teaspoonful of lotion should be added to a glass of boiled, cooled water and applied to the skin as often as required. It can also be used as a cool compress if the skin feels hot to the touch and looks red or angry.

HOMOEOPATHIC MEDICINES

Type	General features	Worse	Better	Remedy
Early stage of nappy rash with abrupt onset of symptoms	Extremely bright red, angry-looking spots that feel hot to the touch. Rash disappears as quickly as it emerged. Symptoms build in severity very quickly. Normally placid babies become fractious, restless and uncharacteristically irritable	Loud noise or disturbance Pressure to affected area Touch Jolting	Moderate warmth Rest Peace and quiet	Belladonna
Nappy rash in babies with poor-healing skin	Moist nappy rash in folds of skin around the buttocks and genital area. Itching and irritation are worse when baby becomes too warm. Skin problems may be combined with misshapen or poor-quality nails	Becoming too hot Chill Damp During the night	Affected area being exposed to fresh air	Graphites
Hot, burning nappy rash that is very sore after urinating	Rapidly developing, hot rash that causes great distress at night. Discomfort interferes with sleep: baby becomes difficult and drowsy during the day. Restlessness, irritability and hypersensitivity	Touch Urinating Becoming chilled Motion	Moderate warmth	Cantharis
Rosy-red, water-logged appearance to nappy rash	Shiny-looking, rather puffy nappy rash that is soothed rapidly by contact with cool air or cold compresses. Baby becomes extremely distressed when overheated. Fidgetiness, irritability and restlessness with discomfort	Touch Hot weather Warm bathing Rest Dampness Warm clothing	Cool air Cool bathing Cool compresses Undressing Motion	Apis

Biochemic tissue salts

Combination Remedy D may ease symptoms of mild nappy rash of recent onset. Crush tablets between two teaspoons until they become a fine powder and rub into your baby's gums. One tablet may be given in powdered form three to six times a day, tailing off the dosage as symptoms improve. If there is no improvement within a few days, it is worth considering a different alternative medical approach.

Herbal preparations

If your baby becomes distressed after passing a stool or urine, giving small amounts of chamomile tea between feeds may soothe and relax him.

If bouts of nappy rash are severe or beginning to occur on a recurrent basis, alternative help, treatment and advice may be obtained from practitioners of any of the following therapies:

- Anthroposophical medicine
- Aromatherapy
- Homoeopathy
- Naturopathy
- Western medical herbalism

Teething

Although some children have little problem when cutting their teeth, others can experience a range of problems from extreme pain, discomfort and inflammation of the gums to associated digestive upsets such as diarrhoea and loss of appetite. Teething can cause hours of misery for both babies and parents alike, often leaving the latter at their wits' end in their search for something that will provide comfort and relief from pain for their distressed child.

Problems are less likely to occur when the first teeth emerge (these are often referred to as milk teeth or incisors) during the first year. Common symptoms that may arise at this stage include a desire to gnaw or chew on something firm, as well as possible dribbling or drooling. However, the most difficult teething phase is usually around the ages of one and three when the first and second molars come through. These may cause more intense distress, with the following being common symptoms:

- Inflammation of the gums.
- Extreme tenderness of the affected area.
- Swelling of the cheek on the painful side.
- Irritability and weepiness.
- Listlessness or malaise.

Self-help measures plus alternative medical approaches can provide an excellent first resort for those who want to avoid resorting to sedative formulations when helping their child through the distress of teething.

However, if the decision of selecting an appropriate alternative approach proves to be an added stress in an already difficult situation, bear in mind that consulting a trained practitioner can diffuse a great deal of the tension. This is also a helpful option to consider if one or two alternative remedies have been tried without success.

Practical self-help

- Painful, inflamed gums can be soothed a great deal by contact with firm pressure. Simply rub the sore area gently, or encourage your baby to chew on a stick of cool carrot or one of the commercially produced biscuits that are designed for this purpose. The latter are very useful because they can be bought with an attached ribbon as a safety feature. This is especially important, since babies should always be watched when they are chewing on anything in order to minimize the potential risk of choking.
- Cool, hard objects are also soothing to sore, hot, swollen gums. Keep a clean flannel in the fridge for your baby to suck on when distressed, or try one of the teething rings with a cavity that can be filled with cold water.

SEEK PROFESSIONAL HELP

- If there is any tendency for your baby to pull or rub at one or both ears.
- If well-established or persistent catarrhal and/or digestive upsets occur in association with teething.
- If pain and discomfort are not significantly eased by using self-help measures.
- If your baby exhibits general symptoms of lethargy, listlessness or a general state of unwellness.

Alternative treatments

For teething it is quite appropriate to give the indicated internal remedy while also applying a soothing preparation to the gums or cheeks.

Topical preparations

Lotions, tinctures or oils can be applied to the inflamed area to soothe and ease pain. Choose from any of the following, bearing in mind that none of the substances mentioned for external use should be taken by mouth.

Aromatherapy oils

Add five drops of Roman chamomile (Chamaemelum nobile) essential oil to 50ml (1¾fl oz) jojoba oil and 'paint' the affected cheek three to four times daily when necessary.

Herbal preparations

• Rub a cooled infusion of catnip or chamomile tea into the inflamed or swollen area.

• Let your child chew on a piece of marsh mallow root, ensuring that you keep a close eye on them so that there is no risk of choking.

Medicines intended for internal use

These ease swelling, reduce inflammation and encourage a speedy resolution of the problem.

Anthroposophical medicines

A homoeopathic potency of chamomile root may be used to ease teething pains in children, especially if they are associated with digestive upsets. Give two pills hourly as needed, or, for very small babies, dissolve the pills in water and give by the teaspoonful.

HOMOEOPATHIC MEDICINES

Type	General features	Worse	Better	Remedy
Teething pains that are especially severe at night	Awful anxiety and restlessness: child screams frantically with intolerance of pain. Child wakes from disturbed sleep in a state of great distress. Pains and distress result in feverish state with hot head and chilled body	During the night Chill Becoming too hot Touch	Moderate warmth Sound sleep	Aconite
Abrupt onset of violent pain and high temperature with teething	Sudden and severe onset of symptoms with extremely bright red, hot, inflamed gums. Symptoms may be more severe on the right side with associated earache. Muscle jerks and spasms in sleep. Extreme irritability and bad temper when in pain	Jarring, sudden movement Touch Becoming chilled Noise Bright light	Lying propped up in a quiet, darkened room Moderate warmth	Belladonna
Frantic, howling and distracted with teething pains	Flushed with pain: one cheek red and the other pale. Colicky pains and loose, green-coloured stools when teething. Angry and frustrated with pain with no chance of being pacified. Throws toys around the room in frenzy	At night Becoming too hot Chill	Moderate temperatures Cool compresses Rocking or being carried	Chamomilla
Delayed, difficult teething with digestive problems	Teething, and other milestones such as walking and talking occur late. Poor stamina and weight problems from difficulty in assimilating calcium	Movement Physical exertion Making an effort	Comfortable warmth Warm bath Resting	Calc phos

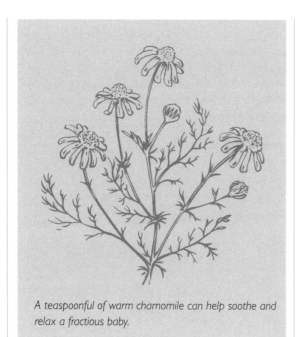

A teaspoonful of warm chamomile can help soothe and relax a fractious baby.

Flower remedies
A few drops of Rescue Remedy may be diluted in a small glass of water and a teaspoonful given as often as is needed to ease distress.

Biochemic tissue salts
Teething pains may be eased by using Combination Remedy R. Alternatively, tissue salt No. 2 may be of help where teething is slow and difficult, with a tendency for catarrhal complications as well. For severe, or acute symptoms, tablets may be taken at hourly intervals, while less distressing pains may be eased by taking four tablets three times a day, tailing off the dosage as symptoms improve.

Herbal preparations
A teaspoonful of warm chamomile or catnip tea may be given at regular intervals to soothe and relax a fractious baby.

Thrush

Although this is a condition that commonly occurs in adults, thrush is also an irritating problem that can affect the mouth or genital area in babies and small children. If your child suffers from oral thrush he is likely to develop sore, white or yellow patches inside the mouth and throat that look slightly raised. The symptoms of genital thrush, on the other hand, are likely to include itching, soreness and general sensitivity of the genital area, with an accompanying white or yellowish-tinged discharge that may resemble cottage cheese in appearance and have a slightly yeasty smell.

Thrush is most likely to arise as a problem after a course of antibiotic treatment, which can interfere with the delicate balance of bacteria in the mouth or the gut. Unfortunately, 'friendly' bacteria are often eliminated during a course of antibiotic treatment, in addition to the bacteria that may be causing infection. If this imbalance occurs, a situation is created where the yeast-like microbe *Candida albicans* can proliferate beyond the locations where it is usually kept in check, such as the gut. If this overgrowth occurs, the symptoms of oral or genital thrush may soon follow.

Practical self-help
• If you are breastfeeding and your baby is suffering problems with thrush, it is best to avoid foods that may make the situation worse. These include sugary foods and carbonated, sweetened drinks, alcohol and fermented products, mushrooms, cheese, pickles and items that contain vinegar, soy sauce, foods that include yeast in their production such as bread, malted items and dried fruit. Include live natural yoghurt and cold-pressed virgin olive oil in regular quantities in your diet. Also consider including supplements that are considered to have specific anti-fungal properties such as acidophilus, caprylic acid, a yeast-free vitamin B complex formulation and powdered garlic tablets.
• Contact with talcum powder, perfumed soaps and bubble baths may aggravate genital thrush. Use gentle, non-perfumed formulas where possible.
• Make sure that no residue of detergent is left behind after your baby's nappies or towels have been washed by rinsing extra thoroughly. Also make a point

of using unscented, non-biological washing powders.

• Try to keep the skin around the genital area as dry as possible by avoiding plastic pants, changing nappies frequently and leaving your child free of nappies for a short time each day to allow the skin to come into contact with fresh air.

• It is possible to avoid spreading infection by keeping your baby's towels separate from other members of the family.

• If the mouth is sensitive or painful as a result of oral thrush, give foods that are fairly bland, cool and nutritious, avoiding anything that is too hot or acidic.

• Breastfeeding mothers should wash their nipples in between feeds in order to avoid encouraging re-infection, and teats on bottles and dummies should also be thoroughly cleaned after use for the same reason.

• Drinks may be given more easily and comfortably through a straw to infants and toddlers who suffer with oral thrush.

SEEK PROFESSIONAL HELP

• If there are any indications of infection or pus formation.

• If your child has not responded to self-help measures, or if thrush symptoms are severe.

HOMOEOPATHIC MEDICINES

Type	General features	Worse	Better	Remedy
Thick white discharge with oral and genital thrush	Discoloured, patchy, 'mapped' tongue with white or grey coating: gums of breastfeeding babies may also be coated in white. Thick, sticky, bland discharge. Itching and discomfort is much more intense at night	Movement Draughts Chill Becoming overheated in bed Night Dampness	Rubbing Cool drinks	Kali mur
Thrush with thick, yellow discharge	Yellow-coated, swollen tongue with oral thrush. Genital thrush with irritating, burning, ropy discharge. Baby is very distressed by contact of clothing around the groin	Contact with cold air Washing Touch Movement Inhaling air	Pressure	Hydrastis
Thrush with alternating watery or thick discharge	Oral thrush with dry, cracked lips and corners of the mouth. Coated, white tongue. Genital thrush with discharge that resembles uncooked white of an egg. Itching, discomfort and irritation are intensified by becoming warm	Touch Heat Sunlight Being cuddled and made a fuss of	Cool bathing Contact with cool, fresh air Resting Rubbing Sweating	Natrum mur
Offensive, greenish discharge with oral and genital thrush	Oral thrush with unpleasant-smelling breath and increased saliva. Enlarged, flabby-looking tongue. Extreme itching with genital thrush that causes great distress and restlessness at night	After feeding Touch Becoming overheated Chill During the night	Moderate warmth Resting	Mercurius

- If your child seems unduly disturbed or distressed by symptoms of thrush.
- If thrush symptoms improve temporarily as a result of self-help measures, but recur on a regular basis.

Alternative treatments

For thrush it is quite appropriate to give the indicated internal treatment while also applying a soothing topical preparation to the skin.

Topical preparations

Lotions, tinctures or creams can be applied to the skin to soothe and heal. Choose from any of the following, bearing in mind that none of the substances mentioned for application to the skin should be taken by mouth.

Aromatherapy oils

A daily bath to which four tablespoons of crystal sea salt has been added is very helpful, or make a massage blend from four drops each of tea tree (Melaleuca alternifolia), lavender (Lavendula angustifolia), niaouli (Melaleuca quinqueneriva), thymus linalol and thymus thujanol added to four teaspoons of carrier oil or gel base. Use four times a day. If symptoms persist, seek the advice of a qualified aromatherapist.

Herbal preparations

Use Calendula lotion or dilute marigold tincture to soothe areas that are subject to irritation and soreness. Apply marigold lotion to affected areas by saturating pads of cotton wool, or swab irritated parts with diluted marigold tincture (one part of tincture should be added to ten parts of boiled, cooled water).

Home remedies

- Apply live natural yoghurt cool from the fridge to the areas affected by genital thrush, or rub it inside your baby's mouth for oral thrush.
- A solution of filtered cider vinegar and water may also be soothing when applied to irritated or sore areas. Add half a teaspoonful of cider vinegar to 150ml (5fl oz) boiled, cooled water.

Medicines intended for internal use

These ease irritation, reduce inflammation and ease discomfort.

If bouts of thrush are severe or beginning to occur on a recurrent basis, alternative help, treatment and advice may be obtained from practitioners of any of the following therapies:

- Anthroposophical medicine
- Aromatherapy
- Homoeopathy
- Naturopathy
- Nutritional therapy
- Traditional Chinese medicine
- Western medical herbalism

Travel sickness

Travel sickness (or motion sickness as it may also be called) can be brought on by the movement of a car, boat or plane. It is a most unpleasant condition that may affect adults as well as children, and can result in nausea, vomiting, disorientation and dizziness.

Practical self-help

- Always discourage reading while being driven in a car, since the combination of the movement and looking down may rapidly bring on feelings of nausea that end in vomiting.
- Looking out of the window at the horizon can reduce dizziness and nausea.
- Children may benefit from being distracted by playing verbal games. These can take their minds off travelling, while avoiding the visual concentration of reading.
- If the anticipation of a journey causes feelings of stress and anxiety, consider taking a short course of vitamin B complex in advance.
- Eat a light, non-fatty meal before travelling (avoid dairy products and fried foods). An empty stomach can intensify nausea.
- Exposure to fresh air can often ease nausea and provide relief after vomiting; always make sure that a car window is kept slightly open, or sit up on deck when travelling by boat.

Alternative treatments

For travel sickness, it is quite appropriate to give the relevant internal remedy while also using a topical preparation.

Topical preparations

Acupressure

Apply firm, steady pressure to the point just below the wrist (inside the wrist three finger widths from the centre of the wrist crease) with three fingers while breathing steadily and slowly in order to relieve nausea. High-street chemists sell towelling wrist bands with a plastic bead attached that are intended to press on the same point.

Medicines intended for internal use

These ease sickness, reduce dizziness and promote relaxation.

Biochemic tissue salts

If anxiety and 'nerves' are a problem when anticipating a journey, symptoms may be eased by taking Combination Remedy F. However, problems associated with sick headaches, nausea, vomiting or biliousness while travelling are more likely to be helped by

HOMOEOPATHIC MEDICINES

Type	General features	Worse	Better	Remedy
Travel sickness with sense of pressure around the head	Nausea is made extremely intense by the slightest movement. Vomiting with excess of saliva and drenching sweats. Awful faint, sinking feeling in stomach. Confused and disoriented with travel sickness	Slightest movement Opening eyes Extreme heat or cold	Cool air Bathing face with cool flannel Uncovering the abdomen Vomiting A good cry	Tabacum
Travel sickness with extreme prostration and chilliness	Nauseating headache with travel sickness. Violent retching with headache and excessive amount of saliva. Becomes very faint when nauseated or sick. Terrible sensitivity to smell of food	Movement Jarring Lack of sleep Stooping Chill Open air Exertion	Indoors Sitting still	Cocculus
Travel sickness with great difficulty in raising vomit	Nauseating headache with travel sickness: pain lodges at the back of the head or over one eye. Chilly and trembly with nausea. Sense of sickness is immediately eased after vomiting. Irritable and oversensitive when unwell	Chill Dry, open air Smell of coffee or tobacco Touch or pressure of clothes Yawning	Having a nap Rest Humid air Warm drinks	Nux vomica
Travel sickness with marked dislike of open air	Nausea is made more intense by hunger or not having something to eat before a journey. Vomiting of green, bitter bile. Giddiness with travel sickness that is felt at the back of the head. Fearful when sick	Movement Cold weather Pressure of clothes Becoming angry	Contact with warm air	Petroleum

Combination Remedy S. Tablets may be taken hourly if symptoms are severe, or three times a day if the situation is less pressing. Always remember to tail off the dosage as soon as there is any indication of improvement setting in.

Herbal preparations

Give your child warm water to sip to which a slice of lemon or fresh ginger root has been added. (If fresh ginger is not available, crystallized ginger may be of help in an emergency.)

Flower remedies

Rescue Remedy may help a great deal with distress or anxiety in anticipation of a journey, or actual distress when travelling. A few drops may be added to a small amount of cold water and sipped as often as required, or a drop or two can be taken on the tongue in an emergency.

Whooping cough

Whooping cough is an extremely contagious viral illness that has an incubation period of approximately one to two weeks. It begins with symptoms that are rather like those of the common cold, including feverishness, runny nose, general malaise and the first signs of a cough. The illness may be distinguished from a cold by the way symptoms do not subside after four or five days, but become more severe as time goes by.

By the second stage of illness your child is likely to have a thick nasal discharge and a distressing cough. By the end of an episode of coughing the characteristic whooping sound is usually heard as your child becomes short of breath. This may also be combined with a tendency to vomit, especially if a meal has been eaten just before a severe bout of coughing has begun. This symptom is the result of the lungs being clogged with thickened mucus that can only be brought up with great effort.

This phase of the illness is likely to cause anxiety in both child and parents, since the child's face may become very flushed due to the effort of coughing, or may also become tinged with blue from lack of oxygen. Any sort of stimulus may aggravate or bring on a coughing bout, such as running, being in a smoky atmosphere, laughing or talking.

The last phase consists of a residual, low-grade persistent cough that may last anything from three to six months. By this stage, however, overall symptoms should have diminished a great deal in severity and frequency.

Generally speaking, it is best to seek the advice of an alternative practitioner if your child is diagnosed as suffering from whooping cough, because it can be an extremely severe illness in young children, often requiring skilled and experienced case management.

Practical self-help

• Above all, it is important to try to reassure your child as much as possible during coughing bouts by talking in as calm and soothing a way as possible. If fear and panic are communicated to your child in what is already a very frightening situation, this can have a negative effect of intensifying your child's feelings of terror and helplessness. Calm reassurance in this situation can help your child relax sufficiently to get over his panic and distress, thus giving a better chance of the coughing bout being over more quickly.

• If your child tends to vomit during a severe or protracted episode of coughing, try to encourage him to eat soon after a coughing bout. By doing so, he has a greater chance of keeping food down than if he eats just before coughing and breathlessness begin. It is also helpful to make sure that the foods offered are as appetizing, light and easily digestible as possible.

• Do not be tempted to give your child a cough suppressant. Although the cough can be very alarming, it fulfils an important function by expelling mucus from the lungs. If this reflex is suppressed, the lungs can become clogged with mucus, making matters worse as breathing becomes increasingly difficult.

• Avoid giving cows' milk products to your child, since they have a tendency to increase mucus production, while also being difficult to digest because of their high saturated fat content. Sugary foods and drinks should also be avoided because of a similar tendency to promote extra mucus.

• If your child feels too unwell to eat, make sure

that fluid intake is kept high by giving plenty of drinks (avoiding milk and sweetened, carbonated drinks for the reasons given above).

• Make sure that babies' faces are kept unobstructed during a coughing bout so that they are able to cough freely. Patting their backs gently while they are held firmly over your knees on their stomachs may also be helpful. Toddlers and young children may also feel comforted by sitting upright on your knees with your hand placed firmly in the small of their back.

SEEK PROFESSIONAL HELP

• If whooping cough symptoms develop in a baby of less than six months old.
• If there are any indications of wheezing, laboured or accelerated breathing.
• If your child complains of chest pain.
• If there are additional symptoms of confusion, drowsiness or severe headache.

Alternative treatments

If there are any signs that your child is not responding to self-help treatment, seek the advice of a trained alternative practitioner without delay.

Medicines intended for internal use

These reduce congestion, ease anxiety and encourage a speedy resolution of the problem with the minimum amount of complications.

Biochemic tissue salts

Episodes of spasmodic, convulsive coughing may be eased by Combination H. The recommended dose for toddlers is two or three tablets three times a day, while older children may be given four tablets three times a day until symptoms improve. Once improvement is forthcoming, the tablets should be tailed off. If no improvement has occurred after using the combination for a few days it is worth considering another alternative approach.

Herbal preparations

• A soothing tea for the chest may be made by infusing 28g (1oz) of thyme in 600ml (1 pint) of hot water. Leave to steep for half an hour, strain, and give warm, sweetened with honey. (Honey should not be given to babies under one year old). Older children may take a tablespoonful four times a day, while infants may be given one teaspoonful of the sweetened tea per day. (However, it is good to be aware that infusions of thyme should be avoided in pregnancy.)

• If your child has been put off eating because of recurrent vomiting as a result of whooping cough, he may benefit from a little powdered slippery elm mixed to a paste with warm water: a little honey may also be added in order to make the mixture more palatable.

Home remedies

• Simmer a washed head of lettuce in 600ml (1 pint) water for approximately half an hour. Strain and give a few sips of the liquid to your child as often as required.

• Slice 450g (1lb) onions and 225g (8oz) garlic finely and place in a covered dish with 600ml (1 pint) sunflower oil. Bake slowly in the oven until the mixture takes on a soft consistency. Once this point has been reached, strain the liquid off and discard

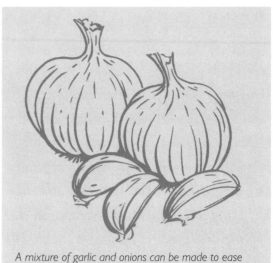

A mixture of garlic and onions can be made to ease bouts of whooping cough in children over two years old.

the onion and garlic pieces. Add 150ml (5fl oz) honey to the flavoured oil and place in a clean glass container with lid. This mixture may be used for children over the age of two, giving a teaspoonful three times a day until coughing bouts improve.

• If your child's stomach is generally sensitive and disordered due to vomiting after coughing spasms, a few sips of grape juice can be very soothing to the digestion.

• Inhaling the steam that rises from sliced garlic floating in a bowl of hot water may ease irritated chests. However, always make sure that your child is supervised when using any inhalant that involves very hot water to avoid the possibility of burns and scalds occurring.

HOMOEOPATHIC MEDICINES

Type	General features	Worse	Better	Remedy
Whooping cough with awful rattling in the chest from excess mucus	Severe congestion in the chest with great effort in expelling mucus during a coughing spasm: child bends backwards while trying to cough up phlegm. Breathlessness before episode of coughing with vomiting afterwards. Needs to sit up in order to breathe more freely	Milky drinks Lying flat Exposure to chill or overheating Motion Fits of anger	After vomiting Sitting upright Expelling mucus Belching	Ant tart
Episodes of coughing with whooping cough that begin as soon as the child goes to bed	Cold sweats, nosebleeds and vomiting accompany distressing coughing bouts. Spasmodic cough is triggered by a sensation of irritation in the throat: it feels as though a crumb is lodged there. Extended bouts of coughing and choking with whooping cough	Lying down Heat After midnight Eating cold food Speaking Singing Stooping Laughing	Contact with fresh air Firm pressure	Drosera
Whooping cough with coughing spasms triggered by stuffy rooms	Awful sensitivity to any feeling of slight irritation in the throat. Swallows all the time in order to rid the throat of mucus. Coughing spasms result in child's face becoming purple-red in colour: ends in vomiting up clear, stringy, sticky mucus	Touch Pressure of clothes Irritation of throat Rinsing mouth Brushing teeth Lying down Warmth	Cool bathing Walking Cool drinks	Coccus cacti
Whooping cough with spasmodic bouts of coughing following each other in quick succession	Unpleasant smothering sensation precedes coughing bout that ends in vomiting stringy mucus. Episodes of coughing begin after eating. Unstable body temperature when unwell: child is overheated when covered, too cold when covers are removed	Change of temperature Inhaling Eating	Steady warmth	Corallium rubrum
Whooping cough with severe bouts of breathlessness that lead to collapse	Episodes of harsh, dry cough quickly become loose and productive. Distressing episodes of coughing with extreme difficulty in breathing: child becomes pale, clammy and exhausted. Craving for fresh air with marked dislike of stuffy rooms	Lack of fresh air Becoming overheated Warmth Speaking	Being fanned Contact with open, fresh air Undressing or loosening clothes After sleeping	Carbo veg

PROBLEMS OF AGEING

Fluid retention

Fluid retention (otherwise referred to as oedema) often arises as a secondary symptom of another medical problem such as coronary heart disease (see pages 334-5), pre-menstrual syndrome (see pages 194-8) or varicose veins (see pages 321-4). It may also develop as a side effect of taking certain drugs, such as lithium, or occasionally the condition may arise in the absence of any obvious cause or trigger.

Symptoms may include any of the following:
- Weight gain.
- Puffy ankles, wrists and fingers.
- Swelling of the thighs and lower back.

If fluid retention becomes a noticeable or persistent problem it is important to seek professional medical advice to establish the nature of the underlying cause. In addition, some of the following practical suggestions may ease a tendency towards the problem.

Practical self-help

- Include regular portions of potassium-rich foods in the diet, since these encourage the body to rid itself of excess fluid. Suitable items include salads, vegetables, raw fruit and freshly squeezed juices.
- Avoid salting meals and eating too many convenience foods that rely on salt as well as a range of other chemical flavourings to produce strong tastes that are considered appetizing. This is important because sodium encourages the body to conserve water. Use a range of fresh herbs instead to make food taste interesting.

HOMOEOPATHIC MEDICINES

Type	General features	Worse	Better	Remedy
Fluid retention with lack of thirst	Puffiness is at its most marked on waking. Affected areas feel taut: swellings look rosy-pink and waterlogged. Marked sensitivity to warmth with fluid retention	Overheated rooms Warm drinks Touch After waking	Contact with cool air Cool bathing Undressing Movement	Apis
Fluid retention that affects the feet in particular	Extreme restlessness and chilliness with fluid retention. Feet become very puffy and swollen. Uneasy feeling with 'restless legs'. Weary, numb feeling in feet	At night Cool conditions Watery fruit and vegetables Alcohol Physical effort	Warmth Warm drinks Gentle movement Sweating	Arsenicum album
Fluid retention with craving for salt	Imbalanced body fluids lead to alternating dryness and overproduction of mucous membranes. Nasal discharges run like a tap, while vaginal dryness can be very severe	Becoming overheated Overexposure to sunlight After a period Emotional stress Touch	Fresh, cool air Cool bathing Sweating Massaging affected area Peace and quiet	Natrum mur

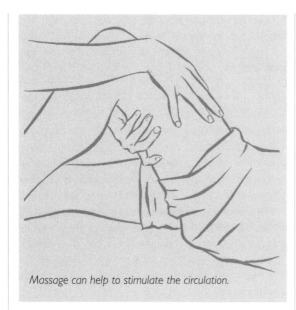
Massage can help to stimulate the circulation.

• If sluggish circulation is a problem, elevate the legs when resting, and make a point of taking regular, gentle exercise, such as walking, on a daily basis as this will ensure proper functioning of the pump action of the calf muscles.

SEEK PROFESSIONAL HELP

If fluid retention is becoming an increasingly severe or established problem.

Alternative treatments

Medicines intended for internal use
These reduce the severity and frequency of the problem.

Home remedies
• Add plenty of fresh parsley as a flavouring to food, since it is an excellent natural diuretic (it encourages the body to rid itself of excess fluid). **NB** This should be avoided if fluid retention occurs in pregnancy.
• Add dandelion leaves (also a diuretic) as an extra green ingredient in salads.
Alternative help, treatment and advice may be obtained from practitioners of any of the following therapies:
• Anthroposophical medicine
• Aromatherapy
• Ayurvedic medicine
• Biochemic tissue salts
• Homoeopathy
• Massage therapy
• Naturopathy
• Nutritional therapy
• Reflexology
• Shiatsu
• Traditional Chinese medicine
• Western medical herbalism

Hot flushes

Hot flushes can affect a large percentage of women as they go through the menopause, and although they need not be a serious problem, many people find them extremely distressing. The severity of hot flushes can vary enormously: a significant percentage experience great discomfort, while others are hardly affected at all.

Certain common symptoms are associated with hot flushes:
• Abrupt and violent waves of heat that wash over the whole body, or are restricted to the head, torso and face. During a flush the skin may become burning hot and deep pink in colour, especially if fresh air is in short supply.
• A vague, indefinable feeling of foreboding or anxiety preceding a hot flush, especially if prone to night sweats. Those who experience night sweats may wake seconds before it occurs, becoming rapidly burning hot and drenched in perspiration once the hot flush sets in. This may occur repeatedly during the night, leaving the sufferer exhausted on waking from poor-quality sleep.
• Panic attacks may also precede or accompany hot flushes. These are likely to be made worse by fear or embarrassment when discomfort is obvious to others.
• Drenching, uncontrollable perspiration accompanying or following a hot flush. This can be one of the most unpleasant symptoms because of the weariness, nausea and chill that remain once the flush has gone.
• Dizziness and headaches.
   The practical self-help measures listed below may be all that is needed to provide a great deal of relief if mild flushes occur on an irregular basis. However,

severe and frequent hot flushes within the context of additional menopausal symptoms are far more likely to be substantially improved during treatment by an alternative medical practitioner.

Practical self-help

• Always wear loose layers of clothing made from natural fibres, such as cotton, linen or silk, that allow the skin to breathe in preference to synthetic fibres, which tend to keep heat in. By wearing layers of clothing, such as a baggy T-shirt under a loose-fitting jacket or cardigan, we can easily remove the top layer if we begin to feel uncomfortably hot. This can be especially helpful when we are not in a position to regulate our surrounding temperature to suit ourselves.

• Night sweats can also be made less traumatic by choosing very loose cotton nightwear. Make a habit of keeping some fresh, dry nightwear by the bedside as well as a towel, sponge and bowl of water, so that you can have a quick sponge down and put on fresh nightwear with the minimum of fuss if a night sweat has occurred.

• If anxiety and panic attacks accompany hot flushes, you can derive great benefit from learning how to relax through an appropriate form of meditation or relaxation technique. Once you can switch on your ability to relax in a stressful situation, you may become liberated from anxiety, and suddenly feel empowered in a situation that previously left you feeling powerless, fearful and totally vulnerable. There is further information on meditation and breathing techniques on page 238.

• Regular, rhythmic exercise can also play a positive role in easing hot flushes, improving circulation and enhancing energy levels as well as improving your sense of well-being. To be most effective, your chosen activity should be vigorous enough to produce a mild sweat, but not to make you breathless (you should be able to conduct a conversation while exercising). Make sure that whatever activity you select does not feel like a chore, but is something that is enjoyable and fun to do.

• Hypoglycaemia (low blood-sugar level) may aggravate your symptoms. In order to keep blood-sugar levels stable, it is best to eat small amounts every couple of hours, rather than leaving long gaps between meals. Avoid items that are likely to give you a sugar 'rush', and see pages 325-6 in the weight gain section for advice on healthy eating. If you are unsure

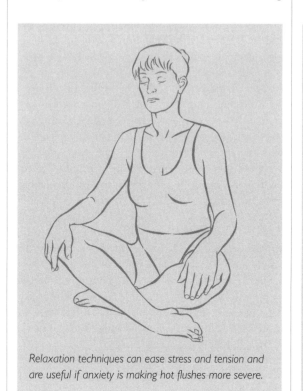

Relaxation techniques can ease stress and tension and are useful if anxiety is making hot flushes more severe.

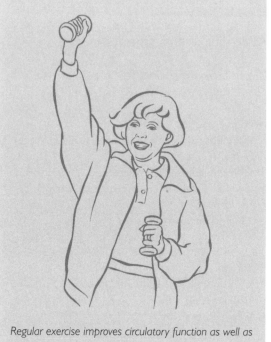

Regular exercise improves circulatory function as well as stimulating energy levels and vitality.

whether erratic blood-sugar levels are a problem for you, the following checklist will give an idea of the most common symptoms:

- Erratic energy levels with short-lived bursts of energy after eating, rapidly followed by drowsiness and tiredness.
- Sleepiness and lack of concentration.
- Confusion.
- Rapid or severe changes of mood.

SEEK PROFESSIONAL HELP

If hot flushes are persistent, severe or frequent within the context of other severe menopausal symptoms.

Alternative treatments

Topical preparations

These include essential oils that can be used in

HOMOEOPATHIC MEDICINES

Type	General features	Worse	Better	Remedy
Severe hot flushes that move in waves of heat through the body	Flushes are brought on by feeling too hot and constricted: especially if clothing is too tight around the neck or waist. Wakes from sleep into symptoms. Hot and bothered during the day, and chilly and clammy at night. Emotionally volatile and unstable with violent mood swings	On waking During the night Tight clothes Badly ventilated surroundings Hot drinks Before a period	Loose clothing Gentle movement Contact with fresh, cool air Cool drinks Eating small amounts often Once a period begins	Lachesis
Hot flushes that are especially severe for becoming heated in bed at night	Awful sensitivity to heat that causes rapid overheating alternating with severe chill. Must push feet out of bedcovers at night in order to cool down. Although skin is burning, it remains dry rather than sweaty. Strong desire to rest during flushes to recover	Standing Overexertion Warmth of bed Stuffy surroundings Becoming chilled Bathing Waking from sleep	Moderate temperatures Rest Lying down	Sulphur
Hot flushes that move in waves from chest to the head	Marked sensitivity to heat around the head which makes the distress of flushes much more severe. Pressured feeling in the head with dizziness and nausea. Anxiety, panic and palpitations occur with flushes as well as an unpleasant sense of disorientation and confusion	Alcohol Movement Warmth Severe chill Bending the head backwards	Keeping as still as possible Exposure of the face and head to fresh air	Glonoine
Flushes with pulsating sensations that move quickly from one part of the body to another	Sensation of heat is localized on the face, ears, neck, hands or feet. Face becomes flushed with pink, rosy circles on cheeks. Recurrent one-sided headaches with menopausal symptoms	Humidity Exertion Chill Touch During the night	Uninterrupted sleep Resting	Sanguinaria

soothing baths and massage to relax and diffuse stress. Choose from any of the following, bearing in mind that none of the substances mentioned for application to the skin should be taken by mouth.

Aromatherapy oils

Adding three drops of Roman chamomile (Chamaemelum nobile), lavender (Lavendula angustifolia) and/or geranium to a bath of warm water can prove helpful.

Medicines intended for internal use

These reduce anxiety, improve well-being and encourage a speedy resolution of the problem.

Biochemic tissue salts

Hot flushes linked to anxiety and nerviness may be eased by tissue salt No. 6. Take four tablets three times a day, or hourly if symptoms are severe.

Herbal preparations

• Hot flushes may be eased by drinking an infusion of sage and motherwort: use a teaspoonful of each herb to a cup of boiling water. Sage should also only be taken for a maximum of a week or two at a time because of the toxic effects of the volatile oil it contains called thujone.

• Hot flushes linked to anxiety and general exhaustion may respond to oriental ginseng. However, the use of ginseng should be avoided in the early stage of acute inflammatory diseases (such as tonsillitis or pharyngitis), since there is a danger that the disease may be driven deeper into the body, leading to additional complications.

• Some doctors will prescribe a product called phytoesterol that contains a combination of extract of hops and rhubarb root. These phytoesterol-rich botanicals appear to reduce the distress of menopausal symptoms such as hot flushes and vaginal dryness in a significant percentage of women.

Home remedies

• Add 75g (3oz) of fresh sage to a bottle of red wine and leave to stand for two weeks. Sweeten to taste with honey, strain and take a liqueur glassful each day to ease night sweats and act as a general tonic.

• Use plenty of chopped mint in cooking and salads.

• Vitamin E capsules have a reputation for easing the misery of hot flushes. Approximately 400IUs should be taken daily, provided there is no history of high blood pressure.

Professional alternative medical help may be obtained from any of the following:

• Anthroposophical medicine
• Aromatherapy
• Ayurvedic medicine
• Biochemic tissue salts
• Homoeopathy
• Naturopathy
• Nutritional therapy
• Reflexology
• Shiatsu
• Traditional Chinese medicine
• Western medical herbalism

Lowered or absent libido

Many people are uneasy about the onset of middle age primarily because of the attendant physical and emotional changes that have a reputation for diminishing the frequency or quality of sexual relationships. Although it is true that certain negative physical symptoms may arise as we get older, it is also important to point out that there is a positive dimension to the ageing process that can enhance the quality of physical relationships. Freedom from the anxiety of unwanted pregnancy, the ability to dispense with contraceptive measures that may have hampered a spontaneous sex life and the increased privacy that occurs once children have left home are a few of the bonuses that may emerge in middle age.

Many people gain increased emotional and sexual confidence in their middle years, becoming more frank or vocal about emotional and sexual needs and preferences. Depending on the quality of your relationship with your sexual partners, this may enhance your sex life. If unresolved emotional strains and conflicts exist, they often find expression in sexual problems, which may emerge with particular strength and vigour in middle age or earlier. If this is the case, joint counselling may help you as a couple identify and come to terms with the underlying causes of emotional conflict.

There are many potential reasons for diminished libido that may include any of the following:
• Long-term or severe depression.
• General fatigue, boredom or lack of physical, emotional or mental energy.
• Painful intercourse from vaginal dryness.
• Lack of self-esteem or self-confidence.
• Relationship problems.
• Lack of communication.
• Side effects of conventional drugs used to treat high blood pressure, allergies or depression.

Alternative approaches can be helpful in treating problems of this nature because of their holistic perspective, which lays great importance on the need to treat physical, mental and emotional problems as part of a greater picture. When they are effective, alternative medicines bring about an enhanced state of well-being and harmony that stimulates libido in its broadest sense (a fundamental sense of vitality and zest for life).

If your symptoms occur infrequently, are mild in nature or are of recent onset, an appropriately selected alternative remedy when used in combination with positive changes in lifestyle may be enough to rectify the situation, but always bear in mind that herbal, biochemic or homoeopathic remedies should not be needed on a long-term basis to maintain an improvement. If this has become necessary, it is best to seek professional advice from a trained alternative practitioner.

Practical self-help
• Consider how much stress you have to deal with on a daily basis. When stress levels are high, sexual appetite and drive is usually the first aspect of our lives to suffer. If anxiety, stress or general tension is a problem, see the chapter on psychological and stress-related conditions for helpful advice on positive strategies for coping.
• Some women are dismayed to find that they uncharacteristically lose interest in or develop an aversion to lovemaking during or after the menopause.

This may happen because of the physical discomfort that may accompany intercourse in the post-menopausal years if the walls of the vagina have become thinned or dry. See the section on vaginal dryness (pages 319-21) for further advice.
• It is helpful to be aware that certain prescription drugs may contribute to problems with impotence or lowered libido. These include beta blockers (drugs used to reduce and stabilize raised blood pressure), some antidepressants and antihistamines. Undergoing surgery that affects the genital area such as hysterectomy may also have an adverse effect on sex drive. If there are viable alternatives to these medical options, it is worth discussing the problem with a sympathetic family doctor.
• Evaluate the quality of your diet and make a point of including nutrients that have a reputation for preserving a healthy libido. These include zinc, which can be obtained from the following foods: oysters, herrings, whole grains, seafood, nuts and seeds and the B complex group, from nuts, whole grains, green, leafy vegetables, fish, yeast extract, soya flour, bananas and brown rice.
• If lowered libido is the result of long-standing emotional problems between you and your partner, counselling may be very helpful in enabling you both to come to terms with the root of the conflict. A counsellor can encourage couples to identify areas of discord in their relationship, thus providing the opportunity to work through these problems in a supportive, non-judgmental emotional environment.
• Lack of pleasure or interest in lovemaking is a frequent symptom of depression. If you suspect that you may be suffering from more than transient depression it is worth consulting your family doctor or alternative health practitioner. See the section on depression (pages 243-4) to identify symptoms.
• Locating and toning the muscles of the pelvic floor can increase sexual pleasure for both partners. In women these muscles can be identified and exercised by stopping and starting the flow of urine by a series of controlled muscular contractions (Kegel exercises).

SEEK PROFESSIONAL HELP
• If lowered libido is persistent, severe or accompanied by symptoms of depression.
• If lowered libido is experienced as a side effect of taking conventional medication.

Alternative treatments

Medicines intended for internal use

These improve energy levels and restore optimum levels of libido.

Alternative help, treatment and advice may be obtained from practitioners of any of the following therapies:

- Anthroposophical medicine
- Aromatherapy

HOMOEOPATHIC MEDICINES

Type	General features	Worse	Better	Remedy
Apathy and indifference with loss of libido	All-pervasive sense of physical and mental exhaustion. Poor concentration and feeble memory as a result of profound tiredness. Weak, relaxed sensation in genital area	Sitting Intercourse Emotional strain Talking Cold draughts	Warmth Short sleep	Phos ac
Lack of self-confidence and diminished sense of self-esteem with low libido	Adopts a domineering and sarcastic manner as a way of concealing insecurity. Burning discomfort in vagina during or after intercourse. Weak erections with related prostate problems	Anticipatory anxiety Stress On waking Eating Digestive discomfort	Stable, moderate temperatures Mental distraction and occupation Gentle exercise in the fresh air Passing water	Lycopodium
Marked aversion to intercourse with absent libido	Depressed, miserable and unhappy with absolute avoidance of sexual activity. Hot, dry, uncomfortable sensations in vagina with thin, gushing vaginal discharge. Absent or premature ejaculation	Warmth of bed At night Contact with cold Exertion and effort	Touch Eating After walking in the fresh air	Graphites
Deep depression with irritability or total indifference to sexual partner	Profoundly, hopelessly depressed with seriously lowered sex drive. Emotional and domestic demands feel overwhelming with resulting anger, irritability and exasperation shown to family members. Hypersensitivity, soreness and itchiness of genital area	Emotional demands and responsibilities During or following the menopause Sitting still Standing Following intercourse	After a sound sleep Vigorous aerobic exercise Fresh air Eating little and often	Sepia
Loss of libido following Caesarean delivery or surgery to genital area	Powerful feelings of violation or humiliation following surgical procedures or invasive tests affecting the genital organs. Awful sensitivity of genital organs with sharp, stinging pains on least touch or pressure. Recurrent cystitis after intercourse	Slight touch or contact Pressure Emotional stress Intercourse	Warmth Rest After eating	Staphysagria

- Ayurvedic medicine
- Homoeopathy
- Massage therapy
- Naturopathy
- Nutritional therapy
- Shiatsu
- Traditional Chinese medicine
- Western medical herbalism

Prostate problems

The prostate is a chestnut-sized gland wrapped around the urethra (the tube that carries urine from the bladder). Because of its location and its tendency to enlarge from middle age onwards, many men find that they experience discomfort and problems with urination as they get older, due to the pressure exerted on the urethra from the swollen gland.

Although younger men can suffer extreme discomfort as a result of inflammation of the prostate (prostatitis), the following problems are more likely to occur in older men:

Benign prostatic hypertrophy (BPH) is often diagnosed in men over the age of forty-five. This condition arises as a result of enlargement of the prostate gland, resulting, in most cases, in problems in passing water. The likelihood of the condition arising increases proportionally with age, with the result that by the age of sixty, 60 per cent of men can expect to experience symptoms of the condition while 70 per cent of seventy-year-olds are likely to be vulnerable to these problems, and so on.

Any of the following may occur as a result of BPH:

- Weak or feeble stream of urine.
- Hesitancy or delay in starting to pass water.
- Starting and stopping in flow of urine.
- A sense of incompleteness after passing water.
- Straining to pass water.
- Dribbling or incontinence of urine.

If irritation of the bladder occurs as a consequence of trying to force the urine beyond the obstruction caused by the enlarged prostate, the following symptoms may arise in addition:

- Discomfort when urinating.
- A powerful sense of urgency in the desire to pass water.
- An increase in the frequency of urination that is especially marked at night.

The risk of developing **cancer of the prostate** appears to increase with age, with the result that it is now a major cause of deaths from cancer in men over the age of fifty-five. However, screening methods have not been shown to have any benefit in reducing the number of people getting the disease, or dying from it.

Factors that may influence the incidence of prostate cancer, the symptoms of which are the same as for BPH, include:

- Hereditary influence: men who have a close relative who has suffered from prostate cancer (a father or brother) have three times a greater risk of developing the condition than others. The risk for those whose more distant relatives have been diagnosed with this condition is six times greater than for a man who has no relatives with the problem.
- Dietary factors may also have a bearing on whether someone is susceptible to developing symptoms of cancer of the prostate or not. Although the incidence of prostate cancer is virtually the same in Chinese,

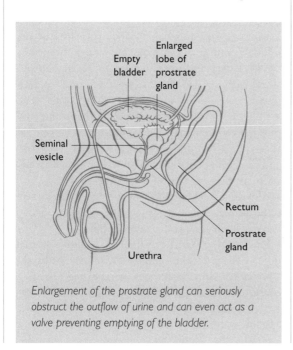

Enlargement of the prostate gland can seriously obstruct the outflow of urine and can even act as a valve preventing emptying of the bladder.

Japanese and American males, the disease is more likely to progress to a point where symptoms become clinically significant in Western males. However, if Japanese men move to the West, their risk of becoming vulnerable to clinical signs of prostate cancer increases within two generations, to the point where it becomes equivalent to the average American male. It has been suggested that one of the environmental factors that may be responsible for this shift is the Western diet.

Symptoms of advanced cancer of the prostate may include any of the following:
- Anaemia.
- Loss of weight.
- Swollen glands.
- Traces of blood in the urine.
- Tiredness.
- Reduced appetite.
- Pain in the bones.

In younger men, **prostatitis** (inflammation or infection of the prostate) may occur. Males between twenty and fifty years of age are likely to be most at risk of developing this problem. Symptoms include any of the following:
- A general sense of malaise or feeling unwell.
- Pain in the lower back, genital organs and thighs.
- Aching between the thighs and genital area or deep pain that radiates between the scrotum and anus.
- Pain on ejaculation.
- Frequent desire to pass water.
- Discomfort or difficulty when urinating.
- Discharge from the urethra, especially after intercourse.

Problems may arise as a result of acute infection (for example, a bacterial infection that travels from the intestines to the urinary system) or may be established as a chronic problem with or without signs of infection. The use of anabolic steroids also increases the risk of developing prostate cancer.

Practical self-help
- A diet that is high in fibre and low in saturated fat appears to be a positive factor in discouraging problems with the prostate gland. Research suggests that the more saturated fat is included in the diet, the higher the chances of developing advanced prostate cancer become. The most problematic foods appear to be red meat, creamy salad dressings, mayonnaise and butter. However, benign fats may be obtained from essential fatty acids in walnuts, pumpkin and sunflower seeds and linseeds, and it has been estimated that everyone should eat at least 30g (approximately 1oz) of these a day.
- A high proportion of vegetables should be included in the diet because of the fibre and zinc content. Zinc has been identified as playing a positive role in controlling the sensitivity of tissues of the prostate to sex hormones, and the prostate may swell due to a decline in the male sex hormones. Vegetables are also valuable because the fibre in them absorbs excess male hormones excreted through bile in the digestive tract.
- Orange, red, yellow and green vegetables are also tremendously important because of their high antioxidant enzyme content. Antioxidants play a vital role in controlling the proliferation of free radicals that can wreak havoc in the body because of their possible association with premature ageing, heart disease and cancer. Because of their potential ability for minimizing the damage that free radicals can cause, antioxidant enzymes have been claimed as vital allies in protecting against cancer and coronary heart disease. The relatively low proportion of vegetables eaten by the average Western male when compared with his Eastern counterpart is regarded as one of the reasons why more advanced symptoms of prostate malignancy appear in Western males.
- Ingredients that are to be found in Far Eastern cuisine, such as soy, rice, kohlrabi and Chinese leaves, are rich in weak plant hormones that may interact with natural male hormones to protect against enlargement of the prostate. As a result, it is worth making an effort to include some of these items in the diet on a regular basis.
- Omit red meat where possible, substituting with pulses, whole grains, skinless chicken and fish. Fish is particularly important because of the potential anticancer benefits fish oil may have, which also protects the health of the circulatory system.
- Although keeping fluid intake up is important, avoid drinks that may irritate the situation further, such as strong tea, coffee and alcohol.
- Pain and discomfort may be eased by using alternating warm and cold compresses, or sitz baths that stimulate circulation in the pelvic area and encourage improved tone of the muscles in this region. To experience a sitz bath, run a comfortably hot bath with enough water to cover the lower half of the body around the hip and pelvic area (around

40°–46°C/104°–115°F) while preparing a basin of cold water. Begin by sitting for half a minute in the hot water, moving to the cold for three seconds. Move from warm to cold water in this way three times, finishing off with the cold. To avoid getting chilled, always ensure that the bathroom is adequately warm, and keep the rest of the body warmly covered. **NB** This technique is best avoided by those who suffer from circulatory problems or high blood pressure.

• Taking exercise is also thought to benefit prostate problems by increasing general circulation. Consider forms of movement that encourage muscular strength and awareness such as yoga, or general activities that encourage brisk movement of the circulation such as walking in the open air.

SEEK PROFESSIONAL HELP

• If symptoms of BPH (see page 313) appear.
• If there are any traces of blood in urine or semen.
• If you experience pain on ejaculation.

HOMOEOPATHIC MEDICINES

Type	General features	Worse	Better	Remedy
Enlarged prostate with dribbling of urine	Discomfort and dribbling of urine are made more intense in bed by lying down. Constant desire to pass water when resting. Interrupted flow: urine stops and starts fitfully from narrowing of urethra	Lying down At night After eating Foods that are high in fat such as pork or cream Overheating	Gentle exercise Standing erect Contact with fresh, open air	Pulsatilla
Enlarged prostate with thin stream of urine that takes a while to pass	Incomplete urination with a troublesome sensation as though a drop of urine constantly remains in the urethra. Frequent desire to pass water with profuse amount of urine or scanty flow that is voided drop by drop. Burning sensation in urethra when not urinating	Sexual activity Touch After urinating When not urinating Surgery to affected area	Rest Warmth	Staphysagria
Inflammation of the prostate with dribbling of urine from coughing or sneezing	Spasmodic pains that extend from genital organs to thighs. Pain and discomfort may only affect or be more intense on the right side. Passing urine is very difficult and painful. Symptoms are aggravated by lying on the back	Contact with cold draughts Coffee Alcohol Stress Lack of exercise Pressure of clothes	Wrapping up warmly Having a nap or resting Lying on the side	Nux vomica
Inflammation of the prostate with stream of urine that is very slow to start	Strains a lot to start passing water. Urine looks murky with deposits that look like sand or gravel. Dribbling of urine when stressed or suffering from anxiety. Frequent desire to pass water is aggravated by movement of travelling	Pressure of tight clothes Overheating On waking Anticipatory anxiety	Gentle exercise in the fresh air Cool compresses When urinating Being distracted from thinking about pain and discomfort	Lycopodium

• If unexplained tiredness, malaise, swollen glands or a general feeling of being unwell develop.
• If weight loss occurs for no obvious reason.
• If aching or discomfort develop in the genitals, thighs, lower back or lower abdomen.
• If urgency or frequency of urination develop in a marked way.

Alternative treatments

For prostate problems it is perfectly appropriate to take the relevant internal remedy while also making use of a topical preparation.

Topical preparations

These include herbal infusions that may be added to bathwater to soothe discomfort and aching.

Herbal preparations

A strong infusion made up of equal parts of the following herbs may be added to a sitz bath (described on page 314): horsetail, couch grass, bearberry and juniper. To make the infusion add 50g (2oz) mixed herbs to 600ml (1 pint) water.

Medicines intended for internal use

These ease pain and reduce inflammation.

Biochemic tissue salts

Problems in retaining urine may be eased by biochemic tissue salt No. 11, while a frequent urge to pass water may respond to No. 2. However, a constant urge to urinate may be more appropriately treated by using tissue salt No. 8. Acute symptoms may require temporary treatment at hourly intervals, while more low-grade or ongoing problems may be better suited to tablets taken three times a day until symptoms improve.

Herbal preparations

The following herbs may reduce the discomfort of an enlarged prostate and ease problems with difficult flow of urine: couch grass, horsetail or saw palmetto. Backache associated with prostate problems may also be eased by infusion of golden rod. However, symptoms that are suggestive of an enlarged or inflamed prostate should be prescribed for by a trained herbalist, and you should also seek conventional medical screening to establish the nature and extent of the problem.

Alternative help, treatment and advice may be obtained from practitioners of any of the following therapies:

• Anthroposophical medicine
• Aromatherapy
• Homoeopathy
• Naturopathy
• Nutritional therapy
• Traditional Chinese medicine
• Western medical herbalism

Stress incontinence

Stress incontinence occurs as a result of weakening and loss of tone of the pelvic floor muscles that support the base of the bladder. In women this slackening may occur due to pregnancy and labour (especially if two or three pregnancies have occurred close together), or may be a part of the general process of ageing. As women become older, the ligaments that support the womb begin to lose their tone and tension. When this happens, the womb tends to sag or droop. This is a very common condition called prolapse of the uterus. If the uterus is protruding from the vagina it is called a procidentia, but this is very rare. In either case the sagging alters the mechanisms that produce the 'anatomical valve', leading to its failure and the leakage of urine — stress incontinence.

Common symptoms of stress incontinence include the following:
• Involuntary leaking of urine when laughing, coughing, sneezing, jogging, jumping or lifting heavy weights.
• A persistent sensation of needing to urinate, even when the bladder is empty.
• If stress incontinence is accompanied by a prolapse

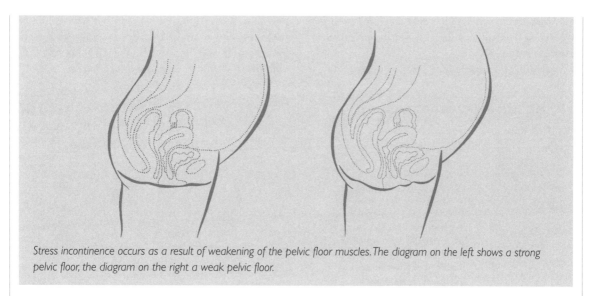

Stress incontinence occurs as a result of weakening of the pelvic floor muscles. The diagram on the left shows a strong pelvic floor, the diagram on the right a weak pelvic floor.

of the womb, there may also be a persistent back-ache and/or difficulty passing water.

Stress incontinence is not a serious problem, but can be embarrassing and frustrating enough to adversely affect the quality and enjoyment of life. Feeling a constant need to pass water or having to wear incontinence pads when exercising can make life less carefree than it should be. However, there are ways of coping with the problem that may improve the situation greatly by putting the sufferer more in control. If symptoms are mild, not associated with a prolapse and occur on an infrequent basis, the self-help measures suggested below may do a great deal to ease the problem. However, if the condition is more severe, it is important to consult a trained practitioner.

Practical self-help

• Exercising the pelvic floor muscles can help ease problems associated with stress incontinence. These muscles may be identified by consciously stopping and starting the flow of urine at will. Once this feels familiar, it will become possible to contract and relax these muscles at other times (sitting at a desk, when driving or watching television). By doing these exercises (sometimes known as Kegel exercises) on a routine, daily basis, the muscles should gradually increase in strength and tone.
• Avoid exercise that involves repetitive pounding, jarring movements on a hard surface, such as jogging or high-impact aerobics. To keep fit, concentrate instead on exercises such as brisk walking, cycling or

swimming that condition the heart and lungs. Yoga postures can also help by encouraging you to become familiar with the strengths and limitations of your body, while also promoting improved muscle strength and tone.
• If stress incontinence is a problem, being overweight can make things worse. Avoid crash dieting or faddy weight-loss plans that are unlikely to encourage you to keep to a healthy weight in the long run, and see pages 325-6 in the weight gain section for advice on sensible weight loss. Eating a healthier, higher-fibre diet will also discourage constipation. Straining at passing a stool can complicate problems with stress incontinence by weakening the muscles of the bladder.
• Where possible, avoid standing for lengthy periods of time and attempt to spend some time each day resting with the feet elevated on a stool.

SEEK PROFESSIONAL HELP

• If the need to urinate is urgent or frequent.
• For severe or persistent symptoms.
• If a prolapse of the womb has occurred.
• If previously mild symptoms begin to deteriorate rapidly.

Alternative treatments

Topical preparations
Herbal preparations
A strong infusion of any of the following herbs may be added to the bathwater in the form of tincture or

infusion: beth root, golden seal and horsetail. **NB** Golden seal should not be taken during pregnancy.

Home remedies

Circulation and muscle tone can be improved in the pelvic area by taking alternating hot and cold sitz baths. To take a sitz bath at home, make sure your bathroom is warm and fill one large bowl with comfortably hot water, and another with cold

HOMOEOPATHIC MEDICINES

Type	General features	Worse	Better	Remedy
Stress incontinence with vaginal dryness	Involuntary dribbling of urine when walking or coughing, but flow is slow to start when urinating at will. General slackness and lack of tone of pelvic muscles. Severe lack of vaginal lubrication leads to avoidance of intercourse. Depressed, antisocial and withdrawn with a marked dislike of sympathetic company	Coughing Sneezing Physical exertion Walking Lying down	Cool, fresh air Gentle motion Peace and quiet Firm pressure to lower back Crossing legs when sitting down	Natrum mur
Stress incontinence with heavy sensation in bladder	Frequent, urgent desire to pass water when anxious. Leaking of urine with sensation of paralysis and weakness in the bladder. General feeling of aching, weakness, and heaviness of muscles leads to permanent desire to lie down	Chill Anticipatory anxiety Overheating Physical overexertion	Fresh air Passing copious quantities of urine	Gelsemium
Stress incontinence with marked discomfort in bladder when lying down	Involuntary dribbling of urine when asleep. Discomfort when walking or resting. Problems with stress incontinence often date from childbirth. Discomfort leads to weepiness and a strong need for sympathy and attention	At night In bed Stuffy, overheated surroundings Resting	Gentle exercise in the fresh air Firm pressure Undressing	Pulsatilla
Gradual, insidious onset of stress incontinence	Involuntary escaping of urine when asleep during the first half of the night. Lack of awareness of even large quantities of urine escaping from bladder when sneezing or coughing. Overwhelming desire to lie down from muscular weakness	Bathing Travelling Coffee Cold, draughty conditions	Warmth Warm, humid weather	Causticum
Frequent need to empty bladder with bearing-down sensation	Disturbed sleep from frequent desire to pass water at night, or urine may leak out involuntarily. General state of exhaustion with sagging, drooping muscles. Lack of libido with depression and general lack of interest in life	Walking Standing for long periods of time Emotional demands	Vigorous, aerobic exercise in the fresh air Warmth In bed Sitting supporting the pelvis with legs crossed	Sepia

water. Sit in the hot water, making sure that it covers the pelvic area, while soaking your feet in the bowl of cold water. Stay like this for three minutes, then sit in the bowl of cold water with your feet in the warm water for a minute. Alternate the treatment like this twice or three times, always ending with your feet in cold water. To avoid getting cold, cover the top half of your body well while bathing the abdomen and feet. **NB** Do not take hot and cold sitz baths if you suffer from high blood pressure or heart problems.

Medicines intended for internal use

These encourage improvement of the problem when combined with additional changes in lifestyle.

Herbal preparations

If symptoms of stress incontinence are aggravated by a tendency to urinary infections, consumption and infusion of horsetail may soothe irritation. Use 28g (1oz) dried herb to 600ml (1 pint) boiling water.

Professional alternative medical help may be obtained from any of the following:
- Anthroposophical medicine
- Biochemic tissue salts
- Homoeopathy
- Naturopathy
- Traditional Chinese medicine
- Western medical herbalism

Vaginal dryness

This troublesome problem commonly occurs as a result of lack of sexual arousal or after the menopause or radiotherapy, and is caused by a thinning of vaginal mucous membrane and loss of lubricating capacity. It occurs after the menopause because the flow of blood to the breasts, clitoris, vagina and vulva that occurs during sexual arousal decreases as we get older. Since this rush of blood is necessary to maintain the suppleness of the mucous membranes of the vagina, once the flow begins to diminish we are likely to become subject to dryness, irritation and infection of the vagina.

Common symptoms of vaginal dryness include the following:
- Pain and discomfort during lovemaking.
- Cracking and bleeding of the walls of the vagina.
- Persistent or recurrent vaginal infections resulting in irritation and itching.

Although these symptoms may sound extremely depressing, it is important to bear in mind that there are practical steps that can improve the situation beyond the use of conventional drugs such as hormone replacement therapy (HRT). Adopting a positive strategy can help preserve an active and pleasurable sex life by reducing or eliminating physical discomfort.

Practical self-help

- The use of strongly scented soaps, vaginal deodorants and soaking for a long time in foam baths should be avoided, since these can aggravate a tendency to vaginal irritation and discomfort.
- If vaginal irritation and general inflammation are a problem, it is important to avoid wearing tight nylon underwear, or close-fitting jeans, leggings or tights that create a humid, warm, environment around the genital area, which encourages vaginal infection and irritation. To discourage this vicious cycle, choose cotton, loose-fitting underwear most of the time, and only wear tight trousers or jeans for a limited period during the day, making sure that the rest of the time is spent in loose, airy clothes.
- Regular sexual activity encourages and maintains lubrication and suppleness of the genital area. Achieving orgasm, with the associated rush of blood and muscular contraction, also plays an essential part in maintaining moisture and flexibility of the vagina. If persistent vaginal dryness makes intercourse less than appealing, making liberal use of a lubricating jelly can do a great deal to ease the situation.

SEEK PROFESSIONAL HELP
- If vaginal dryness is becoming a persistent feature of life.
- If vaginal irritation or inflammation occurs on a regular basis.

• If there is a sign of bleeding from the walls of the vagina after lovemaking.

Alternative treatments

If vaginal dryness occurs, it is quite appropriate to take the relevant remedy internally while also applying a topical preparation to the skin.

Topical preparations

These include lotions, tinctures or creams that can be applied to the skin to soothe and reduce inflammation. Choose from any of the following, bearing in mind that none of the substances mentioned for application to the skin should be taken by mouth.

Herbal preparations

• If vaginal soreness and discomfort are severe, bathing in diluted Calendula or a mixture of marigold and Hypericum tincture will do a great deal to restore comfort to the genital area and discourage the development of infection.

• In addition, a general sensation of vaginal soreness may be soothed by applying Calendula cream to the inflamed area.

• Comfrey oil or ointment soothes vaginal irritation and soreness, as well as encouraging damaged tissues to heal.

Home remedies

• If the vagina feels irritated, inflamed or itchy, apply-

HOMOEOPATHIC MEDICINES

Type	General features	Worse	Better	Remedy
Vaginal tenderness with complete lack of interest in sex	Severe itching and irritation with dryness of the vagina that is aggravated when walking. Discomfort in vagina may be intensified by prolapse of womb and bladder. Complete lack of interest in sex and indifference to sexual partner	Sitting still Touch Emotional demands and pressures	Firm pressure Resting in a warm bed Napping Aerobic exercise in the fresh air	Sepia
Vaginal dryness and discomfort that follow an early menopause caused by a hysterectomy	Painfully sensitive and itchy genital area with stitch-like, stinging pains. Discomfort is much more intense when sitting down. Suppressed anger and resentment with pain	Touch Intercourse Emotional stress Stretching	Warmth Rest	Staphysagria
Vaginal dryness and irritation with a tendency to dry, flaky skin	Dryness and burning of the vagina that is aggravated during and after intercourse. Poor circulation leads to hot flushes and inability to tolerate extremes of heat or cold. Anxiety with digestive problems including heartburn, indigestion and flatulence	Extreme heat or cold Overexertion to the point of exhaustion On waking Pressure of restricting clothes	Moderate temperatures Loosening garments Being distracted or occupied	Lycopodium
Sore, stitch-like pains with severe vaginal dryness that are made much more intense by movement	General state of dryness of skin and mucous membranes with associated problems of stubborn constipation. Burning, irritated feeling in urethra when not urinating. Irritable and short tempered when suffering discomfort	Initial movement after resting (e.g. when rising from a sitting position) Overheating The slightest movement	Keeping as still as possible Cool locally applied	Bryonia

ing liberal amounts of cool, natural yoghurt can do a great deal to make the situation easier.

• A dessertspoonful of common salt added to the bathwater eases vaginal soreness and inflammation, while the equivalent measure of vinegar will discourage irritation.

• Vitamin E oil applied to the vagina encourages lubrication, eases soreness and encourages cracked tissues to heal.

Medicines intended for internal use

These ease soreness, reduce inflammation and irritation.

Herbal preparations

A combination of any of the following may be made into an infusion or decoction: motherwort, marigold, hops, blue cohosh and false unicorn root. These herbs have a balancing effect on female hormones, maintaining oestrogen levels and discouraging adverse vaginal changes. Use 28g (1oz) dried herb (or 50g/2oz fresh) for every 600ml (1 pint) boiling water.

Professional alternative medical help may be obtained from any of the following:

• Anthroposophical medicine
• Ayurvedic medicine
• Homoeopathy
• Naturopathy
• Nutritional therapy
• Traditional Chinese medicine
• Western medical herbalism

Varicose veins

Varicose veins can be an inherited problem, often occurring more commonly in women than men. They develop their characteristic ropy appearance as a result of excess blood seeping into the superficial veins of the legs. These vessels contain valves that work by normally preventing the back-flow of blood into the veins. However, when these valves become less efficient at their job, the increased accumulated back-flow of blood in the vessels leads to the superficial veins becoming twisted, mottled and knobbly in appearance.

Specific factors that may lead to an increased susceptibility to this condition include:

• Being pregnant or recently having given birth.
• Carrying excess weight.
• Standing for long periods of time.
• Doing a sedentary job which involves very little exercise.

We may experience mild, moderate or severe problems with varicose veins that may include any of the following symptoms:

• Alternating aching, throbbing or itching of the skin surrounding or covering the affected vein.
• A swollen, bluish distended appearance to the veins that may be especially noticeable when standing. Vessels most commonly affected are likely to be in the groin, thigh, calf or ankle.
• Feet and ankles that swell at night or swelling and aching of the whole leg.
• Varicose ulcers. These form when the skin surrounding the distended varicose vein becomes inflamed and broken down.
• More noticeable pain, irritation and discomfort of varicose veins leading up to or during a period.

Infrequent or minor problems of this nature may respond well to the general advice given below, in combination with appropriate alternative self-prescribing. However, if varicose veins have arisen as a result of deeper-seated circulatory problems or if varicose ulcers are a severe problem, it is vital to seek help from an alternative practitioner who will attempt to improve the overall situation rather than concentrating on treating isolated symptoms.

Practical self-help

• Support tights or stockings can be useful in providing extra support for varicose veins, easing the aching and discomfort a little. However, if you have a tendency to varicose veins always avoid wearing hold-up stockings, the elasticated tops of which put extra pressure on the upper thigh. Clothes that are extremely tight-fitting around the hips should also be avoided for the same reason.

• Whenever possible avoid standing for extended

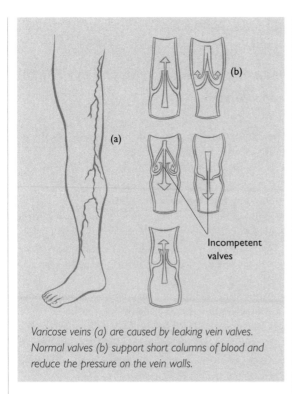

Varicose veins (a) are caused by leaking vein valves. Normal valves (b) support short columns of blood and reduce the pressure on the vein walls.

Incompetent valves

periods of time, and get out of the habit of sitting with crossed legs: try crossing your ankles instead, which puts less pressure on your veins.
• Make a point of resting with your feet raised so that your legs are positioned slightly higher than your body. In this way, swollen, aching veins may feel a little more comfortable.
• Because a tendency to constipation can aggravate varicose veins and lead to haemorrhoids (varicose veins of the rectum and/or lining of the anus) it is very important to ensure that plenty of fibre is eaten on a daily basis. See the sections on haemorrhoids and constipation for further advice (pages 169-71 and 162-5).
• Deep breathing has a beneficial effect on the circulatory system in general and on varicose veins in particular. See the section on anxiety for a description of diaphragmatic breathing (page 238).
• Regular exercise conditions and protects the health of the circulatory system as the veins rely on the pressure provided by the contraction of muscles in the legs to propel the blood through the valves in the blood vessels back to the heart.
• Some nutrients have a reputation for improving the condition of the circulatory system, and as a result, can ease problems with varicose veins. These

nutrients include vitamins C, B_3 and E. Rutin is also important to strengthen the walls of the weakened veins, and may be obtained in supplement form or can be taken in the form of buckwheat.
• If a varicose ulcer develops, make sure that the skin is kept scrupulously clean and cover the affected area with a sterile dressing.
• The profuse bleeding caused by a cut to a varicose vein can be stopped by lying down and lifting the affected part above the level of the heart. A firm dressing can then be applied without any panic.

SEEK PROFESSIONAL HELP
• If pain is persistent or very severe in a varicose vein.
• If brownish discoloration of the skin occurs where circulation is poor.
• If the leg is swollen and aching, especially if the aching is not relieved by rapid elevation.
• If ulceration of the skin develops.
• If the skin over a varicose vein is damaged from a blow or injury and the measures suggested to stop the bleeding in the 'Practical self-help' section (above) do not help. This can result in severe blood loss that requires urgent medical attention to contain the problem.

Alternative treatments
For varicose veins it is quite appropriate to take the relevant remedy internally, while also applying a topical preparation to the skin.

Topical preparations
These include lotions, tinctures, ointments or creams that can be applied to the skin to soothe inflammation and encourage rapid healing. Choose from any of the following, bearing in mind that none of the substances mentioned for application to the skin should be taken by mouth.
Aromatherapy oils
Always seek advice from a qualified aromatherapist and, when given a blend to help, always 'paint' the area affected, never rub the oils in.
Herbal preparations
• Varicose ulcers may respond very well to the application of marigold cream after bathing the area of broken skin with diluted Hypericum and Calendula tincture. Add one part of tincture to ten parts of boiled, cooled water and bathe the inflamed or ulcerated area with this soothing, healing solution.

HOMOEOPATHIC MEDICINES

Type	General features	Worse	Better	Remedy
Constricted sensation in veins with severe discomfort	Bruised, prickling pains with varicose veins and a possible tendency to develop chilblains.	Jarring Movement Touch Pressure Chill During the day	At night	Hamamelis Hamamelis is the most appropriate remedy to consider if specific, characteristic individualizing symptoms are not present
Widespread varicose veins that affect the arms, legs, groin and genitals	Itching, burning pains and a tendency to easy ulceration with varicose veins. Burning pains are eased by contact with cool air and compresses. Cramping, pulsating pains in calf muscles that are especially severe at night. Recurring varicose ulcers bleed easily	Warmth Moist heat Stuffy, airless conditions Becoming chilled Movement	After a good night's sleep Cool, fresh air Being fanned	Carbo veg
Purple, distended veins that may be worse on the left side	Extremely sensitive varicose veins that are uncomfortably heat-sensitive. Discomfort may move from the left to right. Pounding, bursting, throbbing in varicose veins. Movement eases aching and discomfort	Restrictive, tight clothing Keeping still Becoming overheated After sleep During or after the menopause	Cool compresses Contact with cool air Gentle movement Onset of a discharge	Lachesis
Right-sided varicose veins with shifting, changeable pains	Poor circulation with a tendency to chilblains and very cold hands and feet. Varicose veins are aggravated by sitting or standing and eased by gentle exercise. Depressed and weepy when veins are aching and uncomfortable	Becoming chilled or damp Rest Becoming too warm Warm bathing or compresses Heavy clothing or bedcovers	Cool compresses Cool, fresh air Gentle movement Firm support Undressing	Pulsatilla
Extremely painful varicose veins that are sensitive to the touch	Awfully restless legs with a tendency to swollen feet. Constantly moves about in effort to get into a comfortable position. Bruised, aching pains that make the legs feel stiff and tired	Jarring Effort Touch After sleep Cold, damp conditions	Lying with the head lower than the body	Arnica

Calendula cream applied after the diluted tincture can promote efficient and speedy healing of ulcerated skin.
• **NB** Although Arnica may be an appropriate internal remedy for treating symptoms of varicose veins, never apply it in cream form to broken or ulcerated skin since it can intensify inflammation and discomfort of damaged tissue.

Home remedies
• Use alternating hot and cold water to bathe the legs, making sure that you always end with cool water. Although using alternating temperatures of water for bathing in this way is said to improve the circulation, this technique should be avoided by anyone who suffers from high blood pressure or a heart disorder who may find the technique too stimulating.
• A compress of marigold heads may soothe the aching and irritation of varicose veins. In order to make the compress, soak a clean length of soft cloth or gauze in a warm or cooled infusion of marigold (Calendula). Apply it to the affected area and leave it in place as long as it feels soothing or until it has cooled down or warmed up (depending on whether it started off as a warm or cool compress).
• Cool witch hazel may be very soothing when applied to inflamed, aching or very swollen varicose veins.

Medicines intended for internal use
These ease pain, irritation, distension and swelling.
Biochemic tissue salts
General problems with poor elasticity of walls of the blood vessels leading to a history of varicose veins, haemorrhoids or varicose ulcers may respond to tissue salt No. 1. Alternatively, tired, aching legs from varicose veins may be eased by the combination formula Elasto. Either formulation may be given in tablet form three times a day until symptoms show signs of improvement. Once this occurs the dosage should be tailed off.
Herbal preparations
An infusion of hawthorn, yarrow or rosemary can improve circulation and ease the discomfort of varicose veins. To make the infusion add a cup of hot water to a teaspoonful of dried herb. Leave to stand for fifteen to twenty minutes, strain and take three times a day as a hot drink. (**NB** The use of yarrow should be avoided in pregnancy.)
Home remedies
• Foods that may improve sluggish circulation, strengthen blood vessels and aid in the elimination of excess fluid should be included in liberal amounts in the diet. They include citrus fruit, grapes, blackcurrants, spinach, parsley, dandelion and green cabbage. Garlic can also have a positive effect on the circulatory system.
• Lemon juice may be soothing when applied neat to painful or inflamed areas.

Alternative help, treatment and advice may be obtained from practitioners of any of the following therapies:
• Anthroposophical medicine
• Aromatherapy
• Ayurvedic medicine
• Homoeopathy
• Naturopathy
• Nutritional therapy
• Traditional Chinese medicine
• Western medical herbalism

Weight gain

While unwanted weight gain is not exclusively the province of older people, many of us are dismayed to find that although we were able to stay slim in our youth regardless of the amount we ate, once we reach middle age this is no longer the case. This may be due to changes of metabolism that occur after childbearing, or to a general decrease in activity, as, although we are eating the same as before, fewer calories are used, so weight rises.

Establishing how to maintain an optimum weight will vary from one person to another. Generally speaking, subjective impressions can be of more use than relying on charts or tables that offer suggestions of ideal weights. In other words, if your clothes feel uncomfortably tight or you are experiencing the symptoms below, the chances are that you need to take positive action to rectify the situation. However, if you weigh more than the ideal weight for your height suggested by a table, but feel perfectly healthy and comfortable, you may not need to take radical steps as a result.

Symptoms that suggest weight loss may be needed include any of the following:
• Breathlessness when climbing a couple of flights of stairs at a reasonably brisk pace.
• Laboured or difficult breathing after running a short distance.
• Clothing that feels uncomfortably tight or restrictive after a short time.
• Visible signs of excess weight developing on upper arms, hips, thighs or belly.

Apart from making you feel uncomfortable or less confident about your physical appearance, being genuinely overweight can also be linked to a host of potentially serious health problems, including an increased risk of diabetes, heart disease, hypertension (high blood pressure), varicose veins and arthritis. Certain patterns of fat distribution may also have adverse effects on the circulatory system. Research has suggested that a tendency to deposits of excess fat around the stomach and waist points to a greater risk of developing heart disease than for those who carry extra weight on the hips and thighs.

If weight gain has become a problem, seeking help from an appropriate alternative practitioner may be helpful in improving the overall situation. Although it would be misleading to suggest that instant solutions to the weight-loss problem can be provided, it is fair to point out that some alternative practitioners are likely to be able to provide very sound, useful advice about appropriate changes in lifestyle that may help solve the problem. In addition, some alternative medicines may be able to stimulate the whole system to regain an optimum state of balance and harmony, with the possible additional benefit that a recently sluggish metabolism may be stimulated back to its previously vigorous state.

If you have a long-standing weight problem, it is best to seek professional medical help. However, the self-help suggestions may assist you while professional advice is being sought.

Practical self-help
• Firstly, honestly evaluate the quality and quantity of your diet. It is very easy to underestimate the amount of food you eat by relying on general subjective impressions alone. Try the following experiment, and you may be surprised at the results: make

a note of each item of food consumed over a forty-eight-hour period, including all drinks and snacks. Once the results are examined, it may come as a surprise to find that you are eating far more frequently and in larger quantities than you realized. It may also come as a shock to discover that food quality is lower than expected, especially if you have a tendency to snack on crisps, sweets or biscuits.
• It is very important to establish a good-quality eating plan if weight loss is a priority. Foods with a low nutritional status and which contain large amounts of white sugar, flour, preservatives, colourings and flavourings leave us unsatisfied and eager for more. This is particularly true of items containing a large proportion of refined white sugar, such as cakes, biscuits or puddings. Once the craving for sugar has been temporarily satisfied, there is a brief feeling of comfort. However, this is likely to be extremely short lived, rapidly leading to further cravings for more sweet foods, and so the vicious circle continues. If this cycle is established, it is common to be overweight and undernourished, since refined sweet foods provide 'empty' calories that are very low on the scale of nutritional value. However, wholefoods such as grains, pulses, vegetables, fruit and small portions of chicken or fish are far more effective at keeping hunger pangs and cravings at bay, while improving health and promoting weight loss.
• Exchange high-fat, processed foods for fresh ingredients that are high in fibre, vitamins and minerals. Avoid full-fat cheese, cream, butter, margarine, fried or battered items, and convenience foods high in hidden fats and sugar. High-fibre foods that should become a mainstay of your eating plan include regular portions of salad, raw or steamed vegetables, fresh fruit, brown rice, unroasted nuts or seeds and home-made soups incorporating a wide variety of vegetables and pulses. Avoid adding mayonnaise to salads, using a little cold-pressed olive oil and vinegar or live natural yoghurt instead.
• If fluid retention is contributing to a weight problem, avoid 'instant' meals that often contain a high level of sodium as well as a host of other additives and preservatives. Salt should also be removed from the table at mealtimes, since herbs and spices can be relied on to prevent food becoming bland or uninteresting.
• Drastically reduce or even eliminate alcohol from your diet while you are trying to lose weight. Drink

sparkling mineral water instead, with a twist of lemon or lime, or a carbonated soft drink made from fruit juice and herbal flavourings. Avoid diet colas or low-calorie squashes that contain artificial colourings and sweeteners such as aspartame or saccharin.

• Try to eat when there is time to relax and enjoy a meal, rather than eating on the run, when reading or when watching television. Apart from causing unpleasant symptoms such as indigestion, these habits can also lead to overeating or a sense of feeling unsatisfied after a meal. Snacking in the evening when watching television is also a bad idea, since it is easy to lose track of what you've eaten.

• Establish whether you are eating in response to genuine hunger pangs or because there is nothing better to do. Many of us have forgotten to listen to the signals our bodies send us informing us that we are hungry, often mistaking boredom or depression as a need for food.

• Above all, avoid faddy or extreme diets that can aggravate a well-established weight problem. 'Yo-yo' dieting that involves moving rapidly from one extreme diet to the next results in a tendency to put on weight rather than lose it. This happens because the body goes into starvation mode when food intake is reduced, slowing the metabolic rate to make the most of the limited fuel available. As a result, you are likely to lose weight in the initial phase of strict dieting, but will find it increasingly difficult, and weight gain will be rapid once you begin to eat normally again.

• Regular exercise is an important ally in a weight-loss plan. Making time to cycle, take a brisk walk or swim every day, conditions the heart and lungs and stimulates the metabolism. When this is combined with a low-fat, low-sugar, high-fibre eating plan, healthy weight loss should be the result.

• Many people think that regular exercise is likely to increase appetite, thereby encouraging weight gain rather than weight loss. However, the reverse is actually true, since exercise temporarily suppresses appetite, so you should not feel hungry again for a little while after exercise. It is also important to bear in mind that you should wait an hour or two after eating before embarking on any strenuous activity.

• Finally, it is especially important to be realistic about your own optimum weight. Women in particular may attempt to reach an unrealistic body weight once they have reached middle age. It is good to bear

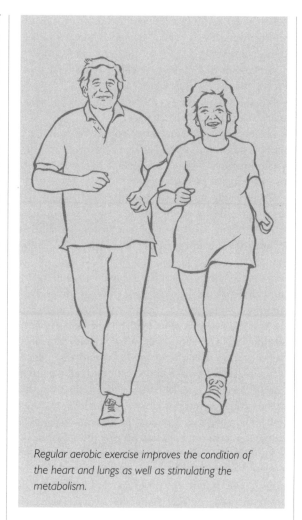

Regular aerobic exercise improves the condition of the heart and lungs as well as stimulating the metabolism.

in mind that there are some advantages to not being underweight, since you are more likely to suffer menopausal symptoms if you are too thin.

SEEK PROFESSIONAL HELP

• If marked weight loss or weight gain have occurred suddenly and for no obvious reason.
• If obesity is a severe, well-established problem that is resistant to sensible self-help measures.

Alternative help, treatment and advice may be obtained from practitioners of any of the following therapies:
• Anthroposophical medicine
• Ayurvedic medicine
• Naturopathy
• Nutritional therapy
• Western medical herbalism

CRONIC CONDITIONS

AIDS and HIV

AIDS (acquired immune deficiency syndrome) was first diagnosed in the early 1980s in the United States and HIV (the human immunodeficiency virus) is known to have been carried by humans since the 1950s. Fierce debate has raged over the question of whether or not infection with HIV is responsible for causing AIDS. It has been strongly argued that once HIV has been passed on through unprotected sexual intercourse or sharing needles for injecting drugs, full-blown AIDS is likely to develop within a predictable period of time. For this reason, testing for potential AIDS consists of determining whether someone is HIV positive. If an HIV-positive diagnosis is made, any conventional medical intervention tends to be delayed until symptoms of AIDS begin to appear.

However, a body of opinion has developed that maintains that HIV does not inevitably lead to death from AIDS. A significant number of patients with HIV have survived without going on to develop AIDS. In one study, HIV could only be detected in approximately 50 per cent of patients sampled, despite the fact that antibodies to the virus could be found in roughly 90 to 100 per cent of the same patients.

From this intriguing perspective, it would appear that if a patient's lifestyle has contributed towards their having a weakened immune response, contact with HIV may be the last straw that tips the balance, leading to AIDS. In other words, the presence of HIV may be seen as one of a number of co-factors in the development of AIDS, rather than the sole cause.

When full-blown AIDS develops, the body loses the ability to fight off infection. As a result, any of the following symptoms may occur:

- Weight loss.
- Extreme weariness and exhaustion.
- High temperature.
- Swollen glands in the neck, armpits and groin.
- Diarrhoea.
- Breathlessness.
- Easy bruising.
- Kaposi's sarcoma (a form of skin cancer characterized by painless purple patches on the face, trunk and limbs).
- Recurrent thrush infections.
- Cold sores and genital herpes.

Apart from contracting HIV, additional co-factors

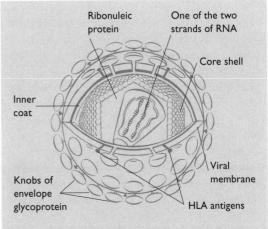

HIV acts by attacking the T4 (helper) T lymphocytes, thus interfering with an essential link in the immune system and opening the way to infections and disorders.

that may put us at risk of developing AIDS may include a combination of the following:
• The practice of anal intercourse with the use of artificial lubricants. The former frequently results in abrasions that can allow the entry of bacterial or viral microbes into the bloodstream. In addition, lubricants manufactured from a petrochemical base may play a role in weakening the immune system.
• Poor nutrition.
• Use of recreational and intravenous drugs.
• Extreme sexual promiscuity with a corresponding history of recurrent venereal infection.
• Emotional and physical stress.

Those who suffer from haemophilia (a disorder that affects men only, characterized by poor blood-clotting ability) have been identified as being at significant risk of developing AIDS from blood products supplied by hospitals, especially contaminated Factor VIII (the clotting agent given to haemophiliacs). All blood products are now screened for HIV, so the risk is substantially reduced.

Practical self-help

• Improving the general quality of life in addition to seeking relevant medical treatment should be the first priority of anyone who feels they may be at risk of developing AIDS. Stress-management techniques have been hailed as useful adjunctive therapy for those who have been diagnosed as HIV positive or who have developed AIDS. These may include learning how to meditate or using relaxation or visualization techniques.
• Nutrition also appears to be a factor of great importance, since those who eat a predominantly junk-food diet high in processed foods, alcohol and caffeine, and also use stimulants such as cigarettes and recreational drugs may find that their immune systems are weakened. To support efficient functioning of the immune system the diet should consist of as many fresh, wholefoods as possible including fresh fruit, vegetables, whole grains, pulses, seeds and six to eight glasses of filtered or mineral water a day.
• Consult a nutritionist for specific advice on supplements. Appropriate nutrients may include vitamin C, vitamin A, vitamin B complex, vitamin E, selenium and zinc.
• Exercise such as brisk walking is thought to relieve stress and encourage improved performance of immune function through stimulation of the lymphatic system.

• Sensible practical precautionary measures include practising safe sex by using condoms, and never sharing needles for injecting drugs.

Alternative treatments

Any of the following may be helpful adjunctive therapies:
• Anthroposophical medicine
• Homoeopathy
• Naturopathy
• Nutritional therapy
• Relaxation techniques
• Shiatsu
• Traditional Chinese medicine
• Western medical herbalism

Allergies

See the advice given for eczema (pages 223-6), asthma (pages 137-40) and hay fever (pages 151-3).

Anaemia

Anaemia occurs when there is a deficiency of haemoglobin in the blood, with the result that not enough oxygen is carried to the tissues of the body. This can be caused by the presence of a number of factors, including severe or protracted blood loss, an inherited tendency to anaemia or the inability to produce an adequate supply of red blood cells.

The most common form of this problem is iron-deficiency anaemia, which can develop as a result of lack of iron in the diet, blood loss or may be associated with another illness or infection. Pernicious anaemia sets in if the body becomes unable to absorb vitamin B^{12}, and can develop in those who have a disorder of the immune system or who are using certain drugs. B^{12} deficiency is common in the elderly due to poor diet, and those who follow a vegan diet may also be at risk.

Megaloblastic anaemia develops from a deficiency

of folic acid and is most likely to occur in the elderly or in pregnancy. On the other hand, sickle-cell anaemia is an inherited condition that is commonly found in those who are of Middle Eastern or African descent. This condition produces symptoms of jaundice (yellow-tinged skin and whites of the eyes), feverishness and exhaustion, and weakness after physical exertion.

Common symptoms of anaemia may include any of the following:
• Weariness.
• Headaches.
• Sleeplessness.
• Dizziness.
• Breathlessness.
• Pale complexion.
• Visual disturbance.
• Puffy ankles.
• Palpitations.
• Chest pains.

Practical self-help

• Iron-deficiency anaemia may be greatly helped by improving the quality of the diet and making sure that plenty of iron-rich foods are included, such as green, leafy vegetables, brewer's yeast, walnuts, raisins, strawberries, apricots, pumpkin seeds, liver and kidneys.
• If pernicious anaemia has arisen as a result of a poor diet (as opposed to an inability to absorb the vitamin), it may respond to the inclusion of dairy foods, liver, kidneys, and eggs in the diet.
• Most forms of anaemia may be helped by including raw, fresh juices such as carrot. In addition, a daily intake of molasses may be of value.
• Increase iron intake by making sure that adequate supplies of vitamin C are taken on a daily basis. Drinking fresh orange juice with a meal is a good way of increasing iron absorption. Also avoid drinking tea before or immediately after a meal, since this can inhibit iron absorption.

SEEK PROFESSIONAL HELP

If you suspect that you may be anaemic, it is extremely important to have a blood test done in order to establish whether action needs to be taken.

Alternative treatments

Any of the following may be of extra support in addition to conventional medical treatment:

• Anthroposophical medicine
• Biochemic tissue salts
• Homoeopathy
• Naturopathy
• Nutritional therapy
• Shiatsu
• Traditional Chinese medicine
• Western medical herbalism

Angina

Angina is the name given to the pain that occurs when the heart muscle is temporarily deprived of oxygen. In an average person, the coronary arteries that convey blood and oxygen to the heart can cope with increased demand due to exertion. However, if someone suffers from coronary heart disease (see pages 334-5) or high blood pressure (see pages 338-40), the performance of the coronary arteries will be adversely affected.

Many people with this problem may not experience any symptoms initially, but if the problem becomes well established or severe, attacks of breathlessness or pain may begin to occur as a result of emotional stress or physical exertion. Characteristically, the pain stops once the activity or stress has ceased, signifying that oxygen requirements are being met once again.

Angina symptoms may include any of the following:
• Pain in the centre of the chest that may radiate to the upper jaw, throat, back and/or arms (the left one in particular).
• Pain that is constricting, dull, or heavy in nature that tends to come on during physical exercise and eases when the demands of physical exertion stop.
• Less commonly, pain that only affects the more peripheral areas of the neck, wrists or arms. Although not as characteristic of angina as the location and nature of the pain described above, this pain is likely

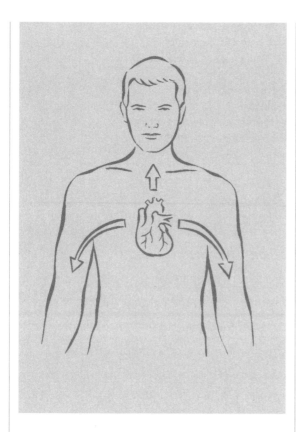

- Marked pallor and clamminess.
- Nausea and/or vomiting.
- Any signs of drowsiness or loss of conscious ness.

Alternative treatments

After confirmation of the condition and discussion of your treatment plan with your doctor, additional help may be obtained from any of the following therapies:
- Acupressure
- Anthroposophical medicine
- Aromatherapy
- Chiropractic
- Flower remedies
- Homoeopathy
- Naturopathy
- Nutritional therapy
- Osteopathy
- Reflexology
- Shiatsu
- Traditional Chinese medicine
- Western medical herbalism

to be caused by angina if it sets in after unusual stress or excitement and improves after rest.
- Dizziness, breathlessness, nausea and clamminess accompanying the pains.

Practical self-help

- If any of the above symptoms occur and you suspect you may be suffering from angina, consult your family doctor, who will be able to confirm the diagnosis and inform you of appropriate treatment.
- Always get urgent medical help if chest pain lasts longer than five minutes after stopping physical exertion, or if episodes of pain and/or breathlessness are increasing in frequency, severity or length.
- For general self-help advice see the section on coronary heart disease (pages 334-5).

SEEK PROFESSIONAL HELP

- If an episode of angina does not respond to rest and relaxation.
- If angina occurs after treatment for a heart attack.
- If any of the following occur:
  - Steady increase in severity of chest pain.

Cancer

Cancer is often called a disease, but it is, in fact, a collective term for about 500 different diseases. Many people may find it difficult to talk openly about cancer because it is a condition that most people instinctively dread. This is often connected to having witnessed the emotional and physical trauma that a diagnosis of cancer can cause in relatives or close friends. Helping a cancer patient cope with the side effects of treatment as well as symptoms of the condition can also encourage the feeling that cancer is an awe-inspiring and frightening illness.

However, it can be immensely positive to appreciate

that cancer can manifest itself in a variety of different ways for a number of different reasons. A diagnosis of cancer has various possible outcomes, depending on the speed of diagnosis, the location of the cancer itself and additional aspects such as hereditary factors and general lifestyle. Once we take this broader picture on board, we are less likely to automatically regard a diagnosis of cancer as a death sentence.

Cancer occurs when abnormal cells develop in the body at a rate where they escalate out of control. Although cells are reproducing on a constant basis in our bodies, sometimes a dividing cell can be produced that is not properly genetically coded. If this mutant cell is allowed to multiply at a fast rate, it is likely to develop into a cancer. When we remain in good health and our white blood cells work efficiently, they should be able to destroy these abnormal cells as they are produced. However, mutant cells can be very elusive and resistant to destruction, and can often try to evade contact from white cells by developing a barrier on their surface.

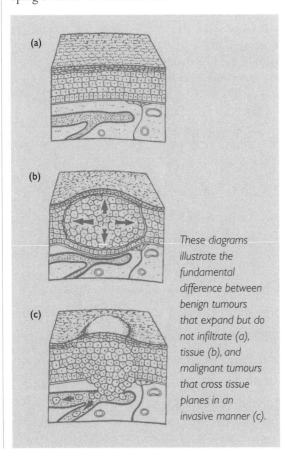

These diagrams illustrate the fundamental difference between benign tumours that expand but do not infiltrate (a), tissue (b), and malignant tumours that cross tissue planes in an invasive manner (c).

Not all cancers develop at the same rate; some can grow rapidly or slowly, dependent on the individual cancer, for example, cancer of the womb has a reputation for slow, insidious growth, while cancer of the neck of the womb (cervical cancer) may develop extremely rapidly. Once a malignant tumour has developed, abnormal cells can migrate to other parts of the body, setting up other sites of mutant cells (often referred to as 'secondaries').

Cancer may take a number of different forms, and names for each sort of cancer will be influenced by the body system or part of the body that has been affected. Carcinomas affect the internal and external linings of the body and many of its organs and body cavities, while sarcomas arise from and invade the bones and muscles. Cancer of the bones is called osteosarcoma, while cancer of the blood is called leukaemia and cancer of the lymph glands, lymphoma. Malignant tumours may develop in any of the following: the brain, kidneys, liver, lungs, ovaries, breasts, bowel, stomach, testicles, womb or the skin.

Early warning signs may include any combination of the following:
• Traces of blood in stools, urine, sputum or vomit.
• Swelling of the abdomen.
• Change in bowel habit for no obvious reason.
• Ulcers or sores that refuse to heal within a few weeks.
• Severe, recurrent headaches with no obvious cause.
• Faintness or dizziness.
• Difficulty in swallowing.
• Nausea and with sudden attacks of vomiting for no detectable reason.
• Persistent cough.
• Breathlessness.
• Persistent heartburn or indigestion.
• Difficulty and/or pain in passing urine.
• Irregular bleeding between periods in women or discharge from the tip of the penis in men.
• Moles that begin to change shape, itch or bleed.
• A lump or puckered area in the breast.
• A detectable lump in the neck.
• Lump on testicles.

Potential triggers or factors that may increase our susceptibility to developing malignancy may include any of the following:
• **Genetic inheritance:** A woman with close female relatives who have suffered from cancer of the breast (mother, aunt and sister) is four times

more likely than the average woman to be susceptible to the same problem. Those who are fair skinned with light-coloured eyes and hair may be more vulnerable to developing skin cancer than those who have inherited dark pigmented skin.

- **Lifestyle:** Our personal and professional environment can also play a major role in making us more vulnerable to illness. Factors that have been identified as being linked to an increased possibility of developing cancer include heavy alcohol intake, significant exposure to radiation or overexposure to sunlight, contact with certain chemicals (such as benzopyrenes used in dry cleaning), smoking, inhalation of asbestos particles, excessive intake of dietary fats.
- **Repressing emotions:** Repressing anger, grief or depression over an extended period of time may also be a co-factor if other triggers are also present. This appears to be due to the way that extended psychological stress can lead to depressed immune function.

Preventative self-help

- If life is becoming unduly stressful it is extremely important to investigate ways of relaxing and unwinding. Appropriate techniques may include meditation, relaxation or imaging techniques. The use of positive imagery has been claimed to have a positive effect in enhancing immune function.
- Vitamin and mineral supplements may help support the efficient functioning of the immune system. Appropriate vitamins include vitamins C, E and A, while trace elements such as the antioxidant enzyme, selenium can also play an important role. Additional useful supplements include zinc, calcium and magnesium. However, advice on the optimum dosage should be sought from a nutritionist.
- Coffee, tea and alcohol consumption should be drastically reduced and smoking eliminated. Smoked and chemically preserved foods should be eliminated from the diet, while the following should be eaten on a regular basis: fresh fruit, vegetables, whole grains, seeds, cold-pressed virgin olive oil and pulses. Small quantities of the following may also be included: fish (unsmoked and unpreserved), free-range poultry, eggs, organic goats'-milk yoghurt. Drinks should include herb teas, freshly pressed fruit juices, mineral or filtered water and grain-based coffee substitutes.

Alternative treatments

Because alternative medical approaches attempt to stimulate the body's defences against disease, they may be especially helpful in situations where illness has set in as a result of the body being unable to destroy rogue or mutant cells. However, it is important to stress that it is not the intention of this book to discourage any cancer patient from pursuing conventional medical treatment, but to offer positive advice on additional therapies that may reduce emotional stress and trauma, encourage a sense of well-being, and ease some of the side effects of conventional treatment. Many cancer patients feel powerless and helpless in the face of the diagnosis of their condition, but alternative medical treatment can help them feel empowered to take positive steps in the direction of recovery. Supportive therapies may include:

- Anthroposophical medicine
- Aromatherapy
- Homoeopathy
- Naturopathy
- Nutritional therapy
- Reflexology
- Shiatsu
- Traditional Chinese medicine
- Western medical herbalism

Chronic fatigue syndrome

This is a controversial condition that may also be referred to as ME (myalgic encephalomyelitis), post-viral syndrome, fibromyalgia or Royal Free disease. Conventional medical opinion has been divided in the past as to whether this condition exists or not, and a variety of opinions have been put forward suggesting possible co-factors that may be responsible for its development. These may include:

- A stressful way of life that does not give a chance

for relaxation and recovery to occur.

• Dependence on stimulants in order to keep the pace. These may include coffee, recreational or prescription drugs, cigarettes or alcohol.

• Reliance on junk foods rather than eating a good-quality, varied diet.

• Recurrent bouts of thrush.

• A history of recurrent infectious illness with repeated treatment by antibiotic drugs. Antibiotics are regarded by alternative therapists to have a compromising effect on the efficient functioning of the immune system.

• Contracting a viral illness that is not given a chance to clear up, and keeps recurring.

• It has also been suggested that a sensitivity to vaccinations may also leave us vulnerable to developing chronic fatigue syndrome, especially if other co-factors are present.

Common symptoms of chronic fatigue syndrome may include any of the following:

• Muscle weakness and pain.

• Joint pains.

• Persistent and recurrent mental exhaustion.

• Poor sleep pattern and quality.

• Glandular swelling.

• Recurrent sore throats.

• Headaches.

• Digestive discomfort and bloating.

• Cramping pains with diarrhoea.

• Fluctuations in mood, including weepiness, anxiety, depression, and panic or irritability when placed under the slightest stress.

Preventative self-help

• It is extremely important to rest as much as possible when in the initial stages of chronic fatigue syndrome. Although exercise is often recommended as an important way of keeping fit and healthy, the usual advice about exercise stimulating energy levels does not apply to those who suffer from this debilitating illness. On the contrary, exercise will probably make matters worse. However, as energy levels build steadily, and provided physical demands remain well within the scope of existing energy reserves, it should be possible to enjoy increasing physical activity, as long as the temptation to overdo things is resisted.

• As energy levels show signs of steady improvement it can be helpful to do gentle stretching exercises to help stimulate the lymphatic system. Always

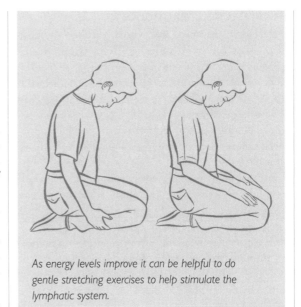

As energy levels improve it can be helpful to do gentle stretching exercises to help stimulate the lymphatic system.

start at a gentle pace, beginning with a few simple yoga postures to loosen up the joints, and encourage muscle strength, stamina and tone.

• Skin brushing can encourage the system to detoxify. Use a natural bristle brush on dry skin before taking a bath or shower. Using firm but gentle movements, brush in an upward direction, avoiding contact with any areas of broken or irritated skin.

• Explore visualization exercises, relaxation techniques and meditation. Make a point of setting aside some time each day in which to relax and concentrate on your breathing (see the advice on diaphragmatic breathing techniques in the section on anxiety, page 238).

• Drink six to eight glasses of filtered or spring water a day, ensuring that as many fresh, whole-foods as possible are included in the diet. Avoid convenience foods, alcohol, strong tea and coffee, and food and drink containing a lot of sugar. See the advice on healthy eating in the sections on influenza (pages 154-6) and weight gain (pages 325-6).

• Consider supplementing with oil of evening primrose and vitamins C, D and E. It has been suggested that those who suffer from chronic fatigue syndrome may benefit from extra zinc if they are found to be deficient in this trace element.

• If chronic yeast infection is also a problem, garlic, caprylic acid and acidophilus may be helpful when taken in supplement form.

Alternative treatments

Alternative therapists are regularly called upon to give help to those suffering from symptoms of chronic fatigue syndrome. Because alternative medical approaches share the central concept that ill health springs from an immune system that has become overwhelmed by physical or mental strain (or a traumatic combination of the two), they provide appropriate therapeutic options for those who suffer from chronic fatigue syndrome. The varied range of symptoms that patients experience need not pose a problem for an alternative therapist, since he or she would in any case identify patterns in symptoms that form a coherent symptom 'picture'. Since alternative approaches as a rule regard energy production as an important indicator of good, poor or indifferent health, they are especially well placed to treat the problems that patients of chronic fatigue syndrome suffer.

However, this is a condition for which case management can be protracted, complicated and subject to relapses or setbacks. For these reasons, self-prescribing with alternative treatments is not recommended. Professional alternative medical help should be sought, and appropriate therapies to consider include:

- Anthroposophical medicine
- Aromatherapy
- Chiropractic
- Homoeopathy
- Naturopathy
- Nutritional therapy
- Shiatsu
- Traditional Chinese medicine
- Western medical herbalism

Coronary heart disease

Before we can understand the nature of coronary heart disease, it is important to gain some understanding of the role played by the coronary arteries. The heart must be supplied with a constant amount of blood, nutrients and oxygen in order to function.

This vital blood supply is transported to the heart muscle by two coronary arteries that keep it nourished via a series of branches covering the surface of the heart. Once fatty plaques form in these arteries, the passages become constricted and compromised in their ability to convey the optimum amount of nutrients and oxygen to the heart. In addition, the narrowing process can cause clotting of the blood that flows through the arteries, so that there is a strong risk of a clot causing an obstruction.

Problems with coronary heart disease often become apparent when the heart beats faster in response to emotional excitement, stress or increased physical activity and requires an increased supply of nutrients and oxygen. If the coronary arteries have become

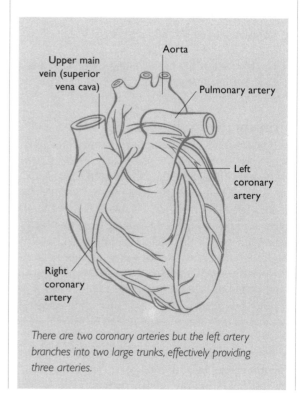

There are two coronary arteries but the left artery branches into two large trunks, effectively providing three arteries.

partially blocked, they are unable to meet the increased demands, and the result is often the pain and breathlessness of angina (see pages 329-30). On the other hand, if a clot has formed in one of the coronary arteries and the blood supply to part of the heart muscle is reduced, the result is likely to be a heart attack (myocardial infarction).

Practical self-help

See the advice given in the section on angina if advanced symptoms suddenly appear. On the other hand, if you feel at all concerned about developing this problem due to a family history of heart disease, the following hints may be of help.

• If you are a smoker, give up the habit as soon as possible. Smoking can be a very difficult habit to break, so consider getting extra help from alternative therapies such as acupuncture or homoeopathy.

• Make sure that fat of any kind makes up no more than 20 per cent of your diet. Be especially careful of saturated fats in full-fat dairy products, eggs or red meat.

• Avoid foods that combine high proportions of fat and sugar, such as cakes, biscuits, ice cream or puddings.

• Eat a high-fibre diet, ensuring that you eat regular portions of raw, fresh fruit and vegetables every day.

• Reduce your salt intake, especially if you have a tendency to high blood pressure.

• When cooking, choose a monounsaturated oil such as cold-pressed virgin olive oil which is believed to convey some protection to the circulatory system, unlike saturated fats such as butter or cream, which appear to do the reverse.

• Increase helpings of oily fish such as mackerel or salmon, and pulses such as lentils.

• It has been suggested that garlic can play a role in reducing blood clotting tendencies as well as onions, fresh ginger and chillies. If the taste of garlic is unpalatable to you, consider taking garlic capsules or tablets.

• Make a point of taking aerobic exercise on a regular basis, ideally three or four times a week. If you have previously led a sedentary, physically unfit lifestyle, begin slowly, avoiding forms of exercise that may be extremely physically stressful at first, such as running or squash. Instead, take up more sustained, gentle but effective rhythmical exercise, such as walking, building up to cycling or jogging.

• If you are overweight, make a point of trying to lose the necessary excess pounds. See page 324 for advice on weight loss.

• If stress levels are proving to be unduly high, consider taking up a form of relaxation technique, meditation or yoga.

SEEK PROFESSIONAL HELP

• If severe chest pain and breathlessness occur that last for more than five minutes.

• If chest pain and distress do not respond to rest and relaxation.

• If any signs of drowsiness, unconsciousness or laboured breathing occur.

Alternative treatments

Once you have had the problem fully checked out by your family doctor, consider any of the following therapies:

• Acupressure
• Anthroposophical medicine
• Aromatherapy
• Homoeopathy
• Massage therapy
• Naturopathy
• Nutritional therapy
• Reflexology
• Shiatsu
• Traditional Chinese medicine
• Western medical herbalism

Diabetes (diabetes mellitus)

Diabetes is a chronic condition that occurs when there is either a deficiency or total lack of insulin being produced by the pancreas, or due to a resistence to insulin caused by the loss of insulin receptors on the surface of the cells. The latter is usually caused by obesity, and the patient will have normal or even increased insulin levels. In either case, glucose (a simple form of sugar) is not adequately absorbed or stored by the body, resulting in too high a concentration of sugar in the blood.

There are two main categories of diabetes. These are:

• Insulin-dependent diabetes. This problem usually occurs in children or young adults where the pancreas produces far too little, or no insulin. The body is forced to break down fat to obtain energy, which if it occurs undetected, can lead to a diabetic coma.

• Non-insulin-dependent diabetes. This form of diabetes usually develops in adults over forty years old. In this situation the insulin-producing cells of the pancreas continue to function but not enough insulin is produced for the body's needs, and often the body is resistant to the effects of insulin.

Symptoms of diabetes may include any of the following:

• Incontinence.
• Increased output of pale-coloured urine.
• Marked thirst.
• Extreme lethargy and exhaustion for no apparent reason.
• Difficulty getting up in the morning.
• Weight loss.
• Cramps in the legs.
• Blurred vision.
• Poor resistance to infection (including recurrent urinary tract infections, thrush or boils).
• Tingling in the feet and hands.
• Impotence.
• Absence of periods.

It is extremely important to establish a diagnosis of diabetes as early as possible to avoid potentially serious complications developing later on, such as chronic kidney failure or diabetic retinopathy. The latter may result in a serious reduction or loss of vision, if diabetes is not treated effectively. Alternatively, peripheral neuropathy may also develop if diabetes is allowed to progress without adequate treatment. Peripheral neuropathy is diagnosed when damage has been sustained to the peripheral nerves of the body. This leads to a gradually developing tingling sensation that begins in the hands and feet, spreading on a progressive basis to the trunk of the body, leading to eventual muscle wastage.

Treatment of insulin-dependent diabetes involves taking regular injections of insulin in combination with a strictly controlled diet to keep blood-sugar levels stable and control weight. However, certain circumstances can increase the body's demand for insulin, such as developing an acute illness like flu: it is important to seek a medical opinion about modifying insulin dosage as soon as possible if an acute infection occurs. Those who suffer from insulin-dependent diabetes also need to take care if they are unduly stressed, become involved in strenuous physical activity or miss regular meals, since these factors can also have a destabilizing effect on blood-sugar levels. Anyone suffering from diabetes should also have extra attention in pregnancy, ideally seeking their family doctor's advice before conceiving in order to arrange for the most efficient management of their condition and to avoid the risk of complications for mother and baby.

Non-insulin dependent diabetes, on the other hand, can be largely contained by sensible dietary modifications, including strict control of carbohydrate intake such as sugar and starches, including those in alcohol. Gentle exercise should be taken on a regular basis and sensible weight loss may also be suggested, since many patients who develop diabetes in later life are also significantly overweight (see the weight gain section on pages 00–00 for advice on healthy eating and weight reduction). Large doses of vitamin C in supplement form should be avoided as these supplements destabilize blood-sugar levels. Once the appropriate measures are taken, many non-insulin-dependent diabetics discover that their condition can be effectively kept under control.

Practical self-help

See the suggestions listed above.

SEEK PROFESSIONAL HELP

• If an acute infection occurs in anyone who suffers from insulin-dependent diabetes.
• If any signs of drowsiness, disorientation, sweating and general incoherence develop in someone who is known to be a diabetic.
• If persistent signs of increased thirst, unusually copious urine output, or extreme fatigue occur for no apparent reason.

Alternative treatments

It must be stressed that diabetes is potentially a very serious illness that requires conventional medical supervision and management, especially when the illness occurs in children. As a result, any of the therapies listed below must be regarded as being helpful supporters to conventional medical treatment and advice:

- Acupuncture
- Anthroposophical medicine
- Aromatherapy
- Homoeopathy
- Massage therapy
- Nutritional therapy
- Osteopathy
- Reflexology
- Relaxation and visualization techniques
- Traditional Chinese medicine

Epilepsy

An epileptic seizure occurs as a result of a burst of excessive electrical activity in the cells of the brain. There are different grades of seizure, depending on the size of the area of the brain affected. If a small part of the brain is involved, this may lead to a localized seizure, whereas an attack that has affected a substantial amount of the brain can lead to a more generalized seizure.

If a generalized problem sets in, it is most likely to occur abruptly and violently. This kind of episode is often referred to as a 'grand mal', and is generally characterized by the casualty falling to the ground in an unconscious state. The muscles become generally stiff, and may begin to jerk in an uncontrollable way until the seizure is over. Once the worst of the episode has passed (this may take between one to four minutes), the muscles relax as the casualty slowly regains consciousness (this may take between five minutes to half an hour). After a seizure, a headache may set in, and there may be a strong desire to fall asleep. Full recovery happens within an hour or two, or may take anything up to a week or so in some cases.

Another kind of generalized seizure is a 'petit mal'. This type of episode commonly affects children and manifests itself as a 'blank' attack that can last for roughly thirty seconds. During this experience, the patient will be unaware of his surroundings. Because petit mal sufferers often look as though they are daydreaming or not paying attention, petit mal episodes may pass without notice by others.

A partial or focal seizure is different in that it is often preceded by an 'aura' (rather in the same way that a migraine sufferer may be able to associate certain changes in perception with the onset of an acute episode). An attack that starts in the temporal lobe of the brain may begin with the patient feeling fearful, associated with a sensation that rises from the stomach to the throat. This may be coupled with a characteristic sound, taste or smell. The focal seizure may be restricted to the experience of an aura as described above, or it may involve peculiar or disoriented behaviour that may lead to the performing of repetitive movements. However, sometimes the seizure spreads through a large area of the brain, culminating in a grand mal episode.

Practical self-help

- However distressing a grand mal seizure appears to be, it is unlikely to be dangerous for the person experiencing the attack provided basic precautions are taken.
- Although it may seem necessary to try to hold the casualty still during a seizure, it is best not to do this since it can cause needless trauma. Instead, make plenty of space around the casualty by moving any nearby objects they might hurt themselves on by thrashing about.
- Make sure that there are no dangerous elements near to hand, such as an open fire. If this is the case, try to move the casualty away from the flames or hot surfaces, so that there is no chance of them becoming burned or injured.
- Do not try to put anything between the patient's teeth in an effort to prevent them damaging their tongue. Unfortunately, by forcing anything in their mouths during a fit it is possible to inadvertently cause trauma to the mouth, or if great force is used, to break a tooth. There is also the possibility that you could get bitten.
- Once the seizure has run its course, put the casualty in the recovery position (see an orthodox first aid book), wiping away any froth from the mouth, and checking that the airway is clear.

• It is not uncommon for a person who has made recovery from a seizure to want to sleep for a while. If they do so, check at regular intervals that their breathing is regular and not laboured.

• If a petit mal or focal seizure occurs you are unlikely to need to do any more than stay with the patient, giving them reassurance when necessary, until they are fully recovered and in touch with their surroundings.

SEEK PROFESSIONAL HELP

• If a grand mal seizure lasts more than three minutes.

• If the casualty appears to recover temporarily but quickly relapses into another seizure.

• If seizures are happening on a more frequent basis despite using appropriate conventional medication.

Alternative treatments

It must be stressed that anyone who is subject to grand mal or regular petit mal seizures requires conventional medical supervision and management. As a result, any of the therapies listed below must be regarded as being helpful supporters to conventional medical treatment and advice:

• Anthroposophical medicine
• Aromatherapy
• Cranial osteopathy
• Homoeopathy
• Naturopathy
• Traditional Chinese medicine

High blood pressure (hypertension)

High blood pressure is a rather insidious condition, since it can give rise to very few or no symptoms at all. As a result, high blood pressure is often only revealed during a routine medical examination. Certain stages of life or drug treatments increase vulnerability to raised blood pressure such as using oral contraceptives or pregnancy. As a result, regular monitoring of blood-pressure levels is always advocated in these situations.

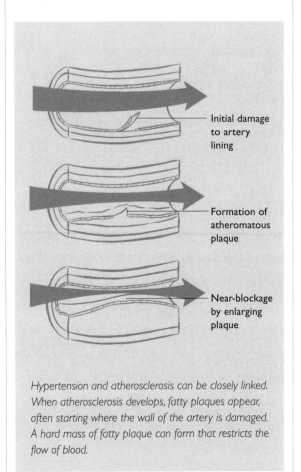

Initial damage to artery lining

Formation of atheromatous plaque

Near-blockage by enlarging plaque

Hypertension and atherosclerosis can be closely linked. When atherosclerosis develops, fatty plaques appear, often starting where the wall of the artery is damaged. A hard mass of fatty plaque can form that restricts the flow of blood.

The major concern related to chronic hypertension is that if the pressure within the circulation is constantly at too high a level it puts too much strain on the circulatory system. As a result, the heart has to do more work to keep the circulation moving. The increased strain on the heart causes heart muscle enlargement to cope with this. This means that the cardiac muscle needs more oxygen and also means that the development of heart attack or angina are more likely. If, in addition, fatty plaques have formed within the coronary arteries, there is a risk that they may become narrowed, and eventually become obstructed completely. If the latter has occurred, the risk of coronary thrombosis (heart attack) is likely to follow. See the section on coronary heart disease for more information (pages 334-5).

In addition, persistently high blood pressure increases the risk of a stroke, because elevated blood pressure encourages the formation of clots in the arteries that supply the brain with blood. Strokes occur when the blood supply to the brain is interrupted, leaving it damaged. The kidneys are also put under greater strain, with an increased risk of kidney failure developing. This creates a vicious cycle, since poorly functioning kidneys lead to increased problems with hypertension, and hypertension leaves the kidneys more vulnerable to damage. Other organs that may also suffer damage from chronic high blood pressure include the brain and eyes.

A 'perfect' blood pressure reading would be somewhere in the region of 120/80, with the higher reading showing the measurement of pressure when the heart is beating, and the lower figure revealing the level of pressure when the heart is at rest. However, fluctuations can arise in blood pressure due to age, amount of stress and being pregnant. As a result, your family doctor is likely to take your case on its own merit, and will only prescribe drugs to reduce blood pressure if readings show a persistently elevated trend for your age and circumstances.

There are two different types of hypertension, 'essential' and 'secondary' high blood pressure. However, 'secondary' high blood pressure is very rare. In the first category, blood pressure may be raised for no obvious reason, while in the second category hypertension is related to another condition, such as a hormone imbalance or kidney disorder.

Hypertension can be symptomless, or the following may occur when blood-pressure readings are particularly high:
• Headaches.
• Palpitations.
• A general feeling of malaise or ill health.

Practical self-help

• If you suspect you have high blood pressure, make a point of having it checked at your doctor's surgery every three to five years. It will be more frequently monitored if you are taking the contraceptive pill.
• If you have purchased a blood-pressure gauge to keep a check on your blood-pressure levels at home, always make a point of taking the measurement after resting, and before eating: one of the most conven-

ient times is usually first thing in the morning.
• If you are a smoker, make efforts to give up the habit. This is important, since smokers with raised blood pressure have an increased risk of additional complications developing. It is also important to bear in mind that a link has been established between the development of coronary heart disease and smoking.
• If you are overweight, follow the advice given in the weight gain section on pages 324-6, since excess weight can also aggravate problems with hypertension, while also increasing your risk of developing heart disease.
• Reduce salty foods in your diet, such as salami, salty fish, crisps, salted nuts and pickles. Avoid cooking with salt and adding extra salt at the table, and remember that convenience foods are a rich source of 'hidden' salt.
• Keep well within, and ideally below your limit of units of alcohol per week.
• Reduce your intake of saturated animal fat, particularly red meat and full-fat dairy products, and increase the amount of fibre in your diet in the form of beans, pulses, whole grains, fruit and vegetables.
• Learn how to meditate, take up yoga, use biofeedback (instruments used to monitor changes in people's physical and mental states) or explore an appropriate relaxation technique if you feel that an inability to deal with stress is contributing to your problems.
• Gentle, regular rhythmical exercise can help maintain the health of the circulatory system. Always seek professional medical advice before embarking on a new course of exercise if you suffer from high blood pressure.

Seek professional medical advice if you suspect you may have high blood pressure.

Alternative treatments

Additional help, advice and treatment may be obtained from professionals working in any of the following therapies:
• Acupressure
• Anthroposophical medicine
• Aromatherapy
• Chiropractic
• Homoeopathy
• Massage therapy
• Meditation

- Naturopathy
- Nutritional therapy
- Osteopathy
- Reflexology
- Shiatsu
- Traditional Chinese medicine
- Western medical medicine

Multiple sclerosis

Multiple sclerosis develops when the myelin sheath (providing covering and protection to the nerves in the brain and spinal cord) becomes swollen and inflamed. If this damage occurs, the passage of electrical impulses and nutrients becomes impaired, leading to impaired performance of the affected nerves, a bit like causing a short circuit in electrical wiring.

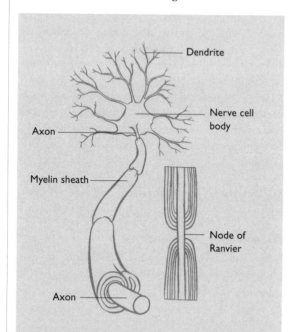

Myelin is a fatty material that acts as a kind of insulate for long nerve fibres (axons) so that nerve impulses can pass normally. Damage to myelin blocks the passage of nerve impulses with serious results.

Symptoms may initially develop in a brief, vague episode that may last no more than a day or so. This may include tingling, weakness or numbness that may affect one side of the body or is restricted to a single limb. Problems of this kind may result in difficulty in walking or carrying objects, and are characteristically aggravated after physical exertion or warm bathing. As the numbness goes, it may be replaced by a sensation of increased sensitivity in the affected area.

Once the first episode has cleared, there may be no further episodes of symptoms. However, there is a risk that similar attacks may occur on a recurrent basis, with less capacity for recovery being shown on each occasion. In addition, weakness and disability may become progressive, with lack of physical co-ordination, numbness and poor vision becoming eventually permanent. However, some multiple sclerosis sufferers find that in between episodes they feel perfectly able to continue their lives and basic activities.

Additional symptoms of multiple sclerosis may include any of the following:

- Unsteadiness.
- Slurring of speech.
- Incontinence or problems with urination.
- Blurred vision.

Practical self-help

- Pay attention to your diet, making sure that it is high in fibre and low in fat. Avoid sugar and stimulants such as tea, coffee, cola and chocolate. For further advice on healthy eating, see the sections on influenza (pages 154-6) and weight gain (pages 325-6).
- Avoid alcohol and smoking, including passive smoking. Always bear in mind that it is especially important to avoid alcohol during episodes of unsteadiness or poor co-ordination.
- The stress that accompanies the diagnosis and experience of MS can be eased by diaphragmatic breathing techniques (see the section on anxiety, page 238) for a description of this and appropriate yoga postures. Yoga also encourages muscular coordination, strength, stamina and flexibility.
- In some cases oil of evening primrose has eased some of the symptoms of multiple sclerosis. Additional helpful supplements may include cod liver oil, vitamin E, vitamin B complex, vitamin C, zinc and magnesium.

- In between acute episodes, it is important to remain as mobile as possible, without engaging in exercise to the point of exhaustion.

SEEK PROFESSIONAL HELP

If acute episodes of multiple sclerosis become more frequent or severe despite appropriate treatment.

Alternative treatment

Although multiple sclerosis is a chronic condition that requires conventional medical supervision, any of the following therapies may be used to provide helpful additional support:
- Anthroposophical medicine
- Chiropractic
- Homoeopathy
- Massage therapy
- Naturopathy
- Nutritional therapy
- Osteopathy
- Shiatsu
- Traditional Chinese medicine
- Visualization and relaxation techniques
- Western medical herbalism

Rheumatoid arthritis

The symptoms of rheumatoid arthritis, unlike those of osteoarthritis (see pages 204-7), can occur at any time of life from childhood onwards. The condition is not associated with ageing or wear and tear on the joints. The joints that are most vulnerable to developing this problem include the small bones of the fingers, wrists, neck, knees and toes.

Symptoms can be very severe and may include any of the following:
- Swelling in, and around the affected joints.
- Redness and general inflammation of the painful joints.
- Flitting sensations of heat or pain, or feelings of heat within specific joints, which may also feel very hot to the touch.

- Vague and generalized feelings of weakness, fatigue and feverishness.

Practical self-help

See general advice given for osteoarthritis on pages 205.

Alternative treatments

See advice given in the osteoarthritis section on page 206-7.

Vertigo

A diagnosis of vertigo may be given where there is a persistent feeling as if the head is spinning or moving. This unpleasant sensation may be combined with nausea and/or vomiting and may be set off by fear of falling.

Symptoms may also be triggered by any of the following: inflammation of the inner ear, travel sickness, high blood pressure or Meniere's disease, where vertigo is associated with tinnitus (see pages 118-19).

Practical self-help

See the advice given for fainting on pages 103-4.

SEEK PROFESSIONAL HELP

- For recurrent or prolonged bouts of dizziness.
- If dizziness is associated with deafness, decreased hearing or tinnitus.

Alternative treatments

- Acupressure
- Anthroposophical medicine
- Aromatherapy
- Homoeopathy
- Naturopathy
- Nutritional therapy
- Reflexology
- Shiatsu
- Traditional Chinese medicine
- Western medical herbalism

A–Z of conditions and medicines

This A–Z lists a variety of remedies from the different medicine-based alternative systems of health care, including herbal, homoeopathic, anthroposophical, biochemic tissue salts and flower remedies as well as dietary supplements to maintain optimum health. Some of the medicines packaged for selling over the counter are named in the following list of conditions, together with information on their legal status and route of sale, indicated by letters in brackets (see below).

There are over 2000 substances making up the complete homoeopathic pharmacopoeia, and these medicines can be used for different conditions. Since these have been detailed in charts throughout the book, they have not been listed in the following A–Z. Instead, the standard available prepackaged homoeopathic medicines in either the 6th or 30th potency have been listed separately on page 344. If you require a remedy that is not mentioned, you can ask your local pharmacy if they have it in stock, or you may have to go direct to one of the manufacturers (see Useful addresses).

Certain ailments discussed in the book have not been listed in this A–Z. This is either because the condition is not suitable for self-prescribing, or because there is not an available prepackaged product specifically manufactured for the condition for general sale over the counter.

See main text for more information and advice about the remedies to take for specific conditions. The suppliers appear in the Useful addresses section. Anthroposophical medicines and biochemic tissue salts do not have the manufacturer listed. This is because Weleda is the only manufacturer of anthroposophical medicines, and New Era is the only manufacturer of biochemic tissue salts (see Useful addresses).

Key to products' legal status
The letters in brackets after the product name show their legal status.

L = this means that the product is a licensed medicine.
PLR = is a product holding a Product Licence of Right.
HR = Homoeopathic Registration Licence.
E = Medicines exempt from licensing.

The above products are medicines registered with the UK's Medicines Control Agency, which means they have been granted licences for both quality and safety. Each of these products will have the letter and a product number on the packaging.

F = Food Law. This covers nutritional supplements, vitamins and minerals and some herbs and comes under the jurisdiction of the UK's Ministry of Agriculture, Fisheries and Food.
T = Toiletry product.

Key to products' route of sale
Most of the products listed are available over the counter in health-food shops or pharmacies or by mail order direct from the supplier (see Useful addresses). Some products are followed by the letter P or POM. P indicates that although no prescription is needed, the product is only available from a pharmacist. POM means that a doctor's prescription is needed to obtain the product.

Homoeopathic medicines

There are hundreds of different homoeopathic medicines available all with a variety of potencies, the majority of which must be obtained from a homoeopathic manufacturer, pharmacy or practitioner. However, the following remedies are readily available in the 6c and 30c potencies at health-food shops, pharmacies or through mail order direct from the supplier.

Aconite	Cantharis	Hamamelis	Phosphorus
Actaea Rac.	Carbo Veg.	Hepar Sulph.	Phytolacca
Allium Cepa	Causticum	Hypericum	Pulsatilla
Apis Mel.	Cina	Ignatia	Rhus Tox.
Argent. Nit.	Cocculus	Ipecac	Ruta Grav.
Arnica	Coffea	Kali. Bich.	Sepia
Arsen. Alb.	Colocynthis	Kali. Phos.	Silicea
Belladonna	Cuprum Met.	Lachesis	Sulphur
Bellis perennis	Drosera	Ledum	Symphytum
Bryonia	Euphrasia	Lycopodium	Thuja
Calc. Carb.	Ferrum Phos.	Merc. Sol.	Urtica Urens
Calc. Fluor.	Gelsemium	Nat. Mur.	
Calc. Phos.	Graphites	Nux Vom.	

NB Most manufacturers also stock homoeopathic first aid kits.

Acne

Anthroposophy
  Aknedoron Lotion (T)
Food Supplements
  including vitamins and supplements, propolis products, vitamin A, selenium, zinc citrate or beta carotene (see list of suppliers, Food)
Herbalism
  HRI Clear Complexion Tablets (Jessup, L)
  Skin Eruptions Mixture (Potter's, L)
  Echinacea Tablets (Potter's, L)
  Echinacea Tablets (Gerard House, PLR)
  Blue Flag Root Compound Tablets (Gerard House, PLR)

Anxiety

Anthroposophy
  Avena Sativa Comp. Drops (PLR)
  Fragador (PLR)
Herbalism
  Kalms (G.R. Lane, L)
  Newrelax Tablets (Potter's, L)

Bedwetting

Herbalism
  Newrelax Tablets (Potter's, L)

Bites and stings

Anthroposophy
  Combudoron Lotion, Ointment or Spray (PLR)
Herbalism
  Tea Tree & Witch Hazel Cream (G.R. Lane, L)
Homoeopathy
  Pyrethrum Spray (A. Nelson, L)

Blisters

Herbalism
  Dermacreme Ointment (Potter's, L)

Boils

Anthroposophy
  Balsamicum Ointment (PLR, P)
  Erysidoron I Drops (PLR, P)

Bronchitis
Anthroposophy
Pyrites 3x Tablets (PLR, P)
Sytra Tea (PLR)
Food Supplements
including propolis products, beta carotene,
ginseng, vitamins B & C, zinc citrate, cat's claw,
Maca (see list of suppliers, Food)
Herbalism
Antibron Tablets (Potter's, L)
Vegetable Cough Remover (Potter's, L)

Bruises
Anthroposophy
Arnica Massage Balm (L)
Arnica Ointment or Lotion (L)
Herbalism
Comfrey Ointment (Potter's, L)
Arnica Cream (A. Nelson, L)
Arnica Ointment or Lotion (Weleda, L)
Homoeopathy
Arnica 6x Tablets (Weleda, PLR)

Burns and scalds
Anthroposophy
Combudoron Ointment or Lotion (PLR, P)
WCS Dusting Powder (PLR)
Food Supplements
including beta carotene, citrus bioflavonoids,
vitamin E, starflower oil, Propex 15ml spray,
propolis products
Herbalism
Comfrey Ointment (Potter's, L)
Dermacreme Ointment (Potter's, L)
Homoeopathy
Burns Ointment (A. Nelson, L)

Candida, see thrush

Catarrh
Anthroposophy
Catarrh Cream (PLR, P)
Oleum Rhinale Nasal Drops (PLR, P)
Biochemic tissue salts
Combination Q (PLR)
Herbalism
Garlic Tablets (Potter's, L)
HRI Garlic Tablets for Catarrh & Rhinitis
(Jessup, L)
Catarrh Mixture (Potter's, L)

Antifect Tablets (Potter's, L)
Lobelia Compound Tablets (Gerard House, PLR)
Catarrheze Tablets (English Grains, PLR)

Chilblains
Anthroposophy
Frost Cream (PLR, P)
Biochemic tissue salts
No. 2 (PLR)
Herbalism
Garlic Tablets (Potter's, L)
Buckwheat Tablets (Potter's, E)
Homoeopathy
Chilblains Ointment (A. Nelson, L)

Colds and influenza
Anthroposophy
Infludo Drops (PLR, POM)
Ferrum Phos Comp (PLR)
Aconite/Bryonia (PLR, P)
Biochemic tissue salts
Combination J (PLR)
Food Supplements
including echinacea, propolis products, zinc
citrate, beta carotene, citrus bioflavonoids & cat's
claw (see list of suppliers, Food)
Herbalism
Peerless Composition Essence (Potter's, L)
Life Drops (Potter's, L)
Garlic Tablets (Potter's, L)
Elderflowers, Peppermint with Composition
Essence (Potter's, L)
HRI Garlic Tablets for Catarrh & Rhinitis (Jessup, L)
Composition Essence (Potter's, L)
Echinacea & Garlic Tablets (Gerard House, PLR)
Homoeopathy
Coldenza (A. Nelson, PLR)

Colic
Anthroposophy
Chamomilla 3x Pills or Drops (PLR)
Biochemic tissue salts
Combination E (PLR)
Herbalism
HRI Golden Seal Digestive Tablets (Jessup, L)
Indian Brandee (Potter's, L)
Olbas Oil (G.R. Lane, L)

Constipation
Anthroposophy
  Laxadoron Tablets (PLR)
  Clairo Tea (L)
Food Supplements
  including starflower oil, organic linseeds, cat's
  claw (see list of suppliers, Food)
Herbalism
  Cleansing Herb (Potter's, L)
  Desal Lax (G.R. Lane, L)
  Senna Tablets (Potter's, L)
  Out of Sorts Tablets (Potter's, L)
  Cleansing Herb Tablets (Potter's, L)
  Gladlax Tablets (Gerard House, PLR)
  Herbulax Tablets (English Grains, PLR)

Coughs
Anthroposophy
  Cough Drops (PLR, P)
  Sytra Tea (PLR)
Biochemic tissue salts
  Combination J (PLR)
Food Supplements
  including propolis products, citrus bioflavonoids,
  beta carotene, zinc citrate (see list of suppliers,
  Food)
Herbalism
  Cough Elixir (Weleda, PLR)
  Antibron Tablets (Potter's, L)
  Vegetable Cough Remover (Potter's, L)
  Lightning Cough Remedy (Potter's, L)
  Herb & Honey Elixir (Weleda, L)
  Horehound & Aniseed Cough Mixture (Potter's,
  L)
  Chest Mixture (Potter's, L)
  Balm of Gilead Cough Mixture (Potter's, L)
  Lobelia Tablets (Gerard House, PLR)

Cramp
Anthroposophy
  Arnica Massage Balm (L)
  Copper Ointment (PLR)
Biochemic tissue salts
  No. 8 (PLR)
Herbalism
  Life Drops (Potter's, L)

Croup
Herbalism
  Vegetable Cough Remover (Potter's, L)

Cuts and grazes
Anthroposophy
  Calendolon Ointment (L)
  Calendula Lotion (L)
  Hypericum/Calendula Ointment (L)
  Balsamicum Ointment (PLR, P)
Herbalism
  Dermacreme Ointment (Potter's, L)
  Tea Tree & Witch Hazel Cream
  Hypercal Cream (A. Nelson, L)
  Hypercal Spray (A. Nelson, L)

Cystitis
Herbalism
  Antitis Tablets (Potter's, L)

Diarrhoea
Anthroposophy
  Melissa Comp. Drops (L)
Biochemic tissue salts
  No. 11 (PLR)
Herbalism
  Spanish Tummy Mixture (Potter's, L)
  Charcoal Tablets (G.R. Lane, L)
  Cranesbill Tablets (Gerard House, PLR)

Eczema
Anthroposophy
  Dermatodoron Ointment (PLR, P)
  Dulcamare/Lyslmachia drops (PLR, P)
  Antimony Ointment (PLR, P)
Herbalism
  HRI Clear Complexion Tablets (Jessup, L)
  Eczema Ointment (Potter's, L)
  Skin Eruptions Mixture (Potter's, L)
  Echinacea Tablets (Gerard House, PLR)
  Blue Flag Root Compound Tablets (Gerard
  House, PLR)

Fever
Biochemic tissue salts
  No. 4 (PLR)

Flatulence
Anthroposophy
  Carbo Betula 3x Tablets (PLR)
  Digestodoron Tablets (PLR, P)
  Digestodoron Drops (PLR, P)
  Biobalm (G.R. Lane, L)
  Carminative Tea (L)

Carvon Tablets (PLR)
Biochemic tissue salts
  Combination E (PLR)
Herbalism
  Charcoal Tablets (Potter's, L)
  Charcoal Tablets (G.R. Lane, L)
  HRI Golden Seal Digestive Tablets (Jessup, L)
  Acidosis Tablets and Mixture (Potter's, L)
  Golden Seal Tablets (Gerard House, PLR)
  Papaya Plus Tablets (Gerard House, PLR)

Fluid retention
Herbalism
  HRI Water Balance Tablets (Jessup, L)
  Prementaid Tablets (Potter's, L)
  Diuretabs (Potter's, L)
  Helonias Tablets (Gerard House, PLR)
  Waterlex Tablets (Gerard House, PLR)
  Buchu Compound Tablets (Gerard House, PLR)
  Cascade (G.R. Lane, L)

Gallstones
Anthroposophy
  Choleodoron Drops (Weleda PLR, P)
Herbalism
  G.B. Tablets (Potter's, L)

Gum disorders
Anthroposophy
  Medicinal Gargle (PLR)

Haemorrhoids
Anthroposophy
  Antimony praep. Ointment (PLR, P)
Herbalism
  Pilewort Ointment (Potter's, L)
  Piletabs (Potter's, L)
  Pilewort Tablets (Gerard House, PLR)
  Piletabs (G.R. Lane, L)
  Heemex (G.R. Lane, L)
Homoeopathy
  Haemorrhoid Cream (A. Nelson, L)

Hay fever
Anthroposophy
  Gencydo Ointment (PLR, P)
  Oleum Rhinale (PLR)
Biochemic tissue salts
  Combination H (PLR)
Herbalism

Antifect Tablets (Potter's, L)
  HRI Garlic Tablets for Catarrh & Rhinitis (Jessup, L)
Homoeopathy
  Pollenna (A. Nelson, PLR)

Headaches and migraines
Anthroposophy
  Bidor 1% Tablets
  Bidor 5% Tablets
Biochemic tissue salts
  Combination S
  Combination F
Herbalism
  Ginger Root Capsules (Potter's, Exempt)
  Feverfew Tablets (Potter's, Exempt)
  Anased Pain Relief Tablets (Potter's, L)
Homoeopathy
  Feverfew 6x Tablets or drops (Weleda, PLR)

Heartburn
Anthroposophy
  Digestodoron Drops (PLR, P)
  Digestodoron Tablets (PLR, P)
  Pinella Tea (PLR)
Biochemic tissue salts
  Combination C (PLR)
Herbalism
  Acidosis Tablets and Mixture (Potter's, L)
  Charcoal Tablets (Potter's, L)
  Papaya Plus Tablets (Gerard House, PLR)
  Golden Seal Tablets (Gerard House, PLR)

Heat/sunstroke and heat exhaustion
Anthroposophy
  Combudoron Spray (PLR)
Food Supplements
  including propolis products, citrus bioflavonoids, starflower oil, cat's claw (see list of suppliers, Food)
Herbalism
  Herbheal Ointment (Potter's, L)
  Tea Tree & Witch Hazel Cream (G.R. Lane, L)

High blood pressure
Food Supplements
  including coenzyme Q10, citrus bioflavonoids, lecithin, vitamins C & E, selenium, magnesium, fish oils and propolis products (see list of suppliers, Food)

Herbalism
  Wellwoman Herbs (Potter's, L)

Indigestion
Anthroposophy
  Digestodoron Drops (PLR, P)
  Digestodoron Tablets (PLR, P)
  Carvon Tablets (PLR)
  Pinella Tea (PLR)
Biochemic tissue salts
  Combination E (PLR)
  Combination S (PLR)
Herbalism
  Acidosis Tablets and Mixture (L)
  Charcoal Tablets (Potter's, L)
  Charcoal Tablets (G.R. Lane, L)
  Biobalm (G.R. Lane, L)
  Papaya Plus Tablets (Gerard House, PLR)
  Golden Seal Tablets (Gerard House, PLR)

Influenza, see colds and influenza

Insomnia
Anthroposophy
  Avena Sativa Comp. Drops (PLR)
  Malvae Comp Tea (PLR)
Herbalism
  Passiflora Tablets (Potter's, L)
  HRI Night Tablets (Jessup, L)
  Valerian Tablets (Gerard House, PLR)
  Somnus Tablets (Gerard House, PLR)
  Natrasleep Tablets (English Grains, PLR)
  Kalms (G.R. Lane, L)
Homoeopathy
  Noctura (A. Nelson, PLR)

Irritable bowel syndrome
Herbalism
  HRI Golden Seal Digestive Tablets (Jessup, L)
  Slippery Elm Tablets (Potter's, L)

Menstrual problems, see periods

Morning sickness
Herbalism
  Ginger Root Capsules (Potter's, Exempt)

Mouth ulcers
Anthroposophy
  Medicinal Gargle (Weleda, PLR)

Nappy rash
Anthroposophy
  Balsamicum Ointment (PLR, P)
Herbalism
  Dermacreme Ointment (Potter's, L)
  Herbheal Ointment (Potter's, L)
  Tea Tree & Witch Hazel Cream

Nausea, see vomiting

Neuralgia
Herbalism
  Anased Pain Relief Tablets (Potter's, L)

Oedema, see fluid retention

Osteoarthritis, see rheumatism

Panic attacks
  Kalms (G. R. Lane, L)
  Rescue Remedy – Flower Remedy

Periods, painful, heavy, absent, irregular
Anthroposophy
  Menodoron Drops (PLR, P)
  Metra Tea (PLR)
  Melissa Comp. Drops (L)
Biochemic tissue salts
  Combination N (PLR)
Herbalism
  Raspberry Leaf Tablets (Potter's, L)

Phobias
Herbalism
  Newrelax Tablets (Potter's, L)

Piles, see haemorrhoids

Pre-menstrual syndrome
Herbalism
  Prementaid Tablets (Potter's, L)
  Diuretabs (Potter's, L)

Prostate problems
Herbalism
  Antiglan Tablets (Potter's, L)
  Protat (Potter's, L)

Psoriasis
Herbalism
    Skin Eruptions Mixture (Potter's, L)
    Psorasolv Ointment (Potter's, L)
    HRI Clear Complexion Tablets (Jessup, L)

Puncture wounds
Anthroposophy
    WCS Dusting Powder (PLR, P)
    Calendula Lotion (L)
    Calendolon Ointment (L)
    Hypericum/Calendula Ointment (L)
Herbalism
    Dermacreme Ointment (Potter's, L)

Relationship break-up
    Kalms (G. R. Lane, L)

Rheumatism
Anthroposophy
    Arnica Massage Balm (L)
    Rheumadoron 1 and 2 Drops (PLR, P)
    Rheumadoron 102A Drops (PLR, P)
    Rhus Tox Ointment (PLR)
    Rheumadoron Ointment (PLR, P)
    Mandragora Comp Drops (PLR, P)
Biochemic tissue salts
    Combination M (PLR)
Food Supplements
    including propolis products, starflower oil, zinc
    citrate, linseeds (see list of suppliers, Food)
Herbalism
    Nine Rubbing Oils (Potter's, L)
    Rheumatic Pain Tablets (Potter's, L)
    Tabritis (Potter's, L)
    Olbas Oil
    Ligvites Tablets (Gerard House, PLR)
    Reumalex Tablets (Gerard House, PLR)
    Rheumasol Tablets (English Grains, PLR)
Homoeopathy
    Rhus Tox Cream (A. Nelson, L)
    Rheumatica (A. Nelson, PLR)

Sciatica and back pain
Anthroposophy
    Arnica Massage Balm (L)
Biochemic tissue salts
    Combination G (PLR)
    Combination A (PLR)
Herbalism

    Sciargo Tablets (Potter's, L)
    Backache Tablets (Potter's, L)
    Kas-Bah Herb (Potter's, L)
    Nine Rubbing Oils (Potter's, L)
    Ligvites Tablets (Gerard House, PLR)
    Reumalex Tablets (Gerard House, PLR)
    Rheumasol Tablets (English Grains, PLR)

Shock
Flower remedies
    Rescue Remedy (Flower remedies suppliers,
    PLR)
Herbalism
    Elixir of Damiana and Saw Palmetto (Potter's, L)
Homoeopathy
    Arnica (see list of suppliers, HR)

Sinusitis
Anthroposophy
    Oleum Rhinale Nasal Drops (PLR, P)
Biochemic tissue salts
    Combination Q (PLR)
Herbalism
    Antifect Tablets (Potter's, L)
    Sinotar (G. R. Lane, L)

Sore throats and tonsillitis
Anthroposophy
    Medicinal Gargle (PLR)
    Cinnabar/Pyrites Tablets (PLR, P)
    Cinnabar 20x Tablets (PLR)
    Bolus Eucalypti Comp (PLR)
Food Supplements
    including propolis products, zinc citrate, citrus
    bioflavonoids, cat's claw (see list of suppliers,
    Food)
Herbalism
    Life Drops (Potter's, L)
    Peerless Composition Essence (Potter's, L)
    Olbas Pastilles (G. R. Lane, L)

Sprains and strains
Anthroposophy
    Arnica Ointment (L)
    Arnica Lotion (L)
    Arnica Massage Balm (L)
    Arnica 6x Tablets (PLR)
    Ruta Ointment (PLR)
Herbalism
    Nine Rubbing Oils (Potter's, L)

Comfrey Ointment (Potter's, L)
Homoeopathy
Strain Ointment (A. Nelson, L)

Stomach ulcers
Herbalism
Acidosis Tablets and Mixture (Potter's, L)
HRI Golden Seal Digestive Tablets (Jessup, L)

Stress incontinence
Herbalism
Newrelax Tablets (Potter's, L)

Teething
Anthroposophy
Chamomilla 3x Pills (PLR)
Chamomilla 3x Drops (PLR)
Biochemic tissue salts
Combination R (PLR)
Homoeopathy
Teetha (A. Nelson, PLR)

Thrush
Homoeopathy
Candida (A. Nelson, PLR)

Tonsillitis, see sore throats and tonsillitis

Toothache
Anthroposophy
Chamomilla 3x Drops and Pills (PLR)
Food Supplements

including propolis products, organic cider vinegar, calcium, vitamin B6, coenzyme, zinc citrate, citrus bioflavonoids (see list of suppliers, Food)
Herbalism
Anased Pain Relief Tablets (Potter's, L)

Travel sickness
Herbalism
Ginger Root Capsules (Potter's, Exempt)
Homoeopathy
Travella (A. Nelson, PLR)

Urticaria (hives)
Anthroposophy
Combudoron Lotion or Ointment (PLR)
Herbalism
Skin Clear Tablets (Potter's, L)

Varicose veins
Anthroposophy
Skin Tone Lotion (PLR)
Biochemic tissue salts
Combination L (PLR)
Herbalism
Varicose Ointment (Potter's, L)

Vomiting
Anthroposophy
Melissa Comp. Drops (L)
Herbalism
Ginger Tablets (Gerard House, PLR)

Bibliography

General Titles

The Alternative Health Guide, Brian Inglis and Ruth West (Michael Joseph, 1983)

The Complete Book of Men's Health, Dr Sarah Brewer (Thorsons, 1995)

The Encyclopaedia of Complementary Medicine: The Complete Family Guide to Alternative Health Care (Carlton Books, 1996)

First Aid Manual: Emergency Procedures for Everyone at Home, at Work or Leisure, The Authorised Manual of St John Ambulance, St Andrew's Ambulance Association, The British Red Cross Association (Dorling Kindersley, 1997)

Gentle Medicine: Thorsons Concise Encyclopaedia of Natural Health, Angela Smyth and Dr Hilary Jones (Thorsons, 1994)

The Handbook of Complementary Medicine, Stephen Fulder (Coronet, 1984)

The HEA Guide to Complementary Medicine and Therapies, Anne Woodham (Health Education Authority, 1994)

The New Macmillan Guide to Family Health, edited by Dr Tony Smith (Macmillan, 1987)

Reader's Digest Family Guide to Alternative Medicine, (The Reader's Digest Association Limited, 1991)

A World Without Aids: The Controversial Holistic Health Plan, Leon Chaitow and Simon Martin (Thorsons, 1988)

Therapies

Anthroposophy

Anthroposophical Medicine: An Extension of the Art of Healing, Victor Batt (Rudolph Steiner Press, 1982)

Anthroposophical Medicine: Healing for Body, Soul, and Spirit, Dr Michael Evans and Iain Rodger (Thorsons, 1992)

Blessed by Illness, Dr L.F.C. Mees (The Anthroposophical Press, 1983)

Fundamentals of Therapy, Dr Rudolph Steiner and Dr Ita Wegman

Living With Your Body, Dr Walther Buhler (Rudolph Steiner Press, 1979)

The Science and Art of Healing, Dr Ralph Twentyman (Floris Books, 1992)

Aromatherapy

Aromatherapy for Common Ailments, Shirley Price (Gaia Books Ltd, 1991)

Aromatherapy for Pregnancy and Childbirth, Margaret Fawcett (Element Books, 1993)

The Art of Aromatherapy, Robert Tisserand (C.W. Daniel, 1977)

The Bloomsbury Encyclopaedia of Aromatherapy, Chrissie Wildwood (Bloomsbury Publishing plc, 1996)

The Fragrant Pharmacy: A Home and Health Care Guide to Aromatherapy and Essential Oils, Valerie Ann Wormwood (Macmillan, 1991)

Holistic Aromatherapy, Christine Wildwood (Thorsons, 1992)

Practical Aromatherapy, Shirley Price (Thorsons, 1994)

Ayurveda

The Book of Ayurveda: A Guide to Personal Well-being, Judith H. Morrison (Gaia Books Ltd, 1995)

Biochemic tissue salts

Biochemic Handbook (Thorsons, 1965)

Dr Schuessler's Biochemistry: A Natural Method of Healing, J.B. Chapman (Thorsons)

Shortened Therapies, William Heinrich Schuessler *Thorsons Complete Guide to Homoeopathically Prepared Tissue Salts,* Dr Peter Gilbert (Thorsons, 1989)

Flower remedies

The Bach Flower Remedies: Illustrations and Preparations, Nora Weeks and Victor Bullen (C.W. Daniel, 1990)

The Bach Flower Remedies Step by Step: A Complete Guide to Prescribing, Judy Howard (C.W. Daniel, 1990)

Collected Writings of Edward Bach, J. Barnard (Ashgrove Press, 1997)

Flower Remedies to the Rescue: The Healing Vision of Dr Edward Bach, Gregory Vlamis (Thorsons, 1990)

A Guide to the Bach Flower Remedies, J. Barnard (C.W. Daniel, 1979)

Healing Herbs of Edward Bach, J. and M. Barnard (Ashgrove Press, 1997)

The Original Writings of Edward Bach, Judy Howard and John Ramsell (C.W. Daniel, 1990)

Homoeopathy

The Complete Homoeopathy Handbook: A Guide to Everyday Health Care, Miranda Castro (Macmillan, 1990)

Everybody's Guide to Homoeopathic Medicines: Taking Care of Yourself and Your Family with Safe and Effective Remedies, Stephen Cummings and Dana Ullman (Gollancz, 1986)

The Family Guide to Homoeopathy: The Safe Form of Medicine for the Future, Dr Andrew Lockie (Elm Tree Books, 1989)

Homoeopathic Medicine at Home, Maesimund Panos and Jane Heimlich (Corgi, 1980)

Homoeopathy, Medicine for the New Man, George Vithoulkas (Thorsons, 1985)

Homoeopathy: Medicine for the 21st Century, Dana Ullman (North Atlantic Books, 1988)

Practical Homoeopathy: A Complete Guide to Home Treatment, Beth MacEoin (Bloomsbury Publishing plc, 1997)

The Science of Homoeopathy, George Vithoulkas (Thorsons, 1986)

Massage

The Aromatherapy and Massage Book, Christine Wildwood (Thorsons, 1994)

An Introduction to Massage, Susan Mumford (Hamlyn, 1995)

The Massage Book, George Downing

Nutritional therapy

The A–Z of Nutritional Health, Adrienne Mayes (Thorsons)

Food and Nutrition, Sheila Bingham (Dent)

Human Nutrition and Dietetics, Davison and Passmore (Churchill Livingstone)

Mental and Elemental Nutrients, Carl Pfeiffer (Keats Publishing, 1975)

Natural Medicine, Stephen Davies and Alan Stewart (Pan)

Nutritional Against Disease, Roger J. Williams (Bantam)

Nutritional Influences on Illness, Mervyn R. Werbach (Keats Publishing, 1990)

Shiatsu

The Book of Shiatsu, Paul Lundberg (Gaia Books Ltd, 1992)

Do It Yourself Shiatsu, Wataw Ohashi (Unwin, 1976)

Shiatsu: The Complete Guide, Chris Jarmey and Gabrielle Mojay (Thorsons, 1991)

Shiatsu Theory and Practice, Carola Beresford-Cooke (Churchill Livingstone, 1995)

Traditional Chinese medicine

Ben Cao Gang Mu, Li Shizhen

The Complete Illustrated Guide to Chinese Medicine, Tom Williams (Element Books, 1997)

The Fountain of Health: An A–Z of Traditional Chinese Medicine, Dr Charles Windridge, consultant editor Dr Wu Xiaochun (Mainstream Publishing Co., 1994)

A Guide to Acupuncture, Peter Firebrace and Sandra Hill (Constable & Co. Ltd, 1994)

Principles of Chinese Herbal Medicine, John Hicks (Thorsons, 1997)

Traditional Chinese Medicine, Sheila McNamara and Dr Song Xuan Ke (Hamish Hamilton, 1995)

Understanding Chinese Medicine: The Web That Has No Weaver, Ted Kaptchuk (Rider, 1983)

Western medical herbalism

The Complete New Herbal, consultant editor Richard Mabey (Penguin, 1991)

The Complete Woman's Herbal: A Manual of Healing Herbs and Nutrition for Personal Wellbeing and Family Care, Anne McIntyre (Gaia Books Ltd, 1994)

The Encyclopaedia of Medicinal Plants, Andrew Chevalier (Dorling Kindersley, 1996)

The Essential Book of Herbal Medicine, Simon Mills (Penguin, 1993)

The Green Witch: A Modern Woman's Herbal, Barbara Griggs (Ebury Press, 1993)

Herbal Remedies: The Complete Guide to Natural Healing, Jill Nice (Piatkus Books, 1990)

The New Holistic Herbal, David Hoffman (Element Books, 1990)

Useful addresses

Practitioner organizations

This list is by no means exhaustive and is only supplied as a helpful guide – the inclusion or exclusion of any organization is not intended either as an endorsement or a criticism.

Acupuncture

British Acupuncture Council
Park House
206–208 Latimer Road
London W10 6RE
Tel: 0181 964 0222

Information

Training: two years' full-time or three years' part-time attendance at recognized colleges to gain MBAcC. Regulatory body for standards of training and code of practice. Students must have five GCSEs and three A levels before being accepted on to the course.

British Medical Acupuncture Society
Newton House
Newton Lane
Whitley, Warrington
Cheshire WA4 4JA
Tel: 01925 370727

Information

Represents medically qualified doctors who have studied acupuncture techniques. Although the training is intermittent, doctors have usually undertaken 100 hours and had 100 cases reviewed to attain accreditation (DipMedAc).

Anthroposophy

Anthroposophical Medical Association
c/o Park Attwood
Bewdley
Trimpley
Worcestershire DY12 1RE
Tel: 0129 986 1444

Information

Only medically qualified doctors can train to become practitioners in anthroposophical medicine. In the UK there is no formally recognized training, so doctors usually undertake their training in Europe, where there are anthroposophical hospitals.

Aromatherapy

Aromatherapy Organisations Council
PO Box 19834
London SE25 6WF
Tel: 0181 251 7912

Information

The AOC is the UK governing body for aromatherapy currently representing thirteen professional associations and ninety-five training establishments. AOC training standards include anatomy and physiology, safety considerations, consultation and referral procedures. Aromatherapists can gain any of the following qualifications: APNT, ESIPF, AMA, IFA, AHPI, ISPA, AAPA, ANM, HAF, RQA, ICA, GCP.

Ayurveda

Ayurvedic Medical Association UK
59 Dulverton Road
Selsdon
Croydon
Surrey CR2 8PJ
Tel: 0181 657 6147

Information

Ayurvedic practitioners study for five years at Indian or Sri Lankan universities to qualify as Doctors of Ayurvedic Medicine and Surgery (DAMS) or Batchelor of Ayurvedic Medicine and Surgery (BAMS).

Association of Accredited Ayurvedic Practitioners
50 Penywern Road
London SW5 9SX
Tel: 0171 370 2255

Information

As for Ayurvedic Medical Association UK.

Chinese herbal medicine

Register of Chinese Herbal Medicine
PO Box 400
Wembley
Middlesex HA9 9NZ
Tel: 0181 904 1357
(answerphone only)

Chiropractic

British Chiropractic Association
Equity House
29 Whitley Street
Reading
Berkshire RG2 0EG
Tel: 0173 475 7557

Information

Training: five years' part-time at recognized colleges, leading to BSc DC. This is the regulatory body for standards of training and code of practice. Students must have five GCSEs and three A levels, including chemistry, biology or zoology.

McTimoney Chiropractic
Association
21 High Street
Eynsham
Oxon OX8 1HE
Tel: 01865 880974

Colonic irrigation

Colonic International Association
16 Englands Lane
London NW3 4TG
Tel: 0171 483 1595

General

British Complementary
Medicine Association
249 Fosse Road
Leicester LE3 1AE
Tel: 0116 242 5406

Information

Forum of practitioner organizations (excluding medical herbalism, homoeopathy, chiropractic, osteopathy and acupuncture). Working to establish professionalism by establishing codes of practice.

The Guild of Complementary
Practitioners
Liddell House
Liddell Close
Finchampstead
Berkshire RG40 4NS
Tel: 0173 473 5757

Herbalism

National Institute of Medical
Herbalists
56 Longbrook Street
Exeter
Devon EX4 6AH
Tel: 01392 426022

Information

Entry qualifications: graduates of recognized colleges/universities with GCSEs and A levels in chemistry and biology. Four years' part-time study leads to MNIMH or FNIMH.

General Council & Register of
Consultant Herbalists
32 King Edward Road
Swansea
South Wales SA1 4LL
Tel: 01792 655886

Homoeopathy

Society of Homoeopaths
2 Artizan Road
Northampton NN1 4HU
Tel: 01604 621400

Information

Entry qualifications: usually a minimum of five GCSEs and two A levels. Three years' full-time or four years' part-time training leads to RSHom or FSHom.

Faculty of Homoeopathy
15 Clerkenwell Close
London EC1R OAA
Tel: 0171 566 7810

Information

Members must be medically qualified and registered with the British Medical Association – training in homoeopathy ranges from short introductory courses to a six-month full-time course, leading to qualifications MFHom or FFHom.

UK Homoeopathic Medical
Association
6 Livingstone Road
Gravesend
Kent DA12 5DZ
Tel: 0147 456 0336

Massage

Massage Therapy Institute of
Great Britain
PO Box 2726
London NW2 4NR

British Massage Therapy Council
Greenbrook House
65a Adelphi Street
Preston
Lancs PR1 7BH
Tel: 01772 881063

Naturopathy

General Council & Register of
Naturopaths
Goswell House
2 Goswell Road
Street
Somerset BA16 0JG
Tel: 01458 840072

Nutritional therapy

British Society for Allergy,
Environmental & Nutritional
Medicine
PO Box 28
Totten
Southampton SO40 2ZA

Information

Admits only medically qualified practitioners.

Register of Nutritional Therapists
Lightwoods
Hatton Green
Warwick CV35 7LA
Tel: 01926 484449

Information

The RNT was formed in 1991 and produced home-study

modules (RNT Update) which have been accepted as an educational standard by the Collegiate of European Certified Nutritional Practitioners as the common European advanced educational standard for nutritional practitioners. This now forms a BSc Degree Course in Applied Nutritional Medicine in Australia and it is hoped that degree courses will follow in the UK. Current qualifications are MRNT and ECNP.

Osteopathy
General Osteopathic Council
Osteopathy House
176 Tower Bridge Road
London SE1 3LU
Tel: 0171 357 6655

Information
In 1993 an Act of Parliment was passed, bringing in Statutory Regulation. By May 2000 all practising Osteopaths will be registered with the General Osteopathic Council (GOC). Those practitioners already registered with the GOC have proved that they are safe, legal and competent and may therefore use the title *Registered Osteopath*.

Osteopathic Information Service
Osteopathy House
176 Tower Bridge Road
London SE1 3LU
Tel: 0171 357 6655 (ext.242)

Information
Osteopaths may have any of these qualifications: MRO, MCO, FCO, MGO, FGO, MNTOS, FNTOS, MLCOM, FLCOM. From 1998 the OIS became the public information arm of the GOC.

Reflexology
Association of Reflexologists
27 Old Gloucester Street
London WC1N 3XX
Tel: 0990 673320

British Reflexology Association
Monks Orchard
Whitbourne
Worcester WR6 5RB
Tel: 01886 82107

Information
No fixed entry qualifications, but advise four GCSEs.

Shiatsu
Shiatsu Society
Interchange Studios
Dalby Street
London NW5 3NQ
Tel: 0171 813 7772

Information
No entry qualifications. Training: minimum three years' part-time training, leading to qualification MRSS.

Research organizations

Acupuncture
Foundation for Traditional Chinese Medicine
124 Acomb Road
York YO2 4EY
Tel: 01904 785120

Complementary and alternative medicine
Research Council for Complementary Medicine
60 Great Ormond Street
London WC1N 3JF
Tel: 0171 833 8897

Homoeopathy
Blackie Foundation
1 Upper Wimpole Street
London W1M 7TD
Tel: 0171 580 5489

Product suppliers
This list is by no means exhaustive and is supplied only as a helpful guide – the inclusion or exclusion of any organization is not intended as either an endorsement or criticism.

Anthroposophical medicines
Available through health-food shops, pharmacies and mail order.

Weleda (UK) Ltd
Heanor Road
Ilkeston
Derbyshire DE7 8DR

Ayurvedic medicines
Mail order only.

Ayurvedic Company of Great Britain
50 Penywern Road
London SW5 9SX

Dabur India Ltd
101–113 Scrubs Lane
London NW10 6QU

Maharishi Ayur-Veda Health Centre
24 Linpole Street
London NW1 6HT

Vedic Medical Hall
6 Chiltern Street
London W1M 1PA

Biochemic tissue salts

Available through health-food shops, pharmacies and mail order.

New Era Ltd
Hedon Road
Marfleet
Hull HU9 5NJ

Dietary supplements

Available through health-food shops and mail order.

Cedar Health Ltd
Pepper Road
Bramhall Moor Estate
Hazel Grove
Cheshire SK7 5BW

G.R. Lane Health Products Ltd
Sisson Road
Gloucester GL1 3QB

Lichtwer Pharma (UK) Ltd
Regency House
Mere Park
Dedmere Road
Marlow
Buckinghamshire SL78 1FJ

Jessup Marketing
27 Old Gloucester Street
London WC1N 3XX

Bio-Health Ltd
Culpeper Close
Medway City Estate
Rochester
Kent ME2 4HU

Nature's Own Ltd
Unit 8, Hanley Work Shops
Hanley Road
Hanley Swan
Worcestershire WR8 0DX

Pharma Vita Ltd
PO Box 3379
London SW11 3ED

Quest Vitamins Ltd
8 Venture Way
Aston Science Park
Birmingham B7 4AP

Vitabiotics Ltd
Vitabiotics House
3 Bashley Road
London

Bee Health Ltd
1 Racecourse Road
East Ayton
Scarborough

Higher Nature Limited
The Nutrition Centre
Burwash Common
East Sussex TN19 7LX

Larkhall Green Farm
225 Putney Bridge Road
London SW15 2PY

Lucas Meyer (UK) Ltd
Unit 46, First Avenue
Deeside Industrial Park
Deeside
Clwyd CH5 2NU

Nature's Best
1 Lamberts Road
Tunbridge Wells
Kent TN2 3EQ
Mail order only. Trained nutritional therapists will answer telephone queries.

Efamol Ltd
Weyvern House
Weyvern Park
Portsmouth Road
Peasmarsh
Guildford
Surrey GU3 1NA

Flower remedies

Available through health-food shops, pharmacies and mail order.

Dr Edward Bach Centre
Mount Vernon
Sotwell
Wallingford
Oxfordshire OX10 0PZ

Healing Herbs Ltd
PO Box 65
Hereford HR2 0UW

Russell & Nelson & Co Ltd
Broadheath House
83 Parkside
Wimbledon
London SW19 5LP

Health foods

Allergycare
Pollard's Yard
Wood Street
Taunton
Somerset TA1 1UP

Blue Green Planet Ltd
PO Box 1454
Slough
Berkshire SL3 9YS

Gluten Free Foods Limited
PO Box 178
Stanmore
Middlesex

Herbal medicines

Available through health-food shops, pharmacies and mail order.

Bio-Health Ltd
Culpepper Close
Medway City Estate
Rochester
Kent ME2 4HU

English Grains Healthcare
William Nadin Way
Swadlincote
Derbyshire DE11 0BB

G.R. Lane Health Products Ltd
Sisson Road
Gloucester GL1 3QB

Gerard House
William Nadin Way
Swadlincote
Derbyshire DE11 0BB

Jessup Marketing
27 Old Gloucester Street
London WC1N 3XX

Lloyds (Portsmouth) Ltd (Mail order only)
51 Albert Square
Southsea
Hants PO5 2ST

Potter's (Herbal Supplies) Ltd
Leyland Mill Lane
Wigan
Lancs WN1 2SB

Herbal supplements

Available through health-food shops, pharmacies and mail order.

Bioforce (UK) Ltd
Olympic Business Park
Drybridge Road
Dundonald KA2 9BE

Peruvian Imports Limited
12 Halifax Road
Bicester
Oxon OX6 7TG

Homoeopathic medicines

Available through health-food shops, pharmacies and mail order.

Ainsworth's
38 New Cavendish Street
London W1N 7LH

Helios Homoeopathics
89–95 Camden Road
Tunbridge Wells
Kent TN1 6QR

Russel & Nelson & Co Ltd
Broadheath House
83 Parkside
Wimbledon
London SW19 5LP

Weleda (UK) Ltd
Heanor Road
Ilkeston
Derbyshire DE7 8DR

TENS (transcutaneous electrical nerve stimulation) pain relief machines

Shire Design Electronics Ltd
The Mill
Mill Lane
Little Shrewley
Warwickshire CV35 7HN

Trade associations

All health-food products including vitamins, supplements, etc.

Health Food Manufacturers
Association
c/o 63 Hampton Court Way
Thames Ditton
Surrey KT7 0LT

Aromatherapy

Aromatherapy Trade Council
3 Latymer Close
Braybrooke
Market Harborough
Leicestershire LE16 8LN

Dietary supplements

Council for Responsible
Nutrition
c/o 63 Hampton Court Way
Thames Ditton
Surrey KT7 0LT

Herbal, homoeopathic, anthroposophical medicines and biochemic tissue salts

Natural Medicines Manufacturers
Association
c/o Old Vicarage Cottage
65 Church Street
Langham
Oakham
Leicestershire LE15 7JE

Herbalism

British Herbal Medicines
Association
Sun House
Church Street
Stroud
Gloucestershire GL5 1JL

Homoeopathy

British Homoeopathic
Manufacturers Association
c/o Old Vicarage Cottage
65 Church Street
Langham
Oakham
Leicestershire LE15 7JE

Consultants

Anthroposophy

Dr Geoffrey Douch (MBBS, MFHom) worked as a general practitioner in the National Health Service for thirty-five years. He is now a consultant in homoeopathic and anthroposophical medicine, has been a member of the Natural Medicines Society's council since 1985 and has served on its Medicines Advisory Research Committee since 1988.

Aromatherapy

Teddy Fearnhamm (IScB/ESIPF France, MRQA, GCP, MIFA) is executive director of L'Institut des Sciences Biomedicales, France and Fellow of the English Societé. She also holds prominent positions in the Aromatherapy Organizations Council, the Register of Qualified Aromatherapists, the Institute of Classical Aromatherapy, the International Federation of Aromatherapists and the Guild of Complementary Practitioners.

Sylvia Baker (SPDipA, MISPA, ISPA, IFA, GCP, RQA(Hon), ESIPF) is Secretary to the Aromatherapy Organizations Council and the Aromatherapy Trade Council and contributes articles on aromatherapy to various journals. She is the Aromatherapy Co-ordinator for the British Complementary Medicine Association, and the Aromatherapy Core Representative for the Care Sector Consortium Project to develop national standards for the profession, and represents the AOC on the UK Forum for Alternative & Complementary Medicine.

Ayurveda

Dr Harish Verma is a Gold medallist in ayurveda from the GND University in Punjab, India. He has over twelve years of training and experience in ayurveda and specializes in bowel and gastro-intestinal disorders, including ulcerative colitis.

Gopi Warrier comes from a family of leading ayurvedic practitioners who run two of the best-known ayurvedic hospitals in India. Although his own training is in management, he has studied privately under leading teachers of ayurveda in India.

Biochemic tissue salts

Suham Sidani (BSc, Pharm.Beruit) is group quality controller and regulatory affairs manager to the Seven Seas Health Care Ltd and New Era Laboratories, manufacturers of biochemic tissue salts. He has served on the Natural Medicines Society's Medicines Advisory Research Committee since its formation in 1988.

Chiropractic

Christopher Turner (CCSP, BCA, AECC, FICS) is registered with the British Chiropractic Association and specializes in sports medicine. He is the media spokesperson for the British Chiropractic Association.

Flower remedies

Julian Barnard has worked with the Bach Remedies for twenty years and has written three books on the subject. As well as editing Dr Bach's collected writings, he lectures on Bach and his discoveries in many countries. He is co-director of Healing Herbs Ltd which has been making flower remedies since 1989.

Homoeopathy

Judith Cresswell (RSHom) is a practising homoeopath with over twelve years' experience. Judith has been a visiting lecturer at several colleges of homoeopathy and is a past chairperson of the Society of Homoeopaths.

Massage

Sean Doherty has been practising since 1981. He holds diplomas in remedial massage, holistic therapy, Thai massage, body psychotherapy and postural integration. He has also studied Chinese massage and cranial sacral therapy. He is currently a Board member of the European Association of Body Psychotherapy.

Naturopathy

Ron Bishop (ND, MRN, DO, MRO, BAcC, MBAcC) has been practising for over twenty-five years and is vice chairperson to the Council for Complementary and Alternative Medicine and is the external examiner for the Anglia University BSc(Hons) degree in Osteopathy at the London School of Osteopathy. He is a member of the General Council and Register of Naturopaths, the British Acupuncture Council, the General Council and Register of Osteopaths and the British Naturopathic Association.

Nutritional therapy

Penny Woolley is the founder and director of the Register of Nutritional Therapists and chairperson of the Collegiate of European Certified Nutritional Practitioners (CECNP). She is responsible for developing the RNT Update (Advanced Educational Home Study Modules) and for the first-ever international university degree courses in Applied Nutritional Medicine.

Roger Groos combines the practices of reflexology, colon hydrotherapy, manual lymph drainage and nutritional therapy into a natural treatment approach to health problems. He is a member of the Association of Reflexologists and has been a Council Member of the Natural Medicines Society since 1990.

Orthodox medicine

Dr Colin Clayton has worked since 1989 as a general practitioner in a Derbyshire practice and attends the minor injuries unit at Ripley Hospital. He believes that modern medicine does not have all the answers to disease and that alternative methods can provide valuable relief from symptoms of minor illness.

Osteopathy

The Osteopathic Information Service was established by the voluntary registering bodies within osteopathy to 'speak with one voice' about osteopathic medicine. Its objectives are to increase awareness and understanding of osteopathy among the general public and the world of medicine at large.

Reflexology

Elizabeth Fraser (MAR) has been a practising reflexologist since 1992 after training and qualifying with the British School of Reflexology.

Shiatsu

Kim Lovelace (MRSS) has been practising shiatsu for five years and is a member of the Board of Directors of the Shiatsu Society. He represents the Shiatsu Society on the UK Forum for Alternative & Complementary Medicine.

Traditional Chinese medicine

A past president of the Register of Chinese Herbal Medicine and a member of the British Acupuncture Council, **Richard Blackwell (BMedSci(Hons), MBAcC, MRCHM)** has been practising for fifteen years and runs a private practice in York. He is Dean of the Northern College of Acupuncture and Research Advisor to the Foundation for Traditional Chinese Medicine.

Western medical herbalism

Andrew Chevallier (MNIMH) is chairperson of the Council for Complementary and Alternative Medicine. An experienced medical herbalist Andrew played a leading role in establishing the degree course in herbal medicine at Middlesex University in 1994, and is now senior lecturer and programme leader of the course.

Index